95

Managing and Treating
Urinary
INCONTINENCE

Managing and Treating *Urinary* INCONTINENCE

by
Diane Kaschak Newman,
R.N.C., M.S.N., C.R.N.P., F.A.A.N.

Co-Director
Penn Center for Continence and Pelvic Health
Division of Urology
University of Pennsylvania Health System
Philadelphia

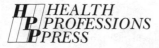

HEALTH PROFESSIONS PRESS

Baltimore • London • Winnipeg • Sydney

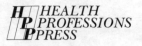

Health Professions Press
Post Office Box 10624
Baltimore, Maryland 21285-0624

www.healthpropress.com

Typeset by Barton Matheson Willse & Worthington, Baltimore, Maryland.
Printed in the United States of America by
Versa Press, Inc., East Peoria, Illinois.

The cases described in this book are based on the author's experience. In all instances, names and identifying details have been changed to protect confidentiality.

Library of Congress Cataloging-in-Publication Data

Newman, Diane Kaschak.
  Managing and treating urinary incontinence/by Diane Kaschak Newman.
     p.   ; cm.
  Includes bibliographical references and index.
  ISBN 1-878812-82-3
  1. Urinary incontinence.   I. Title.
  [DNLM: 1. Urinary incontinence—therapy. WJ 146 N5519m 2002]
  RC921.I5 N488 2002
  616.6'2—dc21   2002017294

British Library Cataloguing in Publication data are available from the British Library.

Contents

About the Author

Diane Kaschak Newman, R.N.C., M.S.N., C.R.N.P., F.A.A.N, Co-Director, Penn Center for Continence and Pelvic Health, Division of Urology, University of Pennsylvania Health System, First Floor Rhoads Pavilion, 3400 Spruce Street, Philadelphia, PA 19104

Ms. Newman is an adult nurse practitioner and a recognized expert in the field of nonsurgical management and treatment of urinary incontinence and related disorders. She is Co-Director of the Penn Center for Continence and Pelvic Health in the Division of Urology, University of Pennsylvania Health System in Philadelphia. Her clinical practice is dedicated to the evaluation, treatment, and management of urinary incontinence and related problems. She treats clients in long-term care, home care, and office practice environments. Ms. Newman participated in several research projects on the effects of behavioral treatment for urinary incontinence.

Ms. Newman received her master of science in nursing from the University of Pennsylvania. She was appointed the Chair of the Committee on Promotion, Organization and Education in Continence for the 2001 World Health Organization's International Consultation on Incontinence. She was also a member of the Project Task Force for the National Association for Continence, Blueprint of Continence Care Guidelines for Assisted Living Facilities, and Co-Chair of the 1996 Update Panel for the Clinical Practice Guidelines called "Urinary Incontinence in Adults," published by the Agency for Health Care Policy and Research, U.S. Department of Health and Human Services. In 1998, the Federal Drug Administration (FDA) appointed Ms. Newman to the Gastroenterology and Urology Device Panel. She is a member of the Centers for Medicare & Medicaid Services' Scope and Severity of Nursing Care Deficiencies guideline panel of experts on long-term care.

Ms. Newman is an internationally known speaker on urinary incontinence and the use of devices and products in the management of incontinence. A prolific writer, Ms. Newman has written and presented more than

75 scientific papers, chapters, and articles in major journals on the subject of assessment, behavioral treatment, and management of incontinence with an emphasis on the nurse's role. She is the author of *The Urinary Incontinence Sourcebook* (Revised edition; 1999, McGraw-Hill).

Foreword

We live and work in a country viewed by many to have the best health care in the world. We have sophisticated centers for treatment of acute illness, the most advanced technology for diagnosing and treating illnesses, and a stunning array of medications from which to choose. So why is urinary incontinence a leading health problem that continues to be underdiagnosed and undertreated or mistreated?

I suspect it's because most nurses and physicians fail to see urinary incontinence as a significant problem, and many patients are embarrassed to talk about it. For more than 16 years, I have produced a radio program in New York City on health issues. I invited Diane Newman to be a guest on my program to discuss urinary incontinence because I knew she approached the topic with openness and care. After some initial dialogue about incontinence, we opened the telephone lines for listener calls and were quickly swamped. People talked about how incontinence limited their lives and how they were afraid to leave their homes because they might not be able to find a bathroom (New York City has few safe, accessible public toilets, and most restaurants limit their bathrooms to customers). They talked about how embarrassing it was to try to talk with family members about the problem (whether the caller or the family member was incontinent) and asked basic questions such as "How long should I be able to go without urinating?"

Although one might conclude that the public is not reluctant to talk about incontinence, note that these callers remained anonymous. My conclusion was that, for the most part, no one talks about urinary incontinence. When given the opportunity, however, people will ask their questions and talk about their concerns because urinary health is very important to them.

Nurses should be leaders in improving the assessment and management of urinary incontinence. We are with patients more than any other provider, and annual Gallup polls continue to document that we are the provider the public trusts most. Yet, we are failing the call to leadership. At one medical center where I worked, we requested that nurses on medical-surgical units ask newly admitted patients if they had any problems with incontinence. More than 30% admitted to having urinary difficulties of some kind. We then did a retrospective chart review and found that less than 1% of patients were discharged with *any* urinary diagnosis, whether it was the primary diagnosis or not. We were not assessing for urinary incontinence, even though it was prevalent among our patients. I'm sure our institution was the rule, rather than the exception. Whether in acute care, long-term care, or home care, we are falling short of what is needed to rectify the situation. While some would argue that staffing shortages make implementation of continence programs impossible, I assert that such a view is indeed shortsighted and reflects an ignorance of what is known about this health problem.

Managing and Treating Urinary Incontinence is an important resource for remedying this disconcerting situation. This book raises our awareness of the extent of the problem across all settings, whether home, acute care, primary care, or long-term care, and the barriers to better care. The book takes an evidence-based, yet practical, approach to providing information about assessment of incontinence, behavioral approaches to its prevention and management, and other treatment options. Illustrations throughout the book add clarity to discussions of bladder functioning and hands-on aspects of care, such as the placement of a pessary.

Effective management of incontinence requires a multidisciplinary approach. This book is *the* most authoritative, comprehensive guide for providers for improving the assessment and management of urinary incontinence. It should be read by every nurse, physician, and physical therapist providing hands-on care or by administrators who need to better understand this costly health problem and to promote excellent continence programs. It should be a required resource for every nursing, medical, and physical therapy curriculum in the country if we are to prepare the next generation of providers to make the assessment and management of incontinence a routine practice.

If nurses are to live up to the public's trust in them, their advocacy for improved continence care for their patients is mandatory. Whether this is done by changing health care systems (e.g., making assessment of urinary incontinence a part of every hospital, nursing home, home care, or primary care admission) or through individual care, one patient at a time, *Managing and Treating Urinary Incontinence* will help nurses to approach this mandate with expertise, understanding, and care.

Diana J. Mason, R.N., Ph.D., F.A.A.N
Editor-in-Chief
American Journal of Nursing

Foreword

Urinary incontinence, overactive bladder, and pelvic floor disorders create a matrix of universal medical problems that threaten the quality of life for men and women of all ages throughout the world. The median prevalence of incontinence in women is now estimated as varying from 14% to 40.5%. Using the definition of the International Continence Society, the median prevalence in women is 23.5%. In men, this varies from 4.6% to 15%. In women, urge and mixed incontinence is estimated to account for a median relative share of 51% of cases, while in men, the combined total is 92%. The symptom syndrome of overactive bladder overlaps somewhat with urge incontinence but is quite separate. Prevalence in the adult population has been estimated as approximately 17%, and of those affected, 35% to 40% will have urge or mixed incontinence. The prevalence of incontinence due to overactive bladder is higher in women than it is in men.

It is obvious from these figures that urinary incontinence and overactive bladder account for an enormous burden for virtually every population in the world. They diminish quality of life, contribute to depression, and interfere with sleep. The direct and indirect costs to society are enormous. Specialists in this area are trying to increase awareness worldwide of these significant problems and to impress upon specialists and primary care providers the importance of identifying these clinical problems. But unless we can evaluate people with these conditions in a more cost-efficient manner and manage them in a way that maximizes quality of life and minimizes morbidity, we have not achieved the desired result.

The author of this well-put-together text, Diane Newman, has been in the forefront of such efforts at recognition as well as intelligent and cost-effective evaluation and management of these and other lower urinary tract dysfunctions for virtually her entire career. She is well respected in this regard by all strata of the health care provider population. As Co-Chair of the 1996 Update Panel for the Clinical Practice Guidelines "Urinary Incontinence in Adults," published by the Agency for Health Care Policy and Research, she co-authored a volume that still stands as a reference work in its field. Her handbook for the general public, *The Urinary Incontinence Sourcebook*, provided a superb overview of the problems of incontinence for the lay public. *Managing and Treating Urinary Incontinence* is put together with the same organizational care and completeness but targets an audience that ranges from primary care providers of all types (nurses, physician assistants, nurse practitioners, family practitioners, and general internists) to specialists in practice or in training who have a special interest in this subject.

This book excels in its description of areas that are typically mentioned by category only in textbooks written exclusively for specialists who are assumed to have a reasonable base of knowledge about these subjects. It embraces areas not seen in other books on urinary incontinence, such as physical and occupational stressors that increase a person's risk for incontinence; the correlation between bladder and bowel dysfunction; and the impact of incontinence in various care settings, such as ambulatory, in-home, and long-term care. It also includes the very latest behavioral treatments and patient education information and provides succinct information on medical and educational options available to professionals. Specialists will find the book remarkably complete about topics related to incontinence and associated voiding dysfunctions. Especially valuable is the extensive chapter on the use of catheters and devices, including the latest information on complications that can occur when managing urinary incontinence with these products. Practical information on these products is usually scattered and not conveniently accessible to the practicing provider. Finally, the chapter on establishing continence services is a much-needed resource in this area of specialty medicine.

There is no substitute for experience when developing a book such as this, and Ms. Newman draws upon her extensive experience as a front line practitioner, consultant, and educator in these fields to provide a very readable, complete, and instructive book.

Alan J. Wein, M.D.
Professor and Chair
Division of Urology
University of Pennsylvania

Preface

Urinary incontinence (UI) and overactive bladder (OAB) are growing health care problems for professionals and a personal concern for more than 17 million Americans, most of whom are women. The symptoms of UI and OAB are often unreported due to the patient's perception that 1) current treatment is not effective, 2) the symptoms are a normal consequence of aging or childbirth, and 3) embarrassment regarding this condition. Nurses often find themselves the first point of contact for patients with these symptoms, as many patients have difficulty discussing this problem with their physician. As a health care provider, the mother of three daughters, and a member of a large, aging family, I am concerned about the lack of open discussion about the problem of UI.

Significant advances have been made in the treatment and management of this problem. In 1992 and 1996, the U.S. Department of Health and Human Services, Agency for Health Care Policy and Research, issued Clinical Practice Guidelines called "Urinary Incontinence in Adults." These guidelines summarized the available research and clinical care recommendations on the assessment and treatment of UI; however, when I ask professional audiences or my health care colleagues if they have obtained a copy of these guidelines, they usually are surprised to learn they exist.

Urinary incontinence is not only a major concern in the United States. The World Health Organization held its Second International Consultation on Incontinence in the summer of 2001 to document the current state of the science of UI and to develop guidelines so that countries throughout the world can develop health care policies that address UI and OAB, are evidence based, and make economic sense.

Federal agencies have funded multiple research projects looking at the use of noninvasive behavioral treatments in ambulatory and long-term care settings. With a surge of increased federal funding for UI research in the mid-1980s, significant development in the understanding of the prevalence, causation, assessment, and treatment of UI came to light. This research has demonstrated that UI is never "normal," not even in older adults, people in institutions, or people with dementia. Research outlines the causes of the problem and how to diagnose UI, concluding that UI is treatable, even cur-able, and can always be managed; however, the fact remains that men and women do not seek treatment. When individuals have come forward and told their doctor or nurse about their problem, many have been told to "live with it." The most common reasons cited for failure to seek treatment are that UI is a normal part of aging or that there is a low expectation of benefit from treat-ment (i.e., "There is really nothing that you can do about it"). My colleagues tell me that they usually don't inquire about UI because, besides recommend-ing an absorbent product, they are unsure of what else to tell people.

As health care providers, we must understand that individuals, espe-cially women, despite their age, do not view UI as abnormal either. Health care providers, doctors, and nurses must take the initiative and ask their clients the all-important question, "Do you leak urine at inappropriate times?" We must begin to address the issues of UI and OAB because we will continue to encounter the problem more frequently in our professional and personal lives. Chances are that in the coming decades, each of us will be in a position of caring for a family member who has a problem of incontinence. We must find the solutions and approaches to this problem now before it becomes an epidemic! Providers need to increase the dialogue about UI with their clients, colleagues, and friends because these conditions are a costly, embarrassing, and distressing problem to society as a whole.

Since the beginning of my nursing career in 1975, I have been involved in the area of urology, the bladder, and the pelvic floor. For 15 years, my ca-reer has focused on incontinence and related problems. I have seen significant changes in this field, but I also believe that nursing continues to do little more than cope with the problem. In 1997, I wrote a book for *consumers,* then found that doctors and nurses consider the book informative. I decided to write a second book specifically for professionals. My goal has been to make it a comprehensive, practical book that could be applied to clinical practice in all settings: acute care, office, home care, and long-term care (LTC). I wanted to share with professionals my endless supply of patient education tools that are invaluable to my practice (reproduced in Appendix A), as most patients do not have knowledge about incontinence or overactive bladder, and they do not usually ask for it. I have included my protocols and patient records because I have found them to be helpful and because they are often requested by col-leagues and audiences during my talks on this topic. These tools and forms (found in Appendix B) can be used in assessment, treatment, and management.

This book is a comprehensive review of the current medical approach to UI and its related condition, OAB. It cites medical and nursing research so that you, the provider, can address the growing problem of UI. For those profes-sionals who attend my lectures and ask, "Where are the protocols, the prac-tice guides that can help me address this problem?," here they are! This book

- Reviews anatomy and physiology of the lower urinary tract and pelvic floor

- Outlines UI risk factors and acute and chronic causes

- Discusses the relationship between bowel function and urinary continence

- Details practical strategies for preventing UI

- Outlines behavioral and drug treatments

- Extensively reviews the current products and devices that can be used to manage UI

- Includes a list of companies that supply these products

For readers unfamiliar with all of the terminology related to urinary and fecal function, incontinence, and devices and strategies used to manage UI, an extensive glossary is provided. Terms appearing in the glossary are italicized the first time they appear in text.

I hope that readers come away from this book better informed and inspired to approach the problems of UI and OAB with greater confidence, empathy, and energy.

Acknowledgments

Thank you to my husband Michael, whose encouragement and strength have seen me through many difficult times. His constant support has sustained me.

Thank you to my three daughters, Carolyn Beth, Michelle Amelia, and Emily Joellis, who are the joy of my life.

Thanks to Michelle for her clerical support.

Special thanks for the editorial support of Mary Magnus and Janet Betten.

1

Introduction

Amelia is 76 years old and has leaked urine, at least when she coughs or laughs, since her last baby was born. In the past, this leakage wasn't an inconvenience; it was only a few drops each time, and she could contain it with a small pad or tissues. Her husband never noticed that she had a problem. Her condition worsened when she broke her hip about 5 years ago and had surgery to replace it. Now, she loses urine on her way to the bathroom, and leakage soaks through her pad to her pants. Amelia compensates by going to the bathroom more often to prevent these incontinence episodes. During the day, this habit is not a problem, but at night, it interrupts her sleep.

Amelia hasn't mentioned this problem to anyone, and she fears her daughters will discover her secret. Her good friend and neighbor, Beth, had the same kind of bladder problem, and her sons sent her to a nursing home in a nearby town because of her urine odor. Amelia doesn't want that to happen to her.

A MISUNDERSTOOD PROBLEM

Amelia's problem is a common one. Urinary incontinence (UI) and overactive bladder (OAB) combined affect 17 million Americans, mostly women. They are also expensive medical problems, requiring $28 billion per year in the United States for management and treatment (Wagner & Hu, 1998). Urine loss can range from small drops, as seen in younger women, to moderate or severe leakage, where urine soaks through outer clothing. Approximately 1 in every 10 people who have UI experiences urine loss in amounts that soak through underclothes or more!

Urinary incontinence is never normal, not even in older adults, people with dementia, or people living in nursing facilities. Although UI is treatable, manageable, and even curable, most people with UI do not seek help for their problem. Surveys have shown that on average, women wait 3 years before seeking treatment, whereas men wait approximately 6 months.

What these people do not realize is that there has been a great deal of medical research looking at the assessment and management of UI. This research has helped doctors and nurses understand the prevalence, cause, assessment, and treatment of UI. New medications are effective and have fewer side effects. Direct-to-consumer advertisement has helped people to become better informed about OAB and available medications. Treatments—particularly behavioral interventions, medications, and, in some cases, surgery—can be successful in 8 out of 10 people (Fantl et al., 1996).

PROFESSIONAL EDUCATION ON INCONTINENCE

The problem, unfortunately, is not just one of consumer awareness. Despite a growing body of information available on incontinence, professional education on urinary and fecal incontinence remains only a small or nonexistent part of the basic training of doctors, nurses, and allied health professionals. Many times, a person who admits to having urinary incontinence is told that the cause is simply old age or typical body change. Self-care practices such as regular toileting, increased fluid intake, reduced caffeine intake, exercise, and weight reduction are some basic ways to prevent or reduce UI, but they are not actively promoted.

In response to this problem, the World Health Organization's Second Consultation on Incontinence recommended compulsory inclusion of incontinence in the undergraduate curriculum of doctors, nurses, physical therapists, pharmacists, and other health care professionals (Newman et al., in press). This group of experts felt that incontinence must be identified and preferably delivered as a separate topic, not fragmented between different modules of the educational curriculum. In addition, in 1992 and 1996 the Agency for Health Care Policy and Research (AHCPR), now known as the Agency for Healthcare Research and Quality (AHRQ), produced Clinical Practice Guidelines called "Urinary Incontinence in Adults" (AHCPR, 1992; Fantl et al., 1996). These guidelines were aimed at health care professionals and were intended to help standardize the assessment and management of urinary incontinence in adults (AHCPR, 1992; Fantl et al., 1996). Although widely quoted, they have failed to inform the practice of medical practitioners or their trainees. In a survey, 50% of physicians who treat bladder disorders (25% of whom were family practice physicians) were not familiar with the AHCPR guidelines (Wein et al., 1998). The concept of using bladder diaries or checking postvoid residual urine as part of basic assessment is still foreign to most gynecologists, family doctors, and advance practice nurses (APNs) not specializing in continence. Specialist education programs with relevant accreditation mechanisms (and planned periodic recredentialing) to safeguard patient interests need to be developed for urologists, gynecologists, specialist nurses, physical therapists, and others.

Although there are a growing number of doctors, nurses, and allied health professionals who are developing expertise caring for incontinent patients, there are no academic or clinical proficiency requirements to be considered a "continence practitioner or specialist." The American Board of Obstetricians and Gynecology has developed courses and credentialing of specially trained *urogynecologists* with separate examinations. These specialists are being trained in academic medical centers that have created a multidisciplinary team that consists of gynecology, urology, gastroenterology, and nursing. This allows the team to treat men and women for all conditions of the pelvic floor: urinary and fecal incontinence, pelvic prolapse, and chronic pelvic pain syndromes. The fear with such credential programs, however, is that incontinence may be seen as the province of an elite group of super-specialists who get further and further away from their colleagues (Newman et al., in press).

The Wound, Ostomy, and Continence Nurses Society (WOCN) developed the first certification program for continence care nurses (Jirovec, Wyman, & Wells, 1998). The Society of Urologic Nurses and Associates (SUNA) certification program for APNs tests knowledge on UI and related urologic disorders. Unfortunately, the number of nurses certified through these two organizations has not been significant.

Nurses are not always positive toward continence education. In one study, 20% of nurses polled thought that nurses working in nursing facilities would be apathetic or resistant to a program on incontinence (Palmer, 1995). Colling (1988) noted that more than half the faculty who teach geriatric content in nursing programs lack any formal education specifically related to UI. In another study, Morishita, Uman, and Pierson (1994) describe UI content that is reportedly taught in most nursing school curricula: The didactic component is only 2 hours in length and clinical experience is left to chance, offering little assurance that practice and feedback are obtained. Specific knowledge about UI, as well as the broader area of gerontological nursing, is not tested in undergraduate programs, which makes adequate coverage of UI content in nursing curricula unlikely.

Part of the problem with UI nursing care is that the care is fragmented and is practiced by several levels of nurses, from nursing assistants or aides to APNs. Because the care is fragmented, so is nursing's approach to basic assessment, treatment, and management strategies. In most institutional health care settings, nurses not only provide direct patient care, they are also responsible for the philosophy, standard, and policy of care while supervising the performance of other nursing staff members (Gallo, Newman, & Sasso, 2001). Although manufacturers have introduced more diverse UI products in the U.S. retail market, nursing strategy for management of UI has centered almost exclusively on containment of urine leakage (i.e., incontinence pads, catheters). Although UI prevalence rates for persons living in long-term care facilities and in their homes are over 50%, prevention techniques and rehabilitative treatments are not routinely initiated by nurses caring for these patients. This is a growing dilemma that will only worsen as the U.S. population ages.

One group of allied health professionals—physical therapists—has targeted women's health as an integral part of the educational curriculum. The American Physical Therapy Association, Section on Women's Health, provides an educational program geared to therapists who are interested in women's health, particularly pelvic muscle disorders such as UI and chronic pelvic pain.

Besides formal training, doctors, nurses, and health care organizations have also established web sites on UI for consumers and health care professionals who are Internet users (Diering & Palmer, 2001; Sandvik, 1999; see Appendix C: Resources). For many professionals, this is a significant source of expanded information on this problem.

Incontinence and OAB are often complex and multifaceted problems, particularly in frail or dependent individuals. These conditions usually require input from a wide variety of providers to be addressed effectively. However, if people do voice their incontinence problems, professionals must be educated on solutions that are individualized and effective. There are many solutions to incontinence, and there are many products and devices that can assist people with managing their problem, so that they can live an active and more enjoyable lifestyle.

Relief for Amelia

Amelia mentioned her incontinence when she visited her family doctor. He felt that a new medication would decrease her incontinence, which he explained was being caused by bladder contractions. At first the medication helped, but after 3 months Amelia noticed that she was having more incontinent accidents. Her doctor suggested she see a specialist at a continence treatment center. The doctor at the center was a urologist who tested her urine for infection and did an ultrasound that showed she was successfully emptying her bladder. He then told Amelia that he would like her to see his nurse practitioner (NP) who specialized in other treatments for UI. Amelia was asked to keep a Bladder Diary for 3 days and to bring it with her to her next visit.

Amelia met with the nurse practitioner, who reviewed her Bladder Diary and diet and pointed out foods and liquids that may be irritating her bladder. She taught Amelia simple techniques for decreasing urinary urgency and told her to keep taking the medication because all of these treatments together would help her problem. After a month, Amelia felt she had more control of her bladder, especially her urgency, and felt she could even ask to cut back on the medication when she next saw her NP.

With better information and resources, professionals could help more people like Amelia regain control and confidence over this critical area of their lives. Here, collected in a single book, is much of what any professional needs to know.

REFERENCES

Agency for Health Care Policy and Research (AHCPR). (1992). *Urinary incontinence in adults: Clinical practice guideline* (AHCPR Publication No. 92-0038). Rockville, MD: Public Health Service, U.S. Department of Health and Human Services.

Colling, J. (1988). Educating nurses to care for the incontinent patient. *Nursing Clinics of North America, 23,* 279–289.

Diering, C., & Palmer, M.H. (2001). Professional information about urinary incontinence on the world wide web: Is it timely? Is it accurate? *Journal of Wound, Ostomy, and Continence Nursing, 27*(6), 1–9.

Fantl, J.A., Newman, D.K., Colling, J., DeLancey, J.O.L., Keeys, C., Loughery, R., Norton, P., Ouslander, J., Schnelle, J., Stoskin, D., Tries, J., Urich, V., Vitousek, S.H., Weiss, B.D., & Whitmore, K. (1996). *Urinary incontinence in adults: Acute and chronic management. Clinical practice guideline* (No. 2. Update; AHCPR Publication No. 96-0682). Rockville, MD: U.S. Department of Health and Human Services.

Gallo, M., Newman, D.K., & Sasso, K. (2001). The evolution of the continence nurse specialist. In L. Cardozo & D. Staskin (Eds.), *Textbook of female urology and urogynaecology.* Oxford, England: Isis Medical Media.

Jirovec, M.M., Wyman, J.F., & Wells, T.J. (1998). Addressing urinary incontinence with educational continence-care competencies. *Image: The Journal of Nursing Scholarship, 30,* 375–378.

Morishita, L., Uman, G.C., & Pierson, C.A. (1994). Education on adult urinary incontinence in nursing school curricula: Can it be done in two hours? *Nursing Outlook, 42,* 123–129.

Newman, D.K., Denis, L., Gartley, C.B., Gruenwald, I., Lim, P.H.C., Millard, R., & Roberts, R. (in press). Promotion, education and organization for continence care. In P. Abrams, S. Khoury, & A. Wein (Eds.), *Incontinence proceedings from the second international consultation on incontinence.* Plymouth, United Kingdom: Health Publication.

Palmer, M.H. (1995). Nurses' knowledge and beliefs about continence interventions in long-term care. *Journal of Advanced Nursing, 21,* 1065–1072.

Sandvik, H. (1999). Health information and interaction on the Internet: A survey of female urinary incontinence *British Medical Journal, 319,* 29–32.

Wagner, T.H., & Hu, T.W. (1998). Economic costs of urinary incontinence in 1995. *Urology, 51*(3), 355–361.

Wein, A.J., Appell, R.A., Blavias, J.G., Bump, R.C., Diokno, A.C., Fantl, J.A., Norton, P., & Resnick, N.M. (1998). *Bladder disorders monitor: Bladder disorders clinical practice consensus report.* Hackensack, NJ: Center for Bio-Medical Communications.

2

The Problem of Incontinence

Urinary incontinence (UI), the involuntary and unwanted loss of urine, is a significant health problem. An estimated 15 million Americans have UI. In addition to UI, the related overactive bladder (OAB; urinary urgency and frequency) also affects millions of Americans. Women may be disproportionately affected by UI. The prevalence of UI has been reported to be higher in women than men (38% versus 19%). The risk of developing OAB increases with age, with a prevalence of 30%–40% in people older than 75 years of age. To put this into perspective, OAB is more common than diabetes and is similar in prevalence to asthma. During 1995, an estimated 6.3 million community-dwelling older adults and 1.2 million nursing facility residents were living with UI (Wagner & Hu, 1998). This is a concern because by the year 2020, more than one in six Americans will be 65 or older, and by the year 2030, nearly one in five Americans will be 65 or older. The most significant rise in the aging population is in the age group older than 85 years, often called the "old-old," whose numbers will more than double by 2030. This group tends to be frail, dependent, and increasingly in need of health care and custodial services. This aging population is already demanding better solutions to the health care problems they face.

Urinary incontinence and OAB affect people of all age groups but are seen more often in older adults. Although age does not necessarily cause UI and OAB, factors that may lead to these conditions are more prevalent in older people. Once UI occurs, it persists in the older adult, especially in someone who is frail and has multiple medical conditions. Importantly, because UI, OAB, and related pelvic disorders (see Table 2.1) are multifactorial problems, they are difficult to distinctively diagnose and therefore treat in a straightforward fashion.

It is difficult to estimate the true prevalence of UI and OAB. Despite the considerable impact of bladder storage symptoms on quality of life, many people never seek medical help and are thus uncounted. The most common reasons that people with UI and OAB do not seek treatment are the (*erroneous!*) beliefs that 1) the symptoms are a normal consequence of aging, childbirth, or both and 2) no treatment is available. Furthermore, the majority of the prevalence studies (and other studies) undertaken in this area have focused only on one symptom, urinary leakage. Frequency and urgency without incontinence

Table 2.1. Associated bladder and pelvic disorders

Condition	Description
Interstitial cystitis (IC)	Severe, debilitating, chronic disorder of the bladder found primarily in women. People with IC have a bladder wall that is tender and easily irritated, leading to uncomfortable symptoms. Symptoms include severe urinary urgency, frequent urination, lower abdominal or perineal pain and pressure, painful sexual intercourse, and, in many cases, urinary incontinence. IC begins gradually and becomes progressively worse. Symptoms may go into remission but usually return.
Prostatitis	Inflammation (swelling) of the prostate gland caused by either a bacterial infection or by the backup of prostate secretions within the prostate gland. Prostatitis may occur in association with sexual activity. Men will have a small, watery discharge from the head of the penis similar to a runny nose and experience symptoms of frequent urination, discomfort when urinating, and urinary urgency.
Chronic pelvic pain (CPP)	Pelvic pain that continues for more than 6 months and is seen more often in adult white women. CPP can be identified clinically by six common characteristics: 1. Duration of 6 months or longer 2. Incomplete relief with most treatment 3. Significantly impaired function at home or work 4. Signs of depression (e.g., early morning awakenings, weight loss, anorexia) 5. Pain out of proportion to pathology 6. Altered family and social roles CPP originates in the region of the lower abdomen and pelvis, although the pain may extend downward to involve the lower extremities or upward to the thoracolumbar area. Changes associated with pain include physical and mental fatigue, depression and anxiety, dyspareunia causing decreased sexual activity, and interruptions in sleep. Other typically reported symptoms include rectal itching, and burning during frequent bowel movements.
Vulvodynia	Chronic vulvar discomfort or pain, especially characterized by complaints of perineal burning, stinging, irritation, or rawness. The most common symptoms are dyspareunia, severe point tenderness on touch, perineal irritation, and vestibular erythema. Women will have complaints of perineal hypersensitivity to clothing and touch. Many women with vulvodynia will also report urological symptoms such as urgency, frequency, and dysuria. These symptoms are similar to those seen with IC.

have seldom been investigated. A further problem in arriving at an accurate prevalence figure is that of defining urgency and frequency.

Prevalence of UI is high, especially in older adults who reside in nursing facilities and those who are homebound. Although prevalence can vary among individual long-term care (LTC) facilities, UI affects approximately 50% of nursing facility residents. Depending on the case mix, rates can be 70% and higher in facilities housing frail adults with functional impairments. The prevalence of UI is considered an indicator of the quality of nursing facility care.

INCONTINENCE IN THE COMMUNITY

An estimated 15%–30% of community-dwelling older adults have UI. The prevalence rate among older women residing in the community is 15%–35% (Fantl, Newman, Colling, et al., 1996). Among middle-age and younger women, prevalence ranges from 12% to 42%, with a mean of 25% (Thom, 1998). Estimates suggest that UI disrupts the lives of approximately 20% of adult women. Incontinence affects between 20% and 34% of adult women in the postpartum period, and 3% of these women experience leakage weekly or more frequently (Wilson & Herbison, 1998). Prevalence rates are 1.5%–5% for men ages 15–60 years and increase to 19% for men older than 60 years (Fantl et al., 1996). Management strategies in dealing with UI differ between men and women. Men are more likely to limit fluids and trips to the bathroom and are more likely to see a physician about their problem. Women more frequently limit fluid intake and wear perineal pads.

Epidemiological and clinical studies of individuals with UI indicate that the condition has considerable impact on overall quality of life and well-being. The inability to control urine is one of the most unpleasant and distressing symptoms a person can experience. The personal consequences of incontinence are numerous. It has been demonstrated that incontinent women have lower levels of emotional well-being than continent women (Wyman, Harkins, & Fantl, 1990).

Urinary incontinence can limit a person's social activities and interpersonal relationships. Depressive symptoms are associated with UI, and in one study the perception of the interference of incontinence with daily activities was the best predictor of depressive symptoms (Dugan et al., 2000). The exact nature of the relationship among UI, depression, and recovery is not clear. However, there are effective treatments for both UI and depressive symptoms in older adults. Clinicians must also engage in preventive measures.

In women, UI is a distressing and disabling condition. It can cause significant morbidity and affects the social, psychological, occupational, domestic, physical, and sexual lives of 15%–30% of women of all ages. It is often the cause of social isolation and physiological problems. Women who experience UI will report anxiety and depression and feel that the abnormal symptoms associated with UI have rendered life intolerable. Some may give up or restrict certain domestic routines and household chores, as well as outside activities such as shopping, traveling, and church attendance. Others will only frequent places where bathroom facilities are known and easily accessible. Women who are physically active and experience urine leakage during these activities will curtail and even stop exercising or dancing. Some will make adjustments in an activity or behavior that causes UI (e.g., change from high- to low-impact aerobics, avoid heavy lifting).

Individuals with UI commonly report a fear of odor and embarrassment. They feel unclean and become obsessed with personal hygiene. Women especially will prematurely turn to absorbent perineal pads to prevent the leakage from becoming noticeable and to avoid odor.

Relationships with spouses and other family members may be affected. Both men and women may avoid sexual intimacy because of the fear of urine leakage during intercourse or interrupting intercourse because of the need to urinate. Men with erectile dysfunction (ED) and incontinence after radical prostatectomy surgery will be disinterested in pursuing treatment for ED until incontinence resolves. Men and women will avoid or curtail activities in an attempt to prevent the possibility of an incontinence episode.

HOME CARE SETTING

Urinary incontinence is seen in 53% of homebound older adults and is a leading reason for caregivers to place a family member in a nursing facility. Urinary incontinence is a frequently seen diagnosis in patients requiring skilled nursing care in the home. Preliminary data from a survey of 8,400 home and hospice health agencies indicated that genitourinary conditions were among the 20 leading diagnoses for patients added to their caseloads (Strahan, 1994). Urinary incontinence is one of the 10 leading diagnoses for homebound individuals and first in total charges to Medicare for nursing services per person served (Ruther & Helbing, 1988). In a study of low-income, older individuals receiving publicly funded home care services, 23% were incontinent of urine and generated greater costs because of paraprofessional and other supportive care (Baker & Bice, 1995). Urinary incontinence tends to be severe among homebound older adults in both frequency and volume (McDowell, Engberg, Rodriguez, Engberg, & Sereika, 1996).

Even though homebound older people tend to have multiple health and functional disabilities, they perceive UI to be a very disturbing problem that further restricts activities. The combination of decreased functional ability and UI is particularly challenging to both professional and nonprofessional caregivers. The magnitude of the problem of caring for incontinent homebound individuals will no doubt increase as the absolute number of older people increases and as maintenance of dependent older people at home becomes more common. Home care providers will need to address this common and costly problem.

The psychosocial impact of UI imposes a significant burden on individuals and their families, caregivers, and health care clinicians. Dependence on caregivers increases as incontinence worsens and as homebound older people use *indwelling catheters* and other supportive devices that increase the risk of infection, morbidity, and mortality. Most people with UI manage using a combination of previous treatment strategies plus their own self-devised strategies. Most have little or no problem finding commercially available absorbent products. Sometimes, though, women refuse to participate in situations outside the home for fear of being incontinent, which can be especially frustrating for family members, particularly spouses (Baker & Bice, 1995; Mitterness, 1987). Urinary incontinence can predispose a woman to admission to a LTC facility. A study that examined reasons for institutional placement found that 44% of family members reported that UI was a significant factor in placing a relative in a nursing facility (Johnson & Werner, 1982). Finally, prolonged incontinence can result in medical complications such as skin irritation, infection, and *decubitus ulcers*.

Incontinence is a relentless source of weariness for caregivers, especially older caregivers. Physical exertion, often called *caregiver burden,* increases day by day. People with functional impairment and UI need to be lifted and turned to prevent skin breakdown, to change incontinence products and bed pads, and to wash away the urine. In addition, incontinence is not only a daytime problem. During the night, a caregiver's sleep is disturbed to assist with toileting and transfers to commodes. In some situations the caregiver's burden is so great that he or she becomes ill. If older partners are frail themselves, they may even die before the incontinent person for whom they are caring.

Denial of incontinence by an older family member is a tricky dilemma for both family members and professionals who may be assisting the family with caregiving. Older people experience a loss of sensitivity to smell as they age. Also, some block out awareness of their incontinence to avoid its implications. If the family confronts the denial head on, they may provoke hostility and humiliation and cause an incontinent individual to further withdraw from acknowledgment of the problem.

INCONTINENCE IN INSTITUTIONS

Long-Term Care

Uncontrolled loss of urine to a degree sufficient to be a problem is the second leading cause of institutional placement of older adults. There are nearly 2 million nursing facility residents in the United States. Among residents of LTC facilities (specifically skilled nursing facilities) in the United States, 50% or more experience UI episodes frequently and 43% have fecal incontinence. Residents who have both are referred to as having *double incontinence.* UI is a primary reason that precipitates or contributes to a person's decision to enter a nursing facility or a family's decision to place an older family member into nursing facility care. Once UI occurs, it appears to persist throughout the resident's stay. Risk factors identified include presence of fecal incontinence, male gender, dementia, and impaired mobility, especially when the person is walking or being moved from one place to another (Palmer, German, & Ouslander, 1991).

Few studies have investigated the incidence of incontinence. One study investigating newly admitted nursing facility residents reported that 24% of women residents who were continent at admission were incontinent 1 year after admission (Ouslander, Palmer, Rovner, & German, 1993). In that study, the development of UI was found to be associated with cognitive impairment, the inability to transfer or walk independently, and poor adjustment to the nursing facility. In a study of 69 hip fracture patients, the incidence of UI in women was 24% (Palmer, Myers, & Fedenko, 1997). Cognitive impairment was found to be an independent predictor of incontinence (Ouslander et al., 1993).

There are many reasons for the occurence of UI in nursing facilities. Restricted mobility is an important factor because nursing facility residents who are placed in *restraints* or use wheelchairs are unable to toilet when needed. Social indifference and cognitive impairment also play a role in the incidence of incontinence in nursing facilities. Many people enter a nursing facility continent but lose their ability to use the toilet soon afterward, usually because they are in a strange environment and the staff fail to take them to the bathroom as often as necessary. Once in the nursing facility, most residents learn to live with UI. Residents will invest more time and effort in protecting themselves from the consequences of urine leakage by "managing" the problem themselves than in seeking treatment (Robinson, 2000).

It appears as though there is a discrepancy between the goals of residents and those of staff for UI treatment preferences in the LTC environment. Residents want treatment that allows them to remain dry but prevents dependence on staff. In a study that surveyed LTC residents, family members, and staff, residents perceived the staff as unwilling and unable to implement UI interventions such as toileting assistance (Johnson, Ouslander, Uman, & Schnelle, 2001). Residents expressed preference for medication and the use of absorbent products as treatments of choice. They viewed toileting or *prompted voiding* programs as fostering dependence. Families preferred medications to absorbent products. Staff felt prompted voiding was a more appropriate UI treatment than either absorbent products or more invasive treatments such as catheters.

Since 1980, federal agencies have focused on the advances made in treating and managing this problem. Federal agencies, specifically the National Institutes of Health, have funded multiple research projects investigating the effectiveness of toileting assistance programs in the LTC setting. Although the value of toileting programs, specifically prompted voiding, has been well documented in the research setting, other elements must be in place if these practices are to be transferred effectively to the clinical setting. Clinical practice guidelines have been developed to outline approaches to assessment, management, and care decisions (American Medical Directors Association, 1996; Fantl et al., 1996).

Although UI is common, especially among older adults, it is not a normal part of aging. Research has shown that, when properly assessed and treated, it can be corrected in about 30% of nursing facility residents and suitably controlled and managed in the rest (Fantl et al., 1996). Problems associated with the delivery of continence care in LTC facilities have been identified

(Lekan-Rutledge, Palmer, & Belyea, 1998; Palmer, Bennett, Marks, McCormick, & Engel, 1994). They include the following:

- Inadequate initial staff education on UI and interventions appropriate for this population

- Lack of assessment or evidence of benefit before placing an incontinent resident on a toileting program

- Lack of individualized continence care; rather, care is at the convenience of the staff

- Lack of any continence care

- Inadequate staffing

- Poor communication and support from administrative staff regarding expectations

- Lack of financial incentives to keep resident dry

Current management practices in nursing facilities are not consistent with recommended guidelines. It is believed that remediable conditions exist in residents of nursing facilities that are not directly related to bladder dysfunction yet have an impact on continence (e.g., inability to transfer, inability to dress, inability to toilet, use of trunk restraints, inability to rise from chair, use of antianxiety/hypnotic medications; Brandeis, Baumann, Hossain, Morris, & Resnick, 1997). However, staff are not actively addressing the problem.

Staff Issues in Caring for Residents with UI   Staff attitudes toward UI play a major role in the way incontinent residents are treated. Ninety percent of the actual care of residents—bathing, dressing, toileting, and feeding—is provided by certified nurse assistants (CNAs), who have limited training and education in the care of older adults. Staff may believe that incontinence is expected in nursing facility residents because UI is a natural part of aging, and they may convey their acceptance of incontinence directly to the resident (Yu, Kaltreider, & Brannon, 1991). Staff also may act out negative feelings toward these residents (Harke & Richgels, 1992; Lekan-Rutledge et al., 1998; Palmer, 1995; Smith, 1998). The resident with UI correctly perceives that the only way to get attention, although many times negative attention, is through incontinence. Staff also feel that it is quicker to change an absorbent pad than it is to toilet a resident. This leads to the usual routine seen in most nursing homes, which is to "check and change."

The hopeless acceptance of UI can make it into a "nonproblem." CNAs are not familiar with interventions such as prompted voiding and therefore are not supportive of treatment. For interventions to be successful in nursing facilities, staff, particularly CNAs, must believe in the value of continence and be committed to achieving it (Wagner & Colling, 1993). One study demonstrated significantly improved outcomes for three clinical problems—urinary incontinence, depression, and pressure ulcers—when gerontological advanced practice nurses (APNs) worked with staff to implement scientifically based protocols (Ryden et al., 2000). In addition to working with nursing facilities to provide resident evaluation as physician extenders, this research indicates that APNs can be an effective link between current research-based knowledge about clinical problems and nursing facility staff. In this study, consistent educational efforts with staff and residents demonstrated that interventions can improve or stabilize the level of UI in many individuals.

Assessment of residents with incontinence is necessary to determine the pathophysiological causes and associated factors that can impede self-toileting. Nurses can perform this evaluation at the bedside. Treatment techniques, specifically behavioral interventions and toileting assistance programs, can be readily incorporated into nursing practice. Most nursing facility staff can easily adapt the use of interventions such as bowel and nighttime voiding management and dietary modifications. Research in the nursing facility has demonstrated the effectiveness of toileting assistance programs; however, very little of this research and few of the resulting documented techniques have been used by facility staff. A statewide assessment of Texas Medicaid nursing facilities (Cortes, Montgomery, Morrow, & Monroe, 2000) indicated that 63% of residents had UI but only 12% had appropriate inclusion of toileting assistance in their care plan. Among those residents for whom a toileting program would be desirable and likely beneficial, 80% did not receive it. The key to success is identifying which residents should be targeted for each specific program. Staff education remains an ongoing issue. Staff must be aware of attitudes and beliefs about the aging process and its impact on the genitourinary system in order to provide effective care.

Impact of State and Federal Regulations   The prevalence of UI is considered an indicator of the quality of nursing facility care (Zimmerman et al., 1995). As part of the state certification survey that nursing facilities must submit to annually to receive federal and state funding, surveyors will look for a completed *Minimum Data Set* (MDS), appropriate *Resident Assessment Protocol* (RAP), and updated plans of care to address UI. The MDS has been found to be reliable when administered by nursing facility staff (Resnick, Brandeis, Baumann, & Morris, 1996). In addition, chronic bladder dysfunction, particularly UI, was identified in guidelines from the Health Care Financing Administration (now called the Centers for Medicare & Medicaid Services facilities) as a primary risk factor for the development of pressure sores (Zimmerman et al., 1995). Therefore, reducing the incidence of or appropriately managing incontinence should reduce the incidence of incontinence-related skin rashes and maceration that are associated with *pressure sore* development.

In recent years, use of the MDS has been expanded, and efforts are being made to compare nursing facilities on MDS-derived quality indicators and to track changes in quality over time. These regulations have changed the atmosphere of long-term care from a custodial to a rehabilitative environment.

Hospitals and Rehabilitation Centers

There are few recent prevalence estimates of incontinence in hospitalized patients. In one report, approximately 24% of patients between 65 and 74 years of age and 48% of patients 75 years and older had at least one episode of incontinence during hospitalization (Palmer et al., 1997). Incontinence is often overlooked in hospitalized older patients. Researchers analyzing Veterans Administration (VA) administrative data found that, although 43% of the patients were incontinent, only 3.4% of cases had incontinence as a discharge diagnosis (Armstrong & Ferguson, 1998). Although acute care hospital stays are generally short, UI is a significant health problem and should not be overlooked. In a geriatric rehabilitation unit, 21.9% of the patients had UI on admission (Resnick, Slocum, Ra, & Moffett, 1996). During the course of rehabilitation, there was a decrease in the incidence of UI to 16%. In this study, UI was highly correlated with limitations in ambulation. Discharge nurses should design a plan that includes referral to a continence nurse or physician specialist for further treatment. Protocols should be developed to direct acute care clinical practice (Bradway, Hernly, & NICHE faculty, 1998).

COSTS AND FINANCIAL ASPECTS

In the United States, society incurs a significant economic burden as a result of UI. The cost (direct and indirect) of caring for incontinent people older than age 65 in the community and in nursing facilities was estimated to be $24 billion annually in 1995 (Wagner & Hu, 1998). This figure is the expenditure for Medicare Part A program costs and reflects the resources spent to treat UI and to mitigate its effects in people older than age 65. The direct costs were estimated as $16.3 billion, including $12.4 billion for women and $3.8 billion for men. Costs for community-dwelling women older than age 65 ($8.6 billion) were greater than institutionalized women ($3.8 billion; Wilson, Brown, Shin, Luc, & Subak, 2001). These costs are predominately for palliative rather than rehabilitative services. Wilson et al. (2001) calculated that, for women, the largest cost category was routine care (70%), followed by nursing facility admissions (14%), treatment (9%), complications (6%), and evaluation and diagnosis (1%). Coverage of treatment costs by third-party payers varies considerably. Because absorbent products are considered hygienic products, they are not reimbursed. Medications prescribed for incontinence are not covered under Medicare. Thus, costs are directly related to the need for increased nursing care from secondary problems such as urinary tract infections, skin breakdown and infection, falls and subsequent injury, psychological distress, and withdrawal (Fantl et al., 1996). It is expected that overall costs for managing UI will increase as the aging population increases.

One study attempted to determine resource consumption within VA facilities for the treatment of UI (Armstrong & Ferguson, 1998). Facilities included those providing acute and long-term care and outpatient care. It was found that a large portion of resource consumption was due to nursing care for clients with UI. Ninety minutes per patient per day was required to clean patients after incontinent episodes ("check and change"), to apply skin products, and to change absorbent pads. An additional 90 minutes of nursing time per patient per day was used to assist patients to the bathroom. Based on these estimates, nursing time cost per incontinent patient per day was estimated to be $119.88. This study indicates that UI may have higher direct costs than was once believed.

REFERENCES

American Medical Directors Association. (1996). *Urinary incontinence clinical practice guideline.* Columbia, MD: Author.

Armstrong, E.P., & Ferguson, T.A. (1998, October). Urinary incontinence: Healthcare resource consumption in Veterans Affairs Medical Centers. *Veterans Health System Journal,* 37–42.

Baker, D.I., & Bice, T.W. (1995). The influence of urinary incontinence on publicly financed home care services to low-income elderly people. *Gerontologist, 35*(3), 360–369.

Brandeis, G.H., Baumann, M.M., Hossain, M., Morris, J.N., & Resnick, N.M. (1997). The prevalence of potentially remediable urinary incontinence in frail older people: A study using the Minimum Data Set. *Journal of the American Geriatrics Society, 45,* 179–184.

Bradway, C., Hernly, S., & NICHE faculty. (1998). Urinary incontinence in older adults admitted to acute care. *Geriatric Nursing, 19,* 98–102.

Cortes, L.L., Montgomery, E.W., Morrow, K.A., & Monroe, D.M. (2000). *A statewide assessment of quality of care, quality of life and consumer satisfaction in Texas Medicaid nursing facilities* (pp. 1–99). Austin: Texas Department of Human Services Long Term Care Office of Programs, Medical Quality Assurance.

Dugan, E., Cohen, S.J., Bland, D.R., Preisser, J.S., Davis, C.C., Suggs, P.K., & McGann, P. (2000). The association of depressive symptoms and urinary incontinence among older adults. *Journal of the American Geriatrics Society, 48,* 413–416.

Fantl, J., Newman, D., Colling, J., et al., for the Urinary Incontinence in Adults Guideline Update Panel. (1996). *Urinary incontinence in adults: Acute and chronic management. Clinical practice guideline* (No. 2. Update; AHCPR Publication No. 96-0692). Rockville, MD: Agency for Health Care and Policy Research.

Harke, J.M., & Richgels, K. (1992). Barriers to implementing a continence program in nursing homes. *Clinical Nursing Research, 1*(2), 156–168.

Johnson, M.J., & Werner, C. (1982). We have no choice: A study of familial guilt feelings surrounding nursing home care. *Journal of Gerontologic Nursing, 8*(11), 641–645, 654.

Johnson, T.M., Ouslander, J.G., Uman, G.C., & Schnelle, J.F. (2001). Urinary incontinence treatment preferences in long-term care. *Journal of the American Geriatrics Society, 49*(6), 710–718.

Lekan-Rutledge, D., Palmer, M.H., & Belyea, M. (1998). In their own words: Nursing assistants' perceptions of barriers to implementation of prompted voiding in long-term care. *Gerontologist, 38*(3), 370–378.

McDowell, B.J., Engberg, S., Rodriguez, E., Engberg, R., & Sereika, S. (1996). Characteristics of urinary incontinence in homebound older adults. *Journal of the American Geriatrics Society, 44*(8), 963–968.

Mitterness, L.S. (1987). The management of urinary incontinence by community-living elderly. *Gerontologist, 27,* 185.

Ouslander, J.G., Palmer, M.H., Rovner, B.W., & German, P.S. (1993). Urinary incontinence in nursing homes: Incidence, remission and associated factors. *Journal of the American Geriatrics Society, 41,* 1083–1089.

Palmer, M.H. (1995). Nurses' knowledge and beliefs about continence interventions in long-term care. *Journal of Advanced Nursing, 21,* 1065–1072.

Palmer, M.H., Bennett, R.G., Marks, J., McCormick, K.A., & Engel, B.T. (1994). Urinary incontinence: A program that works. *Journal of Long Term Care Administration, 22*(2), 19–25.

Palmer, M.H., German, P.S., & Ouslander, J.G. (1991). Risk factors for urinary incontinence one year after nursing home admission. *Research in Nursing and Health, 14,* 405–412.

Palmer, M.H., Myers, A. & Fedenko, K. (1997). Urinary continence changes after hip fracture repair. *Clinical Nursing Research, 6*(1), 8–24.

Resnick, B., Slocum, D., Ra, L., & Moffett, P. (1996). Geriatric rehabilitation: Nursing interventions and outcomes focusing on urinary function and knowledge of medications. *Rehabilitation Nursing, 21*(3), 142–147.

Resnick, N.M., Brandeis, G.H., Baumann, M.M., & Morris, J.N. (1996). Evaluating a national assessment strategy for urinary incontinence in nursing home residents. *Neurourology and Urodynamics, 15,* 583–598.

Robinson, J.P. (2000). Managing urinary incontinence in the nursing home: Residents' perspectives. *Journal of Advanced Nursing, 31*(1), 68–77.

Ruther, M., & Helbing, C. (1988). Health care financing trends: Use and cost of home health services under Medicare. *Health Care Financing Review, 10,* 105–108.

Ryden, M.B., Snyder, M., Gross, C.R., Savik, K., Pearson, V., Krichbaum, K., & Mueller, C. (2000). Value-added outcomes: The use of advanced practice nurses in long-term facilities. *Gerontologist, 40*(6), 654–662.

Smith, D.B. (1998). A continence care approach for long-term care facilities. *Geriatric Nursing, 19*(2), 81–86.

Strahan, G.W. (1994). *An overview of home health and hospice care patients: Preliminary data from the 1993 National Home and Hospice Care Survey* (Advance data from Vital and Health Statistics, No. 256). Hyattsville, MD: National Center for Health Statistics.

Thom, D.H. (1998). Variations in estimates of urinary incontinence prevalence in the community: Effects of differences in definition, population characteristics, and study type. *Journal of the American Geriatrics Society, 246,* 473–480.

Wagner, A., & Colling, J. (1993, Summer). Resistance to change: Understanding the aides' point of view. *Journal of Long-Term Care Administration, 21,* 27–30.

Wagner, T.H., & Hu, T.W. (1998). Economic costs of urinary incontinence in 1995. *Urology, 51*(3), 355–361.

Wilson, L., Brown, J.S., Shin, G.P., Luc, K.O., & Subak, L.L. (2001). Annual direct cost of urinary incontinence. *Obstetrics and Gynecology, 98*(3), 398–405.

Wilson, P., & Herbison, G. (1998). A randomized, controlled trial of pelvic floor muscle exercises to treat postnatal urinary incontinence. *International Urogynecology Journal, 9,* 257–264.

Wyman, J.F., Harkins, S.W., & Fantl, A. (1990). Psychosocial impact of urinary incontinence in the community dwelling population. *Journal of American Geriatrics Society, 38*(3), 282–288.

Yu, L.C., Kaltreider, D.L., & Brannon, D. (1991). Urinary incontinence: Nursing home staff reaction toward residents. *Journal of Gerontological Nursing, 17*(11), 34–41.

Zimmerman, D.R., Karon, S.L., Arling, G., et al. (1995). Development and testing of nursing home quality indicators. *Health Care Financing Review, 16*(4), 107–127.

3

Understanding Bladder Function

The urinary system, composed of the upper and lower urinary tracts, is highly efficient in removing waste products from the blood and excreting them from the body. The *upper urinary tract* includes the two kidneys and two ureters (see Figures 3.1 and 3.2). The paired, fist-sized kidneys filter impurities from the blood and convert them into urine. They also regulate the chemical makeup of the blood and preserve the correct balance between salt and water in the body. Urine is transported from the kidneys through the ureters down to the bladder. In relation to bladder disorders, conditions such as unresolved urinary retention and untreated urinary tract infections can cause upper urinary tract damage.

The *lower urinary tract* is composed of the bladder, prostate (in men only), urethra, internal and external sphincters, and urethral meatus (see Figure 3.3). The bladder fills and expands passively with urine, which is passed via the ureters. In relation to bladder disorders, conditions such as urinary incontinence (UI) usually only affect the lower urinary tract.

BLADDER

The bladder is a hollow, muscular sac that is capable of storing urine for prolonged periods of time. The bladder lies behind the *pubic symphysis* (the center front portion of the pelvic bone) when empty and rises above the level of the symphysis when full, making it easily palpable (Palmer, 1996). It is freely moveable except at the base, where it is continuous with the urethra. The base of the bladder is composed of a triangular fibroelastic muscle known as the *trigone* (see Figure 3.4). The trigone of the bladder, which contains the bladder's sensory nerves, is shaped like an upside-down triangle. The base of the triangle receives the ureters from the right and left kidneys. The apex of the trigone is at the junction where the bladder muscle and the urethra meet (bladder neck).

The wall of the bladder has three layers: an inner mucous layer, a central muscular layer, and an outer fatty layer. The central muscle layer is made up

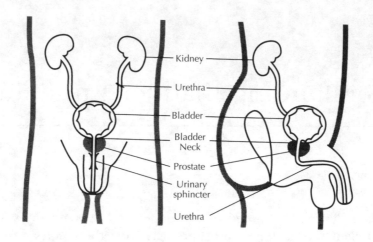

Figure 3.1.   Frontal and lateral views of the male urinary system.

of smooth muscle that is called the *detrusor muscle*. This muscle layer allows for stretching as the bladder fills with urine and then contracts to expel it. Smooth muscle is not under voluntary control but contracts in response to certain reflexes.

The bladder's function is to fill, store, and then empty urine through the urethra. During the filling phase, the bladder muscle (detrusor) relaxes to allow the bladder to accommodate increasing volumes. As the bladder reaches its capacity and becomes distended, the pressure inside (intravesical pressure) increases. The bladder increases to the size of a softball when full. Normally, it can hold about 12–16 ounces (360–480 milliliters) of urine, which is called the *functional capacity* of the bladder. When empty, the bladder lies in folds.

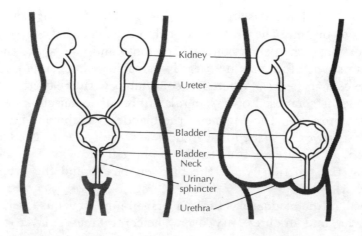

Figure 3.2.   Frontal and lateral views of the female urinary system.

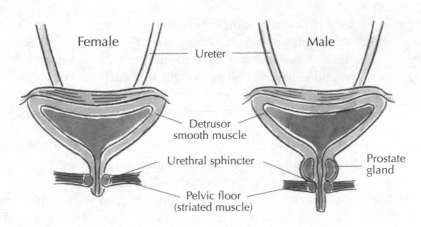

Figure 3.3. Lower urinary system. (Courtesy of Pharmacia)

URETHRA

The urethra is a thin, muscular tube that leads from the floor or neck of the urinary bladder to the outside of the body. It is made up of smooth muscle and, therefore, is not under voluntary control. The urethral orifice or *meatus* is the opening of the urethra to the outside. When not passing urine, the urethral tube is collapsed and held closed by tiny but powerful internal and external sphincter muscles at the neck of the bladder and the urethral meatus, respectively.

In women, the urethra is approximately 1.5 inches in length. The urethra runs from the neck of the bladder along the top of the vagina to the meatus. The meatus is located just between the clitoris and the vaginal opening. The mucosal

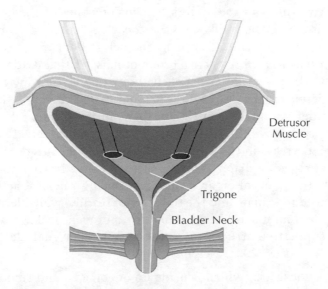

Figure 3.4. The trigone of the bladder. (Courtesy of Pharmacia)

lining of the urethra in women is different from the lining in men in that it contains stratified squamous epithelium, which is subject to effects of the hormone estrogen. After menopause, the lack of estrogen is reflected in poorer quality of collagen, muscle, and skin tone and is thought to contribute to urogenital atrophy, causing symptoms such as incontinence, frequency, and urgency.

In men, the urethra begins at the bladder neck, passes downward through the prostate gland and the urogenital diaphragm, and finally passes along the length of the penis until it ends at the urethral meatus at the tip of the penis. The male urethra is 8 inches long. The uppermost portion (also called the prostatic or sphincteric urethra) is approximately 3 inches long.

The urethra is surrounded by two sphincter muscles, which prevent urine from leaving the bladder. The *internal* and *external urethral sphincters* aid in storage of urine and emptying of the urinary bladder. Control of the inner ring of muscle, or internal sphincter, is involuntary, whereas the outer ring, or external sphincter, is under voluntary control. Unlike the smooth muscles that a person cannot consciously control, the muscles of the external sphincter can relax voluntarily to facilitate emptying of the bladder or contract voluntarily to prevent urine leakage when abdominal pressure is increased, such as during coughing, laughing, or sneezing. The *perineum* is the urogenital diaphragm and consists of superficial muscles that primarily assist with the sexual and urethral sphincter muscles.

PELVIC FLOOR MUSCLE ANATOMY

The *bony pelvis* offers support and protection to the organs and structures located within the pelvis. The bladder itself lies deep in the bony pelvis, as do the lower two thirds of the ureters. The major bones of the bony pelvis—the ilium, the ischium, the pubis, and the coccyx—provide a framework to contain the pelvic organs and to support the pelvic floor muscles.

The *pelvic floor muscles* are a group of muscles that extend from the front (anterior) to the back (posterior) of the bony pelvis, forming a sling that supports the pelvic organs (see Figures 8.2 and 8.3). The pelvic floor muscles are entirely under voluntary control and play an important role in maintaining continence and preventing UI. They can become weakened with childbirth, lack of use, decrease in the hormone estrogen, aging, surgery, and injury. The pelvic and urogenital diaphragm act together. In the resting position they gently support the internal organ structures. During physical activities or when there is a need to urinate and the toilet is not readily available, they tighten by pulling up and in, much like a hammock, to prevent leakage.

The supportive structures of the pelvic floor include (Ashton-Miller, Howard, De Lancey, 2001; Newman, 2000):

1. Endopelvic fascia, which is made up of collagen and smooth muscle, surrounds the vagina and attaches it laterally to the arcus tendineus fasciae.

The arcus tendineus fasciae pelvis in turn is attached ventrally to the pubic bone and dorsally to the ischial spine. The arcus tendineus fasciae pelvis is located on either side of the urethra and vagina. It acts like a suspension bridge and provides the support needed to suspend the urethra on the anterior vaginal wall. It fuses with the endopelvic fascia, where it merges with the levator ani muscle.

2. *Pelvic diaphragm* consists of the levator ani muscle group. The levator ani muscle has three parts: the pubococcygeus, the puborectalis, and the iliococcygeus muscles. The pubococcygeus and the puborectalis muscles form a U-shape as they originate from the pubic bone on either side of the midline and pass behind the rectum. Their fibers create a slinglike band (often referred to as a hammock). This type of muscle is composed of mainly Type I striated muscle fibers (slow twitch muscle fibers) and, therefore, maintains constant tone. The iliococcygeus muscle arises laterally from the arcus tendineus levator ani and forms a horizontal sheet or shelf that spans the opening of the posterior region of the pelvis. The pelvic organs rest on this shelf.

3. *Fibrous urogenital diaphragm* (perineal membrane) is located below the levator ani and spans the anterior portion of the pelvic outlet and connects the perineal body to the pubic bone. The loss of pelvic floor muscle tone and strength can lead to both stress UI and urge UI.

The internal obturator muscle is another important muscle that lines the lower pelvis. It attaches to the obturator tendon within the pelvis and the greater trochanter of the femur. As the obturator muscle contracts it acts as a pulley, lifting the bladder and urethra in to the optimum function. At rest, it maintains the bladder position in the pelvis.

NERVOUS SYSTEM

The functions of the lower urinary system are dependent on an intact, functioning nervous system and brain (see Figure 3.5). The nervous system of the body is divided into a central and a peripheral portion. The *central nervous system* contains the brain and the spinal cord. The *peripheral nervous system* contains the autonomic and somatic peripheral nerves. The *autonomic nervous system* is not under conscious control and is often called the involuntary nervous system. It contains the sympathetic and parasympathetic nervous systems. The *sympathetic nervous system* 1) relaxes the bladder muscle and 2) contracts the internal urethral sphincter to prevent urine from entering the urethra. The *parasympathetic nervous system* 1) stimulates the bladder muscle to contract, causing the urge sensation; and 2) relaxes the internal urethral sphincter, which allows urine to enter the urethra. The *somatic nervous system* is under voluntary control. The somatic nervous system sends a signal

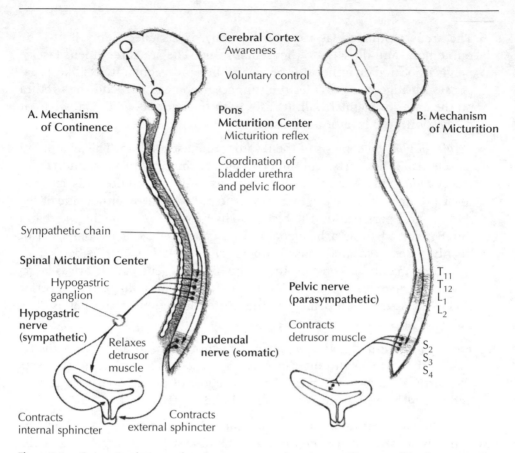

Figure 3.5. Connection between the nervous system and continence. (Courtesy of Empi)

to the external urethral sphincter either to contract, to prevent urine leakage, or to relax, allowing the release of urine. The detrusor (bladder) muscle relaxes as the bladder fills with urine. The pelvic floor muscle and urethral sphincter muscle remain contracted to prevent release of urine. The *pudendal nerve* is part of the voluntary nervous system. This nerve is involved in innervation of the external urethral and anal sphincters and the pelvic and urogenital diaphragm muscles. See Table 3.1 for a summary of nerve activation of the bladder.

Under normal conditions, urine continuously and gradually accumulates as the normal bladder accommodates to increasing volumes of urine with little or no increase in pressure within the bladder (*intravesical pressure*). In the absence of any pathological factors, the sense of bladder filling is not perceived until approximately 50% of the functional bladder capacity is reached. In order to understand bladder disorders, it is important to understand how the bladder empties. At a socially acceptable time and location, voluntary urination (*micturition*) is initiated by a complex set of reflexes organized and facilitated at the level of the brain stem (see Figure 3.6). A signal is sent via the central nervous system to the pelvic nerves initiating a voluntary contraction of the detrusor muscle in coordination with urethral sphincter relaxation and, thereby, voiding is initiated. The steps of the micturition cycle are as follows:

1. The detrusor (bladder) muscle relaxes as the bladder fills with urine. The pelvic floor muscle and urethral sphincter muscle remain contracted to prevent release of urine.

2. As the bladder fills to half its capacity, bladder nerves send messages to the brain and the first sensation of the need to void occurs.

3. Because voiding is voluntary, the individual makes a conscious decision to toilet or to delay voiding. If toileting occurs, the pressure in the bladder (detrusor) muscle rises, causing the bladder to contract and the urethral sphincter and pelvic muscle to relax.

4. Voiding occurs.

   In order for the individual to maintain continence, the bladder pressure must be less than the pressure within the urethra. However, under certain conditions, an involuntary contraction of the detrusor muscle ("spasm") may

Table 3.1. Normal bladder function nerve activation

Storage

Nervous system	Nerve	Originates	Innervates	Function
Voluntary (Somatic)	Pudendal	S2–S4	Pelvic floor muscles	Contracts external urethral sphincter (maintains closure) or relaxes urethral sphincter, allowing the release of urine
Involuntary (Sympathetic)	Hypogastric	T11–L2	Detrusor muscle and internal urinary sphincter	Relaxes detrusor muscle (allows filling) and contracts internal sphincter (maintains closure to prevent urine from entering the bladder)

Emptying

Nervous system	Nerve	Originates	Innervates	Function
Involuntary (Parasympathetic)	Pelvic	S2–S4	Detrusor muscle	Stimulates the detrusor muscle to contract (causing the urge sensation) and relaxes the internal sphincter to allow urine to enter the urethra (causing emptying)

From *The Fundamentals of Pelvic Floor Stimulation*. St Paul, MN: Empi. Adapted by permission.

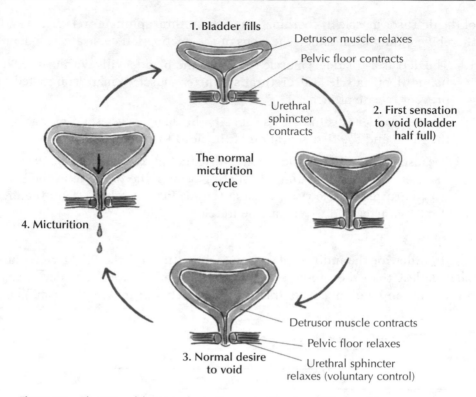

1. Bladder fills
Detrusor muscle relaxes
Pelvic floor contracts

Urethral
sphincter
contracts

**2. First sensation
to void (bladder
half full)**

**The normal
micturition
cycle**

4. Micturition

Detrusor muscle contracts
Pelvic floor relaxes
Urethral sphincter
relaxes (voluntary control)

**3. Normal desire
to void**

Figure 3.6.   The steps of the normal urination cycle. (Courtesy of Pharmacia)

spontaneously occur at any point during bladder filling. This phenomenon will raise the pressure within the bladder precipitously, and, if sensation is intact, will result in a perceived sensation of impending micturition and urinary urgency. This precipitous rise in bladder pressure may result in the unexpected involuntary expulsion of urine through the urethra (i.e., UI). Urinary frequency occurs as a result of reduced functional bladder capacity, or, rarely, as a result of an organically diminished bladder capacity. It can also be due, at least partly, to a coping mechanism adopted by the individual to avoid leakage of large volumes of urine by maintaining a relatively low volume in the bladder through frequent urination.

Men and women have different habits when they void. Men stand and often void in public with other men. They contract their abdominal muscles to aid in complete bladder emptying. Women tend to void in private and must relax to open the external sphincter. They will sit or squat over a toilet seat to void. This position is important as women compress their abdomen to empty the bladder.

NIGHTTIME FUNCTION

Nocturia is defined as the number of voids recorded from the time the individual goes to bed with the intention of going to sleep, to the time the individual wakes with the intention of rising. Nocturia is caused by *nocturnal polyuria* (NP), which causes the largest amount of urine production to occur at rest and usually at night. During the day, fluid accumulation occurs in extra-cellular spaces followed at night by increased renal perfusion and excretion of excess fluid. Chronic medical conditions such as congestive heart failure, venous stasis with peripheral edema, hyperglycemia and excess urine output, obstructive sleep apnea, and diuretics, as well as evening and nighttime fluid consumption, are causes of NP (Colling, Owen, & McCreedy, 1994). NP can also be caused by low bladder capacity secondary to OAB, benign prostatic hypertrophy (BPH), urethral obstructions, atrophic vaginitis, low bladder compliance, and even bladder cancer. If urine is lost during sleep, this is called *nocturnal enuresis* (nighttime incontinence).

During the night, there is a lower level of physical activity, and body fluid moves more quickly from one part of the body to another, causing an increase in the amount of urine in the bladder. Treatment could be something as practical as fluid restriction, giving diuretics at 2:00 P.M. rather than 6:00 P.M. or 7:00 P.M., afternoon naps with elevation of the legs, compression stockings, or treatment with the vasopressin analogue desmopressin (DDAVP), which increases reabsorption of fluid in the kidneys (Newman, 1999). For the treatment of low bladder capacity due to overactive bladder, anticholinergic therapy and behavior modification are generally the treatments of choice.

AGING AND CHANGES IN THE URINARY SYSTEM

The physiological, psychological, and environmental changes that accompany aging do not directly cause the bladder to malfunction, but they do predispose older adults to an increased risk or incidence of disorders. The following normal age-related changes occur in the urinary system:

- There is a 30%–40% loss of functional cells (nephrons) in the kidneys.

- There is a decrease in the kidney's ability to filter blood and concentrate urine.

- The sensory nerve tracts from the bladder through the spinal cord and to the brain often "wear out," creating breaks in the neural pathway. There is "short-circuiting" of nerve firing, and messages may not completely reach the brain. In general, the nervous system takes longer to respond to sensory stimuli. This causes the bladder urge sensation (which tells the person to void) to be delayed. Because of the degenerative changes in the nervous system, the interval between the time the urge to void is felt and actual voiding is shortened. This shortened warning period is called *urgency*. This urgency, which in most people is sudden and strong, causes the individual to rush when attempting to toilet.

- Because of this incomplete nerve pathway, there is an increase in *bladder spasms,* or detrusor overactivity, resulting in small, frequent contractions that create the urge to void before the bladder is full. These bladder contractions, over which the person has no control, cause urine leakage (urge UI) on the way to the bathroom.

• The bladder does not empty completely (*urinary retention*) because the capacity of the bladder is decreased. This is the reason why older adults need to void often in small amounts (urinary frequency). The urine that remains in the bladder after the person has voided (*postvoid residual*) may become infected with bacteria. Hence, there is an increased incidence of urinary tract infection.

• Aging causes an increase in *nocturia,* typically defined as an average of more than 2 voids per night. One nocturnal void per decade above 60 years of age can be added and still be considered normal.

Because many losses accompany old age, an individual may use incontinence as a means of regaining control, getting attention, or showing anger. However, although UI is common among older adults, bladder disorders are not a normal part of aging or of living in a residential facility. Therefore, when properly assessed and treated, bladder dysfunction can be corrected in about 30% of residents of extended care facilities and suitably controlled and managed in the rest.

REFERENCES

Ashton-Miller, J.A., Howard, D.S., & DeLancey, J.O.L. (2001). The functional anatomy of the female pelvic floor and stress continence control system. *Scandinavian Journal of Urology and Nephrology, 207* (Suppl.), 1–7.

Colling, J., Owen, T., & McCreedy, M.R. (1994). Urine volumes and voiding: Patterns among incontinent nursing home residents. *Geriatric Nursing, 15,* 188–192.

Newman, D.K. (1999). *The urinary incontinence sourcebook* (2nd ed.). Los Angeles: Lowell House.

Newman, D.K. (2000). *Continence for women: Research-based practice.* Washington, DC: Association of Women's Health, Obstetric and Neonatal Nurses.

Palmer, M.H. (1996). *Urinary incontinence.* Gaithersburg, MD: Aspen Publishers.

4

Causes of Incontinence and Identification of Risk Factors

Urinary incontinence (UI) can be described as any involuntary loss of urine from the bladder via the urethra, whatever the cause, that is not controlled by the individual. In addition to incontinence, associated lower urinary tract symptoms (LUTS) may be present that include urgency, frequency, nocturia, postvoid dribbling, nocturnal enuresis, straining to void, and hesitancy and weak stream. The variety of causes and types of UI have led to a number of attempts at classifying the problem. In addition to the underlying physiological origins, in many clients UI is associated with psychological, functional, environmental, and social factors. Incontinence is also a symptom that, especially in older adults, can be caused by two or more interrelated factors. Because UI is such a prevalent problem in adults, understanding its causes is imperative. Assessment of UI in all care settings is necessary and, in the case of nursing facilities, is required by federal regulations. To perform a thorough assessment, the clinician must understand the underlying causes of UI, be able to differentiate between transient and persistent UI, and identify those clients at risk. This chapter discusses current definitions for the different types of UI, its underlying pathophysiology, and related risk factors. Emphasis is on UI in older adults.

TYPES OF INCONTINENCE

There are two classifications, or types, of UI: 1) transient or acute, and 2) persistent or chronic. The distinction between transient and persistent UI is clinically important. Persistent UI refers to incontinence that continues over time and is unrelated to an acute illness.

Transient Incontinence

Transient incontinence, often referred to as acute incontinence, appears during an illness or specific medical problem. Any neurological or acute illness in-

Table 4.1.   Causes of acute and reversible incontinence

D	Dehydration
	Delirium
	Diapers
R	Retention
	Restricted mobility
I	Infection (acute symptomatic UTI)
	Inflammation (atrophic vaginitis/urethritis)
	Impaction (fecal)
P	Polypharmacy
	Polyuria (hyperglycemia, hypercalcemia—rare)

From Kane, R., Ouslander, J., & Abrass, I. (1994). *Essentials of clinical geriatrics* (3rd ed., p. 154). New York: McGraw-Hill; adapted by permission from McGraw-Hill Companies.

terrupting the nerve pathways between the brain and the central nervous system adversely affects the bladder, urethra, internal and external sphincters, and pelvic floor muscles. Perception of the need to urinate, or the sensation of a full bladder, diminishes or completely disappears. Two mnemonics—DRIP and DIAPPERS (see Tables 4.1 and 4.2)—prompt the clinician to search for factors that, when addressed, might resolve transient or transiently exacerbated UI. In acute UI, the causes of incontinence are potentially treatable. Once the underlying disorder is reversed or treated, the incontinence usually disappears. Table 4.3 highlights predisposing conditions and solutions for resolving acute UI. The causes of transient UI are outlined in more detail in the following text.

Dehydration   Dehydration is the most common fluid and electrolyte problem among older adults. It is caused by an excess loss of water, failure

Table 4.2.   Causes of transient incontinence

D	Delirium
I	Infection—urinary (symptomatic)
A	Atrophic urethritis/vaginitis
P	Pharmaceuticals
P	Psychological conditions, especially depression
E	Excessive urine output (e.g., congestive heart failure, hyperglycemia, elevated blood sugar)
R	Restricted or decreased immobility
S	Stool impaction

From Resnick, N.M., & Yalla, S. (1998). Evaluation and management of urinary incontinence. In P. Walsh, A. Retisk, T. Stamey, & E. Vaughn (Eds.), *Campbells urology* (7th ed., p. 1045). Philadelphia: W.B. Saunders; adapted by permission.

Table 4.3. Predisposing conditions causing the development of transient urinary incontinence

Condition	Approach
Stool impaction—can cause urge incontinence and may induce fecal incontinence as well.	Disimpaction restores continence in most instances if this was the cause. A bowel regimen must be implemented that would include use of increasing fiber in diet, with use of stool softeners and laxatives if diet changes are not successful. Adequate mobility and fluid intake should also be considered.
Limited or restricted mobility—can aggravate or precipitate UI because of inability to respond promptly to the urge to void.	Can frequently be corrected or improved by treating the underlying condition (e.g., arthritis, poor eyesight, Parkinson's disease, or orthostatic hypotension). A urinal or bedside commode and scheduled toileting often help resolve the incontinence that results from hospitalization and its environmental barriers (e.g., bed rails, restraints, and poor lighting).
Increased urine production from *metabolic conditions* such as hyperglycemia, hypercalcemia, Paget's disease, venous insufficiency with edema, and congestive heart failure. Many of these conditions cloud the sensorium and induce a diuresis with polyuria (e.g., hypercalcemia, hyperglycemia, and diabetes insipidus).	Treatment of the underlying condition. Implement bladder retraining to assist with frequency and urgency.
Atrophic urethritis or vaginitis—can cause atrophic changes of the lower genitourinary tract (bladder and urethra).	Estrogen replacement therapy, especially topical application of estrogen
Prostate cancer treatment (surgery and radiation) in men—disruption of sphincter mechanisms may or may not be permanent.	Behavioral interventions, including pelvic muscle exercises, bladder re-training, and neuromuscular electrical stimulation
Medications—can impair bladder and urethral function. Examples include	
• Caffeine—causes aggravation or precipitation of UI	Reduce intake of caffeine-containing liquids and food products.
• Alcohol—has a diuretic effect causing increased urine production, urinary frequency, frequency, delirium, and impaired mobility	Restrict alcohol intake.

(continued)

31

Table 4.3. *(continued)*

Condition	Approach
• Diuretics—cause polyuria, frequency and urgency for several hours (up to 6) after taken	If clinically possible, discontinue or change therapy.
• ACE (angiotensin-converting enzyme) inhibitors—antihypertensives with a common side effect of cough, which can worsen stress UI	Dosage reduction or modification (e.g., flexible scheduling of rapid-acting diuretics to allow accommodation to sudden increase in urine volume).
• Anticholinergic agents—cause urinary retention and impaction.	
• Antidepressants—cause anticholinergic actions, sedation	
• Sedatives/hypnotics/CNS depressants—cause sedation, delirium, immobility, muscle relaxation	
• Narcotic analgesics—cause urinary retention, fecal impaction, sedation, delirium	
• Calcium channel blockers—cause relaxation of the detrusor muscle and urinary retention, can increase urine production at night and constipation	
• α-adrenergic agonists—present in many cold and over-the-counter preparations, these cause urinary retention	
• α-adrenergic blockers—cause smooth muscle relaxation of the bladder neck and urethral relaxation and leakage	
Urinary tract infection—can cause dysuria and urgency and, in an older person, impair the ability to reach the toilet in time, causing urge UI.	Treat underlying infection. In clients who have recurrent infections, suggest acidification of urine. Cranberry juice inhibits bacterial adherence to mucosal surfaces.

to recognize the need to increase water intake, or impaired water ingestion (Lavizzo-Mourey, 1987). Dehydration causes an increase in the concentration of urine, which irritates the bladder muscle and urethra, resulting in urinary frequency, UI, or both. During an illness, dehydration may mask the urge sensation. The individual's response to bladder sensations may be slow or ignored until the urge sensation becomes uncontrollable. In many cases, a UI incident is the first indication to an ill person that a bladder problem exists. When hydration occurs, the UI may be resolved.

Dehydration is a significant problem in long-term care (LTC) residents. The mean amount of fluid consumed by residents averages 1,200–1,500 milliliters (ml) per day (Kayser-Jones, Schell, Porter, Barbaccia, & Shaw, 1999). The daily water requirement is 30 ml/kilograms (kg) of body weight. It has been estimated that dehydration is present in 33% of LTC residents (Colling, Owen, & McCreedy, 1994). Warning signs of dehydration include dark, foul-smelling urine; dry mouth; falling; weakness and fatigue; decreased urine output; headache; weight loss; muscle cramps; and increased confusion.

Delirium   Delirium and mental confusion will alter a person's awareness of the urge to urinate. Mental confusion occurs frequently in people recovering from a medical illness, surgery, and the like. In older adults, acute confusion may be caused by a urinary tract infection (UTI). Once the confused state is resolved and the person is able to recognize and respond to the urinary urge sensation, UI typically resolves also.

Retention   Urinary retention, should be considered in any person who suddenly develops UI. Among other causes, urinary retention is an adverse effect of prescription and over-the-counter (OTC) drugs that have anticholinergic properties (e.g., Benadryl). Urinary retention can also be caused by urethral obstruction (e.g., enlarged prostate, urethral structure).

In men, one of the most common urological causes of UI is prostatic enlargement. As men age, the prostate gland enlarges. More than 50% of 60-year-old men and more than 90% of 85-year-old men have microscopic evidence of benign prostatic hyperplasia. Of these men, approximately 50% will have enlargement of the prostate gland and will experience urinary symptoms. The enlarged prostate can cause obstruction at the bladder neck, with narrowing and compression of the urethra. This can lead to incomplete bladder emptying or urinary retention. Blockage or an obstruction in the urethra secondary to urethral stricture can lead to retention or temporary overflow incontinence. Treatment depends on the cause of the obstruction and the severity of the medical condition.

Restricted Mobility   Restricted mobility, the impaired ability to use the legs, arms, or upper/lower body, and other physical disabilities are obstacles to using the toilet and can worsen urinary urgency and frequency, leading to urge incontinence. Especially for older people, physical limitations present difficulties when the person attempts to self-toilet. Recovery from surgery, serious illness, and bed rest also limit physical mobility and present additional toileting challenges. Inability to independently toilet can lead to UI during some stage of a person's incapacity. Environmental factors often accentuate immobility and cause a sudden onset of UI. If toilet facilities are not easily reached and accessible, if a portable bedside commode or urinal is not at hand, or if no one is near to provide assistance in getting up and walking to a bathroom, sitting on a toilet, or using a bedpan, toileting may be impossible. Physically restraining nursing facility residents or homebound people by using various straps and ties, as well as geri-chairs and chemical restraints such as sedating drugs, also increases the potential of an acute episode of incontinence. Mobility problems and decreased function place an older person at risk for acute and chronic UI and are emphasized throughout this chapter.

Infection   Infection, specifically a UTI, can cause a sudden onset of incontinence. Bacteria irritate the mucous membranes of the bladder wall and urethra, triggering urinary urgency, UI, and occasional pain or burning when urinating. UI is often an older person's only symptom of an infection. Other symptoms of UTI in the older adult include change in temperature; dysuria; change in cognition; alteration in urine color, smell, and consistency; and hematuria. A bladder dysfunction, such as an overactive bladder, aggravates UTI.

UTI is a greater risk for women than for men because the female urethra is shorter in length and is closer in proximity to the anus, allowing contamination with fecal bacteria. UTI is also more common in older women because of changes in the urinary tract that occur with age and less efficient immune systems. A common problem seen in older women, especially those residing in nursing homes, is *bacteriuria*. Bacteriuria is defined as a growth of 100,000 or more colony-forming units per milliliter of a specific bacterial organism and can be caused by estrogen deficiency. A decrease in estrogen in the pelvis and perineum will lead to atrophic changes, disappearance of colonizing lactobacilli, an increase in vaginal pH, and subsequent colonization with uropathogenic bacteria. Most residents in long-term care will have bacteriuria without symptoms of infection (called asymptomatic bacteriuria). UTIs are the most common source of bacteriuria in nursing facilities, and the use of an indwelling catheter increases the risk of bacteriuria by 60% (Muder, Brennan, Wagner, & Goetz, 1992; Rudman, Hontanosas, Cohen, & Mattson, 1988).

It is believed that cranberry (juice or tablets) has several therapeutic properties, including the prevention of bacterial adherence to mucosa. One randomized, double-blind, placebo-controlled trial demonstrated that cranberry juice has a more significant effect in eradicating bacteria from urine than in preventing the occurrence of UTI (Avorn et al., 1994). Other means of preventing UTIs are provided in Appendix A: How to Prevent Bladder Infections.

Inflammation Inflammation of the vaginal and perineal mucosa from a decrease in the hormone estrogen has a detrimental effect on the bladder and pelvic muscles. The tissues of the vagina and urethra become thinner, drier, and possibly weaker and more susceptible to irritation. This deficiency weakens pelvic floor and urethral tissue, causing atrophic vaginitis/urethritis—a dry, red, and inflamed condition in a woman's vulval and urethral area. This inflammatory condition may cause frequency and urgency, which can precipitate UI. It is also common for women with UI who manage their urine leakage by wearing perineal pads to develop vaginal yeast infections.

Atrophic vaginitis/urethritis is frequently missed in frail older women, especially those living in LTC facilities or those who are homebound. Usually routine pelvic examinations are neglected in these women. Topical estrogen for atrophic urogenital changes should be considered.

Impaction Impaction secondary to bowel dysfunction may be a cause of an acute onset of temporary UI. Constipation or fecal impaction increases pressure on the bladder, changing its position within the pelvic area and causing either UI or urinary retention. Once normal bowel movement is restored, the person is able to void and UI can be resolved.

Polypharmacy Polypharmacy, or the use of multiple drugs, is frequent among many older adults. An adult older than age 65 takes an average of two to three drugs per day. Many of these medications have UI as a possible side effect. Thus, the more drugs an individual takes, the greater the potential for UI. Prescription drugs as a cause of UI among older adults is often overlooked by the clinician prescribing them. Table 4.3 outlines medications that can alter bladder function.

Polyuria Polyuria is seen in hyperglycemia and volume-expanded states that cause excessive urinary frequency and nocturia (e.g., congestive heart failure [CHF], venous insufficiency). In hyperglycemia, the body attempts to rid itself of excess glucose through diuresis, causing increased fluid volume in the bladder. In CHF, fluid mobilization may occur at night while there is less stress on the heart. As diuresis occurs, the individual may have UI as a result of an excessive volume of urine, inability to wake in time, and inability to reach the toilet.

Chronic Incontinence

The majority of people with UI have experienced problems for several years. *Chronic incontinence* occurs because of persistent, long-term abnormalities of the structure or function of the lower urinary tract (Newman, 1999). When UI develops in functionally independent older people, it is commonly related to a defect or dysfunction of the bladder (filling phase) or the bladder outlet (emptying phase), including

Filling Phase—dysfunction in the bladder

- Bladder overactivity or hypersensitivity (the bladder contracts when it should not)
- Bladder underactivity (the bladder fails to contract when or as well as it should)

Emptying Phase—dysfunction in the outlet (urethra and sphincters)

- Urethral obstruction, usually resulting from an enlarged prostate or stricture (narrowing of the urethra)

- Urethral incompetence, wherein the resistance is too low, resulting in urine leakage

These dysfunctions produce the most common types of UI: stress, urge, or mixed symptomatology of stress and urge. Chronic UI is classified into five groups: stress incontinence, urge incontinence, mixed, overflow incontinence, and functional incontinence (see Table 4.4). Common diagnoses associated with persistent UI are outlined in Table 4.5. The symptomatology, underlying pathophysiology, and incidence of chronic UI are discussed in the following text.

   Stress Incontinence   *Does your client report leakage of small amounts of urine when coughing, sneezing, or during physical activity? Have you ever heard someone say, "I laughed so hard I wet my pants"?*

   These symptoms are associated with stress UI. In stress UI, the problem lies with a damaged or weakened urethra and urethral sphincter (see Figure

Table 4.4.   Summary of classifications of persistent UI

Type	Description
Stress	Small amount of urine leakage that occurs with effort or exertion or on coughing, laughing, sneezing, physical activities, exercise, or any action that increases intra-abdominal pressure
Urge, or overactive bladder	Sudden urge to pass urine and the inability to delay voiding after sensation of bladder fullness (urge) is perceived. Symptoms include moderate to large amounts of leakage, urine loss on the way to bathroom, "key-in-lock syndrome," urgency, and frequent urination.
Mixed	A combination of any of the above.
Overflow	Sudden overflow of urine when pressure inside the bladder exceeds the pressure of a urethral obstruction. Symptoms include small, frequent voidings; post void dribbling; hesitancy; and straining to void.
Functional	Urine loss resulting from inability to reach bathroom because of physical disabilities or psychological problems that do not allow self-toileting.

Table 4.5. Common diagnosis and definition of terms

Diagnosis	Definition
Atonic bladder	A bladder that is not able to contract and empty properly, usually because of damage to the nerves that control the bladder. As a result, the bladder fills with urine and remains full, and excess urine that cannot fit in the bladder flows over and dribbles out through the urethra, causing overflow incontinence.
Detrusor overactivity (also called overactive)	Hyperactivity or overactivity of the bladder muscle, caused by nerve impulses, often resulting in urge incontinence
Detrusor sphincter dyssynergia (DSD)	Lack of coordination between the bladder and the pelvic floor muscles. Normally when a person attempts to empty the bladder, the pelvic floor muscles relax, allowing the urethra to open. Then, the bladder contracts and pushes the urine through the urethra. With DSD, the pelvic floor muscles contract instead, clamping in on the urethra and interfering with the flow of urine.
Detrusor hyperactivity with impaired bladder contractility (DHIC)	A condition characterized by frequent but ineffective involuntary detrusor contractions. A person either is unable to empty the bladder completely or can empty the bladder completely only with straining as a result of poor contractility of the detrusor. This abnormality of the bladder was first diagnosed in nursing facility residents.
Neurogenic bladder	A bladder that functions incorrectly because of nerve innervation abnormalities

4.1). Urine loss is usually accompanied by a loss of support of the urethrovesical junction (angle between the bladder and urethra). Increased intra-abdominal pressure causes an increase in bladder pressure and results in urine loss when bladder pressure exceeds urethral pressure. Urine escapes because the bladder outlet is inadequate and does not stay closed tightly during the increases in bladder pressure. Loss of urine occurs immediately following certain activities that cause a *Valsalva maneuver* (increase in intra-abdominal pressure). Urine loss also may occur when getting out of bed in the morning as the abdominal muscles push down on the bladder. In response to stress UI, the individual usually will start a pattern of frequent urination because a stress UI episode is more likely to occur with a full bladder.

Stress incontinence usually produces only drops or small amounts of urine leakage; however, the severity of leakage may change, depending on the specific activities that cause the urine loss. Minimal urine leakage can occur with relatively vigorous activities: coughing, laughing, and sneezing. Moderate urine leakage can occur with activities such as rising from a sitting to standing position, swinging a golf club, or walking across a room. Severe urine leakage can occur with more severe physical exertion such as lifting heavy objects and aerobic exercise. Sometimes the leakage is not related to any given activity. Specific types of stress UI are outlined in Table 4.6.

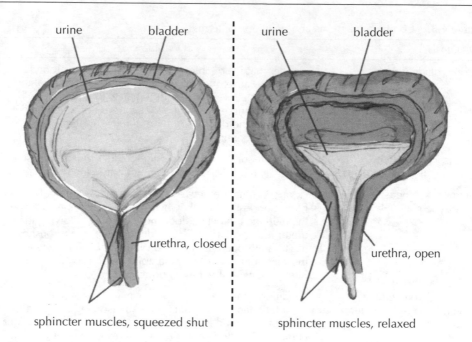

Figure 4.1.   Weak sphincter muscles as seen with stress UI.

Excessive weight, constipation, or nerve injuries in the lower back can cause stress UI in both men and women. In one case–control study, constipation and straining at stool were more common in women who developed stress UI (30%) and pelvic organ prolapse (61%; Spence-Jones, Kamm, Henry, & Hudson, 1994). However, stress UI is predominantly seen in women and has many causes, including weakness of, or damage to, the bladder outlet, the urethra, or the pelvic floor muscles that surround and support these structures. Stress UI is often associated with multiparity (having delivered a child more than once) or direct anatomical damage to the urethral sphincter, which may lead to severe, continuous leakage. Childbearing stretches and relaxes a woman's pelvic floor musculature and may damage nerves in the pelvic area and tissue in the bladder's neck. As many as 35% of childbearing women experience postpartum stress UI for 6–12 months after delivery.

Table 4.6.   Types of stress UI

Diagnosis	Definition
Type I	Mild incontinence in which the bladder and urethra are in normal position and leakage only occurs with coughing, laughing, straining, and so forth
Type II	Moderate incontinence in which the bladder and urethra are protruding into the vagina
Type III—intrinsic urethral (sphincter) deficiency	Severe incontinence in which the urethra does not work at all

A decline in estrogen levels at menopause and pelvic organ prolapse cause stress UI in middle-age women. A woman's estrogen level lowers after menopause and drops dramatically when the ovaries and uterus are removed in a hysterectomy. This further weakens pelvic floor and vaginal area muscles and tissues, increasing the likelihood of stress incontinence.

Women with pelvic organ *prolapse* will complain of a "fallen uterus," one that has shifted within the abdominal cavity. The position of the uterus, bladder, and bladder neck within the abdomen has a direct effect on the control of urine. Pelvic muscle exercises can be used to strengthen the pelvic floor muscles to help prevent or improve pelvic organ prolapse and resulting stress UI (see Chapter 8). However, it is estimated that at least 50% of young women are unable to identify the correct muscle for these exercises (Bump, Hurt, Fantl, & Wyman, 1991). This is also a difficult exercise to teach to postmenopausal women.

Approximately 5%–15% of men experience UI after prostate cancer surgery, especially in the first 3–6 months after the operation. The removal of the prostate during radical prostatectomy eliminates the support given to the bladder neck by the prostate and exposes the external urethral sphincter to the full task of maintaining continence. Therefore, postprostatectomy incontinence is primarily caused by sphincter incompetence. In these men, urine leakage occurs mostly after exercise or physical exertion. Fatigue of the striated muscle of the pelvic floor leads to increased loss of urine during the second half of the day. Often UI is temporary, but sometimes it is a prolonged condition that causes anxiety and disruption in a man's life.

Urge Incontinence   *Does your client complain about the inability to make it to the bathroom in time without losing urine? Have you ever heard someone say, "When I gotta go, I gotta go"?*

These symptoms are associated with urge UI, often referred to as overactive bladder. Urine loss occurs when the detrusor muscle of the bladder wall involuntarily contracts during bladder filling, forcing urine through the urethra. Ordinarily, when a person feels the urge to urinate, a detrusor contraction can be inhibited through cortical control or contraction of pelvic muscles. The person with urge UI senses the urge to void, but is unable either to inhibit detrusor contraction or to prevent loss of urine by adequate closure of the outlet. In most but not all cases, uninhibited bladder contractions (detrusor overactivity) can be documented as causing the UI through urodynamic tests.

Typical symptoms of the overactive bladder include an increased number of micturitions (urinary frequency, usually greater than eight voids per day), a strong and sudden desire to void (urinary urgency), and, if the urge cannot be suppressed, urge UI. An additional symptom is nocturia three to four times per night with subsequent nocturnal enuresis. With detrusor overactivity, usually an event will "trigger" the urine leakage, and there is usually a delay between the precipitating event and the urine loss. A very common trigger is "key-in-the-lock" or "garage door syndrome," terms that characterize a sudden urge to urinate with subsequent leakage when attempting to open a door. Other triggers include urine leakage in response to the sound of running water, washing dishes or clothes, placing hands in warm water, anxiety, or exposure to cold. A person may be aware of the need to urinate and yet cannot seem to get to the toilet before having an incontinence episode.

Urinary urgency or leakage triggered by certain events is probably due to a conditioned reflex—a reflex that gradually developed in the body by the frequent repetition of a specific stimulus (e.g., if you burn your finger when touching a hot stove you will not touch it again). If approaching a door or opening a "garage door" continues to cause urgency and UI, then the person will subconsciously begin to associate putting the key in the lock or opening a door with the urge to void, and eventually it will happen uncontrollably.

People suffering from overactive bladder (OAB) typically have to empty their bladders frequently and, when they experience a sensation of urgency, may leak urine if they are unable to reach the toilet quickly or if the sensation of urgency is very strong. The volume of urine lost with accidents varies tremendously and does not seem dependent on bladder volume. Urine loss may be greater than 100 ml because the bladder may empty completely and involuntarily. The individual will complain that the urine just "gushes" out, wetting underwear and even outer clothing. Sleep may be disturbed because the need to void may awaken the person. People with OAB and urge incontinence will develop certain behaviors such as *toilet mapping*, which involves locating toilets in advance of travel or only visiting places where they know the toilet location.

Urge UI is the most common pattern of UI in older people. It is estimated that between 60% and 70% of older adults have urge UI. Causes of urge UI include medical conditions such as stroke, which impairs inhibition of bladder contractions (neurogenic detrusor overactivity), and local factors such as UTI or bladder tumors, which can cause bladder irritation leading to urge UI. Urge incontinence with detrusor overactivity is the most common type of UI encountered among residents in nursing facilities. In these individuals, UI is often associated with impaired cognitive or physical function or both. It is frequently difficult to determine whether the detrusor overactivity or the functional disability is the predominant cause of the UI.

Mixed Incontinence   At history taking, at least 40% of people with incontinence report a combination UI including both stress and urge symptoms. Usually these individuals are diagnosed as having mixed incontinence. A common picture is the middle-age or older woman who has been experiencing stress UI since her last child was born and is now having urge UI episodes secondary to decreased ambulation. Together, these three types of UI account for more than 80% of UI in community-dwelling older adults.

Overflow Incontinence   *Does your client complain about urine "dribbling" or a feeling of "bladder fullness?"*

The cause may be overflow incontinence, which occurs when the urethra is narrowed or blocked by an obstruction such as a prolapsed (sagging or dropped) pelvic organ, a stricture, an enlarged prostate, chronic constipation, or neurological disease. An enlarged prostate is common in men and causes overflow incontinence. The prostate blocks the urethra and the bladder does not empty completely during voiding. Overflow incontinence can be precipitated by the use of OTC cold remedies that cause the urethral sphincter to constrict and close.

Urethral obstruction with subsequent overflow UI is associated with symptoms of hesitancy, poor or weak urinary stream, and postmicturition dribble. Men report straining while urinating, with small volumes voided. When blockage is present, a full bladder cannot empty and may leak small amounts of urine all day. A common complaint is continual urine leakage or postmicturition dribble. When toileting, the individual may have difficulty starting the urine stream and, once started, the stream is weak. People with overflow UI always complain that they feel as though their bladder never empties. However, some individuals with overflow UI may not be aware that they are leaking urine because the sensation of bladder fullness is diminished and the stream of urine is weak.

There are several causes of overflow incontinence. Diabetes and drugs such as narcotics, antidepressants, and smooth muscle relaxers may increase the capacity of the bladder, but they dull the sensation of the need to urinate. Trauma to the spinal cord affects the central nervous system, impairing the ability to control the urinary cycle. Peripheral neuropathy reduces the bladder's ability to contract and release stored urine. All of these problems can cause urinary retention (incomplete bladder emptying) and overflow incontinence.

Functional Incontinence   *Have you had a client's spouse, daughter, or son complain to you about their loved one's poor toileting habits or inability to get to the toilet?*

Functional incontinence involves a person's inability or unwillingness to use toilet facilities because of decreased mental awareness, decrease or loss of mobility, or personal unwillingness to go to the toilet. The diagnosis of functional incontinence is problematic because it implies a normal lower urinary tract, which may not be present in older individuals. Functional UI is rarely seen in the absence of bladder or neurological abnormality, and assigning this diagnosis may result in failure to appropriately investigate the patient's condition, leading to misdiagnosis.

More than 25% of UI cases found in acute care hospitals and LTC facilities have some component of decrease in function or mobility. Some hospitals have very poor and inconvenient bathroom facilities. Staffing problems, as well as Medicare and insurance company policies regarding length of hospitalization and medical treatment, do not place an activity such as toileting, which is an activity of daily living, as a high priority. Nursing facilities may manage UI with absorbent products such as adult briefs. Individual client needs and assessment of voiding patterns and toileting habits are not usually part of the client assessment process in LTC facilities; however, it is important to remember that many people who suffer from impaired cognitive function or mobility are not incontinent.

Common factors contributing to functional incontinence include

- Restricted mobility or dexterity—inability or difficulty in getting to the bathroom or in toileting because of physical disability

- Environmental barriers—inconvenience of bathroom or toilet equipment, stairs, lack of handrails, and narrow doorways that do not accommodate wheelchairs or walkers

- Mental and psychosocial disability—lack of awareness of the need to urinate, confusion over the location of the bathroom, or individual toileting habits that cause a person to be completely unaware of the need to urinate

- Drugs that affect awareness, mobility, or dexterity

Individuals with conditions such as spina bifida or spinal cord injury (paraplegia) do not have the urge sensation to urinate when the bladder contracts involuntarily. This condition, often referred to as detrusor overactivity or *neurogenic bladder dysfunction,* can lead to incontinence. Neurogenic bladder dysfunction represents one of the most common problems in individuals with a variety of neurological impairments. These impairments include, but are not limited to, traumatic and nontraumatic lesions of the spinal cord, demyelinating disease, and diabetes mellitus. Neurogenic voiding problems generally manifest clinically as either UI (failure to store) or urinary retention (failure to empty) or a combination of both. There are four types of neurogenic bladder dysfunction (Newman, Smith, & Goetz, 1992): flaccid or atonic bladder, spastic or reflex bladder, uninhibited bladder, and sensorimotor paralytic bladder.

Flaccid or Atonic Bladder   Flaccid or atonic bladder, which is frequently seen after an acute spinal cord injury, is a result of the phenomenon of spinal shock. During the stage of spinal shock, which may persist for several weeks to several months after injury, all reflex activity below the level of injury ceases. This includes detrusor contraction, which is normally stimulated through the voiding reflex and found in the second through fourth sacral segments of the spine (S2–S4). Because the detrusor fails to contract in response to even high levels of filling, the result is acute urinary retention. As spinal shock subsides, reflex detrusor function should return, except when the actual site of the injury involves the S2–S4 segments or cauda equina. When the spinal reflex is permanently disrupted by an injury to this area, the atonic or flaccid bladder persists, resulting in chronic urinary retention. Overflow incontinence may occur if retention is not periodically relieved through intermittent catheterization. Stress incontinence may also be seen when injury to the sacral cord and nerves coming from this area results in a flaccid external sphincter. People with multiple sclerosis may also experience urinary retention as a result of flaccid bladder, if scarring involves the S2–S4 area. Whether this condition is temporary or chronic depends on the extent to which remyelination occurs.

Spastic or Reflex Bladder   Spastic or reflex bladder occurs in clients with lesions in the spinal cord above the S2–S4 segments. In this condition, the voiding reflex is intact but hyperactive, because the normal inhibiting influence of the cerebral centers is blocked at the level of the spinal lesion. Voiding will occur frequently and uncontrollably as a result of bladder spasms and a lack of sensation. The bladder capacity is decreased because the detrusor is maintained in a state of nearly constant contraction. The strength of detrusor contractions is inadequate to promote complete emptying. Emptying may be further impaired if *detrusor–sphincter dyssynergia* (DSD) is present. Dyssynergia occurs when reflex bladder contractions are accompanied by simultaneous spasm of the urinary sphincters. Very high bladder pressures may be generated, which predisposes these individuals to reflux of urine into the ureters and ultimately kidney damage. People with complete spinal cord injury above the S2–S4 area, or those with multiple sclerosis plaques in the upper cord, commonly present with a spastic or reflex bladder.

Uninhibited Bladder   Uninhibited bladder may be viewed as a milder form of the spastic bladder previously discussed. Lesions in the cerebral cortex of the brain, such as may occur in stroke, brain tumor, head injury, or multiple sclerosis, cause this type of bladder dysfunction. Changes in the brain with age may also result in impairment of function in a high percentage of older people. Cortical damage impairs the ability to inhibit the sacral voiding reflex efficiently. Often, bladder sensation is retained so that urgency is felt, but the important inhibiting signal is weak or absent, and urgency and urge incontinence can result. This condition is identical to detrusor overactivity and can be used to describe an uninhibited bladder of neurogenic or idiopathic origin. Urinary frequency is common in this type of bladder dysfunction, but emptying is generally adequate.

Sensorimotor Paralytic Bladder   Sensorimotor paralytic bladder occurs in diseases of the peripheral nervous system, which can attack the local nerve supply to the bladder. This is especially common in people with diabetes mellitus, which can affect both sensory and motor pathways. Even if sensation alone is deficient, the bladder may become overdistended because an adequate cue to toilet is never experienced. Motor damage leads to inefficient bladder emptying, and overflow incontinence can develop. Similarly, extensive pelvic surgery can disrupt peripheral nerves.

IDENTIFYING INDIVIDUALS AT RISK

The reasons why people develop UI are unclear, although a multitude of risk factors, especially in the older adult, have been proposed. A person's UI may be directly connected to defined internal and external predispositions. These predispositions, or risk factors, affect the anatomy and physiology of the lower urinary tract. Studies have tried to evaluate the risk factors for UI. Daily UI episodes have been associated with increasing age, history of hysterectomy, higher body mass index, smoking, diabetes, chronic obstructive pulmonary disease (e.g., asthma, emphysema), and poor overall health (Brown, Seeley, Fong, Ensrud, & Grady, 1996). Documented risk factors associated with UI are wide ranging and are described here in decreasing order of their impact on continence.

Age

There is consistent evidence that the frequency of UI increases with age, especially in women. Pelvic muscle relaxation accelerates rapidly after menopause and may progress with aging in general. This relaxation of the pelvic floor causes prolapse of pelvic organs in women. Stress UI is believed to be more common in women ages 45–54 years, whereas urge UI increases with age between 35 and 64 years.

Sex and Race

Throughout their life spans, women are twice as likely to develop UI as men. It has been suggested that Caucasian women have a shorter urethra, weaker pelvic floor muscles, and a lower bladder neck than African American women, thus making them more likely to have stress incontinence (Duong & Korn, 2001). However, parity and socioeconomic factors may also contribute to the difference. There are no data on the relationship between race and UI or OAB in men, but being African American may be a significant predictor of urge UI in women (Graham & Mallett, 2001).

Childbearing

Pregnancy, vaginal delivery, and episiotomy are the most common precipitating events causing UI in women. Half of all women pregnant for the first time experience UI, especially during the last trimester. The incidence of incontinence at 9 weeks postpartum has been reported as 21% for spontaneous birth and 36% for forceps delivery (Meyer, Schreyer, DeGrandi, & Hohfield, 1998). Overall, 30% of women will develop stress UI within 5 years after their first vaginal delivery. Risk for future stress UI is four times higher for women who develop stress UI during pregnancy and postpartum (Viktrup & Lose, 2001). Bladder dysfunction may become more severe with each additional pregnancy. Vaginal birth, especially when the infant is large or the second stage of labor is protracted, imposes pressure, stretch, and shearing risk to the muscles and nerves of the pelvic floor (Sampselle, 2000). Vaginal delivery can also cause neuromuscular damage to the pelvic muscles.

Damage sustained from vaginal delivery primarily occurs during the second stage of labor. When the baby's head encounters the muscular floor of the pelvis, the mechanical process of extension of the head, along with further descent of the baby, causes significant stretching and compression of the nerves to the urethrovesical junction and levator ani muscles. Further extension of the baby's head through the urogenital opening causes distention of the pubococcygeus muscle, with similar soft tissue trauma to muscle and nerves, as well as breaks in the adjacent endopelvic fascia that supports the urethra. Crowning of the head produces significant perineal descent, which stretches the pudendal nerves whose perineal branch innervates the urethrovesical junction and proximal urethra.

Urinary incontinence that occurs immediately after childbirth has been associated with several risk factors that occur during delivery: use of forceps, episiotomy, and pudendal anesthesia. Women who have only borne one child and who develop UI in the immediate postpartum period usually regain continence within 3 months. However, it has been suggested that continence function regained in the first postpartum period declines yearly as a result of additional trauma (e.g., additional births), the effects of aging, or the loss of estrogen following menopause.

Menopause

With menopause, the depletion of estrogen hormone receptors found in the lower urinary tract of women contributes to UI. Estrogen depletion increases the atrophy rate of the muscosal tissue that lines the urethra and vagina (Ulmsten, 1995). This deterioration and a decline in mucus production within the urethra weaken the urethra's ability to maintain a tight seal, especially when intra-abdominal pressure increases with a Valsalva maneuver. Symptoms of urgency, frequency, dysuria, and UI may occur.

Pelvic Muscle Weakness

Pelvic muscle weakness causing pelvic organ prolapse can occur in women with aging. Poor pelvic support of the bladder and urethra by weak muscles can cause prolapse of these organs; as a result, they lie below their normal positions, leading to defects in the transmission of pressures. When the muscles of the pelvic floor are weak or lax in the absence of a prolapse, the *proximal urethra* (the portion of the urethra closest to the bladder) lies below the pelvic floor. Consequently, the urethral pressure does not rise in correspondence with the rise in the bladder pressure, causing stress UI.

Depression

Symptoms of depression are more likely to be reported by adults with UI, and adult women with bladder control problems indicate more emotional distress than continent adults. Adults with UI were more apt to report depression if UI interfered with their daily lives (Dugan et al., 2000).

Impaired Mobility

Impaired mobility that is seen with chronic degenerative disease such as arthritis and osteoporosis can lead to the inability to self-toilet. Confinement to a bed or a use of a wheelchair as a result of a disease such as Alzheimer's disease, hip fractures that do not heal properly, or other surgical complications places individuals at increased risk for developing UI. In addition, there appears to be a relationship between UI, urinary urgency, and falling (Tinetti, Inouye, Gill, & Douchette, 1995). For example, the presence of an urge UI episode at least once a week was independently associated with a 34% increase in fracture risk (Brown, Vittinghoff, et al., 2000).

Polypharmacy

Multiple medications have been previously discussed as causes of acute UI. However, older people who take numerous medications are at increased risk for developing long-term UI as well.

Pelvic Surgery

Pelvic surgery, especially in women who have undergone hysterectomy, increases the risk of UI. Studies have indicated that at least 40% of women who have undergone a hysterectomy will develop UI (Brown, Saways, & Thom, 2000). In men, UI may occur and persist after prostate cancer surgery.

Smoking

Smoking increases the risk of developing all forms of UI, and stress UI in particular, depending on the number of cigarettes smoked (Fantl et al., 1996). It is thought that smoker's cough (more violent and frequent than that of a non-smoker) promotes the earlier development of stress UI (Bump & McClish, 1994). There may also be an association between nicotine and increased detrusor contractions.

Obesity

Obesity has been identified as a risk factor for UI in women in cross-sectional and case-controlled studies (Dwyer, Lee, & Hay, 1988; Wingate, Wingate, & Hassanein, 1994). The UI seen in obesity may be secondary to increased pressure on the bladder and greater urethral mobility. Also, obesity may impair blood flow or nerve innervation to the bladder. Maintaining normal weight through adulthood may be an important factor in the prevention of the development of UI. A significant decrease in symptoms of stress UI were seen in morbidly obese women following weight reduction induced by surgery (Deitel, Stone, Kassam, Wilk, & Sutherland, 1988).

Physical and Occupational Activity

Certain physical activities cause increased pressure in the abdomen thus increasing downward pressure on the bladder. It is thought that at least 50% of women who exercise regularly are at risk for developing stress UI (Bo, Stein, Kulseng-Hanssen, & Kristofferson, 1994; Nygaard, DeLancey, Arnsdorf, & Murphy, 1990). College athletes participating in high-impact activities are more likely to report the symptoms of stress incontinence during exercise than those participating in low impact exercise (Nygaard, Thompson, Svengalis, & Albright, 1994). Usually, women wear a tampon or perineal pad, limit fluid intake, change their sport, or stop exercising altogether to cope with the incontinence. Men report stress UI when swinging a golf club. Sports associated with causing increased pressure on the bladder include combat sports (karate, judo), team games (basketball, volleyball, handball), horseback riding, body building with heavy weights, and track and field (jumping and running). Activities with little risk include swimming, bicycling, walking, rowing, low-impact aerobics, and others in which at least one foot touches the floor at all times.

Work Environment

Very little is known about the occupational impact of UI. Certain provocations may cause stress incontinence; Davis and Goodman (1996) described nine infantry trainees who had never borne children and who developed stress incontinence and pelvic floor defects for the first time during airborne training that included parachute jumping. Sherman, Davis, and Wong (1997) reported that one third of 450 female soldiers reported incontinence during physical exercise, but only 5% reported the incontinence as significantly impacting their work. Fitzgerald, Palmer, Berry, and Hart (2000) surveyed women who worked for a large academic center. Of the 1,113 women surveyed, 21% reported UI at least monthly. Incontinent women were significantly older and had a higher body mass index than continent women.

Women in blue-collar jobs (e.g., factory, sales) may have limited breaks and restricted access to a bathroom. Many of these jobs require heavy lifting, bending, walking, or standing, thus placing the women at greater risk for incontinence, urgency, and frequency. Increased publicity has focused on the importance of employers providing rest breaks and the right for employees to use these breaks (Linder & Nygaard, 1998). A 1995 lawsuit by workers at a Nabisco plant in California cited bladder and urinary tract infections that stemmed from "being forced to wait hours for permission to use the restrooms." Women resorted to wearing adult briefs (i.e., diapers) when supervisors ordered them to urinate in their clothes or face suspension (Linder, 1998).

To address the issue of toileting in the workforce, the Occupational Safety and Health Administration (OSHA) has defined for the workforce environment "toilet facility," "toilet room," "urinal," and "water closet" (OSHA Regulation 1910-141). OSHA interpretation of the regulation states that employees must make toileting facilities available to employees and avoid imposing unreasonable restrictions on employee use of these facilities so that workers will be protected from possible health risks (e.g., UTIs), which can result if the person is unable to use a toilet when needed (OSHA, 1998). Certain states (e.g., California, Kentucky, Nevada, Colorado, Oregon) have regulations mandating rest, relief, and relaxation for employees.

Chronic Disease

Chronic diseases that cause peripheral neuropathy or decreased mobility may place a person at risk for developing UI (Adams, Lorish, Cushing, & Willis, 1994). Urinary incontinence in older men and women is associated with cognitive impairment and impaired mobility (Fantl et al., 1996; Hunskaar, Ostbye, & Borrie, 1998).

Alzheimer's disease is a neurological disorder that causes certain memory, speech, intellectual, and muscular functions, including those of the lower urinary tract, to deteriorate (Skelly & Flint, 1995). As the stages of dementia progress, the ability to perform personal care functions diminishes. Urinary incontinence occurs in the later stage of Alzheimer's disease because of the changes in the neurological pathways between the brain and bladder.

Urinary incontinence and other types of bladder dysfunction can occur after a *stroke,* usually within the first few days. A stroke may cause impaired mobility, perceptual problems, or communication dysfunction together with specific physiological bladder disturbances, such as detrusor overactivity, any of which may predispose a person to incontinence. Many individuals experience a lack of sensory awareness of the need to void or inability to control bladder emptying.

Parkinson's disease and rigidity of muscles contribute to the inability to ambulate to the toilet and self-toilet. Muscle weakness affects the sphincter muscles, particularly the rectal sphincter, causing urinary and fecal incontinence. In one study, stroke and Parkinson's disease each were associated with an increased risk of subsequent UI in men and women (Thom, Haan, & Van den Eeden, 1997).

For people older than age 65, the classic symptoms of *diabetes mellitus*—excessive thirst, blurred vision, extreme hunger, dramatic weight loss, drowsiness, irritability, and mood swings—include two urinary symptoms, frequent urination and frequent UTIs. As the diabetes progresses, the individual develops neuropathy, causing urinary retention and a reduced sensation of the need to void.

Multiple sclerosis (MS) causes urinary dysfunction in the form of a neurogenic bladder in about 80% of people with the disease. The loss of bladder control may be temporary, improving as the symptoms of the disease improve. One of the most significant bladder problems associated with MS is urinary retention. The person may not be aware that the bladder has not emptied completely by voiding. Instead, the person may experience urgency, frequency, nocturia, and/or UI. Another cause of UI is involuntary bladder contractions that cause urination without control.

CONCLUSION

This chapter has outlined the causes of UI with identification of risk factors. UI is seen in all practice settings by caregivers and in all client age groups. Many clinicians accept the UI without investigating the underlying reason for the problem. If the clinician can identify those clients at risk for UI, intervention and treatment can be provided. Also, having a common language for understanding the reason for the UI makes the effort to find solutions that much easier.

REFERENCES

Adams, C., Lorish, C., Cushing, C., & Willis, E. (1994). Anatomical urinary stress incontinence in women with rheumatoid arthritis: Its frequency and coping strategies. *Arthritis Care Research, 7*(2), 97–103.

Avorn, J., Monane, M., Gurwitz, J.H., Glynn, R.J., Choodnovsky, I., & Lipsitz, L.A. (1994). Reduction of bacteriuria and pyuria after ingestion of cranberry juice. *Journal of the American Medical Association, 271,* 751–754.

Bo, K., Stein, R., Kulseng-Hanssen, S., & Kristofferson, M. (1994). Clinical and urody-namic assessment of nulliparous young women with and without stress incontinence symptoms: A case-control study. *Obstetrics and Gynecology, 84*(6), 1028–1032.

Brown, J.S., Saways, G., & Thom, D.H. (2000). Hysterectomy and urinary incontinence: A systematic review. *Lancet, 356,* 535–539.

Brown, J., Seeley, D., Fong, J., Ensrud, K., & Grady, D. (1996). Urinary incontinence in older women: Who is at risk? *Obstetrics and Gynecology, 87,* 715–721.

Brown, J., Vittinghoff, E., Wyman, J., Stone, K., Nevitt, M., Ensrud, K., & Grady, D. (2000). Urinary incontinence: Does it increase risk for falls and fractures? *Journal of the American Geriatrics Society, 48*(7), 721–725.

Bump, R.C., Hurt, W.G., Fantl, J.A., & Wyman, J.F. (1991). Assessment of Kegel pelvic ex-ercise performance after brief verbal instruction. *American Journal of Obstetrics and Gynecology, 165*(2), 322–327.

Bump, R.C., & McClish, D.M. (1994). Cigarette smoking and pure genuine stress inconti-nence of urine: A comparison of risk factors and determinants between smokers and nonsmokers. *American Journal of Obstetrics and Gynecology, 170*(2), 579–82.

Colling, J., Owen, T., & McCreedy, M. (1994). Urinary tract infection rates among incon-tinent nursing home and community dwelling elderly. *Urologic Nursing, 14,* 117–119.

Davis, G.D., & Goodman, M. (1996). Stress urinary incontinence in nulliparous female sol-diers in airborne infantry training. *Journal of Pelvic Surgery, 2*(2), 68–71.

Deitel, M., Stone, E., Kassam, H.A., Wilk, E.J., & Sutherland, D.J.A. (1988). Gynecologic-obstetric changes after loss of massive excess weight following bariatric surgery. *Jour-nal of the American College of Nutrition, 7*(2), 147–153.

Dugan, E., Cohen, S.J., Bland, D.R., Preisser, J.S., Davis, C.C., Suggs, P.K., & McGann, P. (2000). The association of depressive symptoms and urinary incontinence among older adults. *Journal of the American Geriatrics Society, 48,* 413–416.

Duong, T.H., & Korn, A.P. (2001). A comparison of urinary incontinence among African American, Asian, Hispanic and white women. *American Journal of Obstetrics and Gy-necology, 184*(6), 1083–1086.

Dwyer, P.L., Lee, E.T.C., & Hay, D.M. (1988). Obesity and urinary incontinence in women. *British Journal of Obstetrics and Gynaecology, 95,* 91–96.

Fantl, J.A., Newman, D.K., Colling, J., et al. for the Urinary Incontinence in Adults Guide-line Update Panel. (1996). *Urinary incontinence in adults: Acute and chronic management. Clinical practice guideline* (No. 2. Update; AHCPR Publication No. 96-0682). Rockville, MD: Agency for Health Care Policy and Research.

Fitzgerald, S., Palmer, M.H., Berry, S.J., & Hart, K. (2000). Urinary incontinence: Impact on working women. *AAOHN Journal, 48*(3), 112–118.

Graham, C.A., & Mallett, V.T. (2001). Race as a predictor of urinary incontinence and pelvic organ prolapse. *American Journal of Obstetrics and Gynecology, 185*(1), 16–120.

Hunskaar, S., Ostbye, T., & Borrie, M. (1998). The prevalence of urinary incontinence in elderly Canadians and its association with dementia, ambulatory function, and institu-tionalization. *Norwegian Journal of Epidemiology, 8*(2), 177–182.

Kane, R.L., Ouslander, J.G., & Abrass, I.B. (1994). *Essentials of clinical geriatrics* (3rd ed.). New York: McGraw-Hill.

Kayser-Jones, J., Schell, E.S., Porter, C., Barbaccia, J.C., & Shaw, H. (1999). Factors con-tributing to dehydration in nursing homes: Inadequate staffing and lack of professional supervision. *Journal of the American Geriatrics Society, 47,* 1187–1194.

Lavizzo-Mourey, R.J. (1987). Dehydration in the elderly: A short review. *Journal of the National Medical Association, 79,* 1033–1038.

Linder, M. (1998, February 22). Viewpoint: A fight for restroom rights. *The New York Times.*

Linder, M., & Nygaard, I. (1998). *Void where prohibited: Rest break and the right to urinate on company time.* Ithaca, NY: Cornell University Press.

Meyer, S., Schreyer, A., DeGrandi, P., & Hohfield, P. (1998). The effects of birth on urinary continence mechanisms and other pelvic floor characteristics. *Obstetrics and Gynecology, 88,* 470–478.

Muder, R.R., Brennan, C., Wagner, M.M., & Goetz, A.M. (1992). Bacteremia in a long term care facility: A five year prospective study of 163 consecutive episodes. *Clinical Infectious Disorders: An Official Publication of the Infectious Diseases Society of America, 14,* 647–654.

Newman, D.K. (1999). *The urinary incontinence sourcebook* (2nd ed.). Los Angeles: Lowell House.

Newman, D.K., Smith, D.A., & Goetz, G. (1992). Neurogenic bladder dysfunction causing urinary retention. *Journal of Home Health Care Practice, 4*(4), 45–60.

Nygaard, I.E., DeLancey, J.O., Arnsdorf, & Murphy, E. (1990). Exercise and incontinence. *Obstetrics and Gynecology, 75*(5), 848–851.

Nygaard, I.E., Thompson, F.L., Svengalis, S.L., & Albright, J.P. (1994). Urinary incontinence in elite nulliparous athletes. *Obstetrics and Gynecology, 84*(2), 183–187.

Occupational Safety and Health Administration Regulations, 29 C.F.R. §141 (1910).

Resnick, N., & Yalla, S. (1998). Evaluation and management of urinary incontinence. In P. Walsh, A. Retisk, T. Stamey, & E. Vaughan (Eds.), *Campbell's urology* (7th ed.). Philadelphia: W.B. Saunders.

Rudman, D., Hontanosas, A., Cohen, Z., & Mattson, D.E. (1988). Clinical correlates of bacteremia in a Veteran's Administration extended care facility. *Journal of the American Geriatric Society, 38,* 726–732.

Sampselle, C.M. (2000). Behavioral intervention for urinary incontinence in women: Evidence for practice. *Journal of Midwifery & Women's Health, 45*(2), 94–102.

Sherman, R.A., & Davis, G.D. (1997). Behavioral treatment of exercise-induced urinary incontinence among female soldiers. *Military Medicine, 162*(10), 690–694.

Skelly, J., & Flint, A. (1995). Urinary incontinence associated with dementia. *Journal of the American Geriatrics Society, 43,* 286–294.

Spence-Jones, C., Kamm, M.A., Henry, M.M., & Hudson, C.N. (1994). Bowel dysfunction: A pathogenic factor in uterovaginal prolapse and genuine stress incontinence. *British Journal of Obstetrics and Gynaecology, 101,* 147–152.

Thom, D.H., Haan, M.N., & Van den Eeden, S.K. (1997). Medically recognized urinary incontinence and risks of hospitalization, nursing home admission and mortality. *Age and Ageing, 26,* 367–374.

Tinetti, M., Inouye, S., Gill, T., & Doucette, J. (1995). Shared risk factors for falls, incontinence. and functional dependency. *Journal of the American Geriatrics Society, 273,* 1348–1353.

Ulmsten, U. (1995). On urogenital ageing. *Maturitas, 21,* 163–169.

U.S. Department of Labor, Occupational Safety and Health Administration. (1998, April 6). *Interpretation of 29 C.F.R. 1910.141(c)(1)(i): Toilet Facilities.* Available on-line at http://www.osha-slc.gov/OshDoc/Interp_data/I19980406.html

Viktrup, L., & Lose, G. (2001). The risk of stress incontinences 5 years after first delivery. *American Journal of Obstetrics and Gynecology, 184*(2), 20–27.

Wingate, L., Wingate, M.B., & Hassanein, R. (1994). The relationship between overweight and urinary incontinence in postmenopausal women: A case controlled study. *Journal of the North American Menopause Society, 1,* 199–203.

5

Bowel Dysfunction and Its Relationship to Urinary Incontinence

Bowel dysfunction is commonly seen in older adults with urinary incontinence (UI). Bowel regularity or irregularity has an impact on the bladder and its ability to empty. Therefore, it is important for the clinician to investigate any bowel disorder that is identified in a UI evaluation. The most common types of bowel dysfunction are fecal incontinence, chronic constipation, fecal impaction, and diarrhea. These conditions can occur together or alone. For example, severe constipation can contribute to fecal incontinence and fecal impaction. A presenting symptom of fecal impaction is fecal incontinence, wherein liquid stool eventually trickles around the impaction and leaks out.

The embarrassment surrounding bowel dysfunction results in significant underreporting. Therefore, determining the prevalence of these disorders is problematic. The standard definition of constipation is fewer than three stools per week, which indicates a 2%–3% prevalence of constipation in older adults. However, approximately 50% of older adults use over-the-counter laxatives, and more than 3 million prescriptions are written for *cathartics* yearly (Nelson, Norton, Cautley, & Furner, 1995). Every year, Americans spend $200 million on laxatives, and there are more than 70 commercially produced laxative products (Johanson, 1998).

Fecal incontinence is one of the most common reasons for placing an older person in a nursing facility. Some 15%–60% of people living in residential facilities are estimated to have some degree of bowel disorder, mainly constipation and fecal incontinence (Chassagne et al., 1999). Constipation is more prevalent among older adults, women, Black people, individuals with low income or low levels of education, and people who are not physically active (Johanson, 1998). Taboos regarding bowel function and feces create social and psychological problems for people with fecal incontinence and other bowel disorders that are even greater than those associated with UI and overactive bladder. For many older adults, especially those who are homebound or residing in a nursing facility, constipation and fecal incontinence represent a humiliating regression in bodily function, severely impairing activity and socialization.

This chapter reviews the most common bowel disorders that older adults with urinary incontinence may experience: fecal (anal) incontinence, constipation, fecal impaction, and diarrhea. The clinician should have

- Knowledge of the anatomy and physiology of the lower rectum in relation to the normal bowel

- Awareness of common bowel conditions seen in older adults

- Knowledge of stool type by rectal examination

- Ability to discuss constipation, fecal incontinence, and fecal impaction management options

- Critical synthesis of evidence-based practice and relevant literature

ANATOMY AND PATHOPHYSIOLOGY OF THE BOWEL

Normal anorectal function includes storage and appropriate evacuation of stool. Certain requirements must be met to achieve these functions. The continence component requires normal perception and discrimination of bowel contents, as well as colonic and rectal accommodation (presence of stool).

The large intestine is a hollow muscular tube about 5 feet in length. It is divided into the cecum, colon, and rectum. The *cecum* comprises the first 2 or 3 inches of the large intestine. The *colon* is subdivided into the ascending, transverse, descending, and sigmoid colon (see Figure 5.1). The large intestine has many functions, all related to the final processing of intestinal contents, or feces. Very little, if any, digestion takes place in the large intestine, whose most important function is the absorption of water and electrolytes. Approximately 600 milliliters of water is absorbed daily from intestinal contents. The longer the fecal mass stays in the colon, the more water can be absorbed. The movement, or *peristalsis,* of intestinal contents in the large intestine is slow. Mass peristalsis, which is a contraction involving a large segment of the colon, moves the fecal mass into the sigmoid colon, where it is stored. Soft, formed stool is delivered to the rectum at regular intervals, typically one to three times per day, especially after breakfast.

The sigmoid colon bends toward the left as it joins the rectum (see Figure 5.1). (This is the rationale for lying on the left side when receiving an enema.) This junction, called the *rectosigmoidal junction,* plays an essential role in maintaining fecal continence and normal defecation. Not only does this angulation provide a mechanical break for material leaving the colon, but there is also evidence that the sensory response to sigmoidal distention modulates rectal sensation.

The last portion of the large intestine is the *rectum,* which extends from the sigmoid colon to the anus (about 6 inches). The last inch of the rectum is called the *anal canal.* It contains the internal and external anal sphincters, which play an important role in regulating defecation. Muscle contractions in

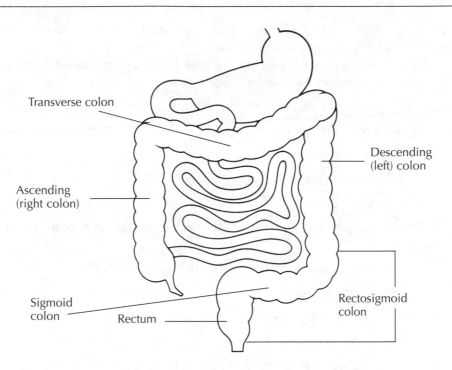

Figure 5.1. Anatomy of the large intestine, frontal view. (Courtesy of Hollister)

the colon push stool toward the anus. By the time stool reaches the rectum, it is solid because most of the water has been absorbed.

The nerve supply to the large intestine contains both *parasympathetic* and *sympathetic nerves.* In general, stimulation of the sympathetic nerve fibers inhibits activity in the gastrointestinal (GI) tract. It also excites the internal anal sphincter. Thus stimulation of the sympathetic fibers can totally block movement of feces through the GI tract both by inhibition of the wall and closure of the two anal sphincters. Stimulation of the parasympathetic nerve fibers causes an increase in bowel activity and in the defecation reflexes. Awareness of rectal distension is dependent on both intact nerve pathways and a normal mental status. Normal sensory awareness includes the ability to discriminate among gas, liquid, and solid contents as well as the ability to recognize rectal distention from stool.

Two distinct anal sphincters are important in maintaining continence. The internal sphincter is a thin (2- to 3-centimeter) smooth muscle sphincter, which is largely responsible for resting tone in the anal canal. The internal sphincter is normally closed, thus preventing the passive seepage of stool. The external sphincter is composed of voluntary (striated) muscle. The external sphincter surrounds the internal sphincter, and its main function is to preserve continence during the urge to defecate and during rises in abdominal pressure such as occur during physical activity. As the feces approach the anus, the internal anal sphincter is inhibited and, if the external anal sphincter is relaxed, defecation will occur. Because the external anal sphincter is under voluntary control, normal defecatory function is a learned behavior that is amenable to behavior modification.

Defecation is a reflex involving the muscles of the anal canal and terminal bowel. The stages of defecation are as follows:

- A comfortable and upright seated position is assumed
- Abdominal pressure rises
- Rectal pressure rises
- Relaxation of anal sphincter pressure occurs
- Internal anal sphincter pressure falls
- External anal sphincter pressure falls—rectal pressure is now higher than anal pressure
- The puborectalis muscle portion of the pelvic floor muscles relaxes
- The pelvic floor descends
- The anorectal angle increases
- Defecation occurs

Entry of the fecal mass into the rectum distends the rectal walls and stimulates mass peristaltic movements of the bowel, which move the feces toward the anus. Normal defecation occurs only when intra-abdominal pressure increases through a contraction of the chest muscles and simultaneous contraction of the abdominal muscles (Valsalva's maneuver or straining). At the same time, the puborectalis muscle relaxes, allowing voluntary passage of stool. The defecation reflex may be halted by voluntary contraction of the external anal sphincter. When this is done, the defecation reflex dies out after a few minutes and usually will not return for several hours.

A key factor in the defecation process is access to toilet facilities. Repeated inhibition of the defecation reflex is common in people who are immobile and need assistance to toilet. If the urge to defecate occurs and a caregiver is unavailable, the person will inhibit the urge, thus allowing stool to further solidify. Water continues to be absorbed from the fecal mass, causing it to become firmer, so that subsequent defecation is more difficult and constipation may result. If the stool is not passed in a timely manner, the continued absorption of water may cause it to become impacted.

FECAL INCONTINENCE

Fecal incontinence is defined as the involuntary or inappropriate passing of liquid or solid stool and can also include the incontinence of flatus (gas). Fecal incontinence is a leading cause of nursing facility placement, and its prevalence in nursing facilities is reported to be higher than in the community. Nelson, Furner, and Jesudason (1998) found that 47% of nursing facility residents had fecal incontinence. Dementia, restricted mobility, diarrhea, and male gender have been identified as risk factors for fecal incontinence (Johanson, Irizarry, & Doughty, 1997). In adult women, the most common cause of fecal incontinence is obstetrical or surgical trauma, usually a direct injury to either the anal sphincter or the pudendal nerves (Jackson, Weber, Hull, Mitchinson, & Walters, 1997). People with long-standing constipation can develop fecal incontinence because the sensation of the movement of feces into the rectum does not occur. Table 5.1 outlines common causes of fecal incontinence.

Fecal or anal incontinence can be described as mild, when there is loss of small amounts of gas or liquid stool; or major, when there is intermittent, involuntary loss of large amounts of solid stool. People with mild fecal incontinence may pass small amounts of stool that is visible on the underclothes, which is referred to as *fecal staining*. Mild anal incontinence may occur with a normal anal sphincter and can be caused by anorectal conditions such as hemorrhoids, colitis, or irritable bowel syndrome. Poor mental activity caused

Table 5.1.   Common causes of fecal incontinence in adults

Causes	Examples
Sphincter or pelvic floor muscle damage	Obstetric trauma (vaginal delivery) Chronic straining with stool Direct trauma or injury
Diarrhea states	Inflammatory bowel disease Intestinal diarrhea Infectious diarrhea Laxative abuse Irritable bowel syndrome
Iatrogenic/postsurgical	Posthemorroidectomy Sphincterotomy for fissure or anal stretch
Anorectal pathology	Rectal prolapse Anal or rectovaginal fissure
Neurological disease	Spinal cord injury Multiple sclerosis Spina bifida Parkinson's disease Alzheimer's disease/dementia Peripheral neuropathies (e.g., diabetes, chronic alcoholism)
Overflow diarrhea	Fecal impaction Institutionalized or immobile elderly
Environmental	Poor toilet facilities Inadequate care Lack of toileting by staff
Idiopathic	Unknown cause

by dementia or depression can also predispose to incontinence, as can limitations of mobility. Major anal incontinence is usually the result of neuromuscular damage to the anal sphincter mechanism. People who report fecal/anal incontinence may be referring to soiling, diarrhea, poor hygiene, or minor anal abnormalities such as hemorrhoids. Some people soil their clothes without knowing that they are about to have a bowel movement.

The combination of fecal incontinence and UI, called *double incontinence,* is well known and is seen in the long-term care setting as a result of poor mobility and cognitive impairment. Double incontinence may be also a result of peripheral neurological lesions such as repeated obstetrical injuries or severe chronic constipation. Fecal incontinence without UI occurs in only 2% of long-term care residents (Chiang, Ouslander, Schnelle, & Reuben, 2000). The reason both types of incontinence may occur at the same time is that the digestive tract and the lower urinary tract are closely connected, and anything that affects one of them can affect the other. Both systems share common nerves and are supported by the pelvic muscles and other structures that play a vital role in maintaining continence. Therefore, anything that causes damage or trauma to the nerves that supply the rectum or pelvic floor will cause urinary and fecal incontinence. Diseases or injuries that affect the spinal cord or the nerves or muscles can affect both systems. Having both urinary and fecal incontinence is so difficult to manage that people with double incontinence live in a constant state of anxiety and may totally withdraw from society.

Rectal sensation warns of imminent defecation and helps a person discriminate between formed and unformed stool and gas. Impaired rectal sensation may deprive a person of this useful information and result in incontinence. Probably one of the most common causes of fecal incontinence is damage to one or both anal sphincters. The external sphincter is responsible for delaying bowel emptying once the rectum fills and the urge to empty the bowel is felt. People with a weak or damaged external anal sphincter muscle typically experience urgency and must rush to the toilet as soon as the need to defecate is felt; if the toilet is not reached in time, urge fecal incontinence can occur. The weakened sphincter muscle is unable to squeeze hard enough to prevent the seepage of stool.

Among older people, the most common cause of fecal incontinence is neither loss of mobility nor dementia but simply the natural effects of aging on the body. Muscles and tissues weaken, lose their elasticity, and become lax. Changes in muscle strength, muscle mass, and muscle and nerve reflexes affect the anorectal area. The strength of the external anal sphincter and pelvic muscles decreases with aging. Thus, some older adults cannot retain gas or stool, especially liquid stool, as well as or for as long as they once could. Also, the older adult may not be able to reflexively close the anal sphincter quickly enough to avoid a fecal incontinence accident. Compared to continent people, incontinent older adults have less rectal sensation and less sphincter strength. In older adults living in nursing facilities, acute diarrhea and fecal impaction are the main causes of fecal incontinence.

CHRONIC CONSTIPATION

A decrease in the normal frequency of bowel movements is often associated with increased difficulty in defecation. As mentioned previously, constipation is defined as having fewer than three stools per week. It has been estimated that at least 17% of the adult population will be constipated at some point in their lives. Usually an individual's definition of constipation is considerably broader, however, and includes straining at stool, painful defecation, dry hard stools, small stools, and incomplete or infrequent stool evacuation. The prevalence of constipation increases with age, and constipation is more common in women than in men, in non-Whites than in Whites, and in those with lower family income and lower levels of education (Kumar et al., 1992). The steepest increase in reported prevalence rates of constipation occurs in the sixth decade and ranges from 4% to 30%. Older adults are five times more likely than younger adults to report problems with constipation.

Two types of constipation are functional constipation and rectosigmoidal outlet delay. *Functional constipation* refers to slow transit of stool and is seen in at least 40% of older adults. The definition of functional constipation requires that a person have more than two of the following four parameters for 1 year or longer:

1. Fewer than three stools per week

2. Hard, pelletlike stools on 25% of bowel movements

3. Straining at defecation 25% of the time

4. Sense of incomplete evacuation after 25% or more of bowel movements

Rectosigmoidal outlet delay occurs in cases of anorectal dysfunction. This type of constipation is characterized by prolonged defecation—usually more than 10 minutes. The person will report a need to press in or around the anus with a finger to aid in defecation (digital stimulation). Usually, if more than 3 days pass without a bowel movement, feces may harden or may become pelletlike. The person may have difficulty or even pain during elimination and may use excessive straining to pass the stool. Risk factors for constipation include age, recent abdominal or perianal surgery, general anesthesia, limited physical activity, inadequate diet or fluid intake, history of constipation or laxative abuse, and drugs known to cause constipation.

Constipation may present as a change in bowel habit or as overflow fecal incontinence. People suffering from constipation may present with acute changes in cognition, urinary retention, UI, and fecal impaction. If the person also has UI, once constipation is resolved, improvement in urine leakage usually occurs. Constipation is a symptom, not a disease, but prolonged constipation can lead to urinary retention and incontinence. Also, repeated straining to expel hard stool that occurs over many years can eventually lead to pelvic muscle weakness, weakening of the anal sphincter, and rectal prolapse (Resnick, 2001).

Many people have misconceptions concerning normal bowel habits. Many times older people become overly concerned with having a daily bowel movement, and constipation may be imaginary. Older individuals are more likely to describe themselves as constipated if they had to strain during defecation or had incomplete evacuation, difficulty or pain with defecation, or hard stools. They believe that a bowel movement is necessary every day. These people need to be taught that bowel patterns can vary and that having a bowel movement every other day or every third day may be normal. Also, an individual may express concern that if wastes remain in the bowel, they are absorbed and can shorten the person's life. Therefore, these individuals take large amounts and many different types of laxatives to have daily movements and to get rid of "harmful wastes."

People with constipation commonly use laxatives, enemas, and other invasive procedures such as manual removal of fecal impaction. These interventions are not without risk and may produce undesired side effects such as cramping, bloating, dehydration, diarrhea, rectal bleeding, anal irritation, and fecal incontinence. Heavy dependence on laxatives can become habit-forming because long-term use of laxatives interferes with the colon, decreasing peristalsis. Mineral oil coats the intestines; blocks absorption of vitamins A, D, E, and K; and also may interact with other medications. Milk of magnesia can increase peristalsis and prevent complete and adequate absorption of vitamins and minerals. Habitual use of enemas leads to loss of normal bowel function. Bowel retraining programs have been shown to be successful in reducing constipation in the chronically constipated person who is at risk for injury from overuse of laxatives and enemas. Ignoring or suppressing the urge to defecate contributes to constipation (Sanburg, McGuire, & Lee, 1996).

FECAL IMPACTION

Fecal impaction occurs when stool that has not been passed builds up over days and becomes hardened in the rectum. This condition is not very common but may occur in frail, ill, older adults. Fecal impaction may present as diarrhea, fecal incontinence, or both in the geriatric population; the stool proximal to the obstructing fecal mass becomes liquefied and oozes around the mass. This condition, sometimes called fecal oozing or fecal staining, commonly presents with semisolid fecal soiling many times daily. Approximately 25%–30% of impactions are high impactions, which may not be easily diagnosed by rectal examination.

Impaction is caused by a combination of factors that include poor rectal sensation, immobility, inadequate fluid and food intake, drug side effects, and inability or delay in recognizing or responding, or inappropriate responding, to the urge to defecate. If fecal impaction is left untreated or unremoved, it can cause intestinal obstruction, ulceration, and urinary problems. Usually the person is unable to pass this large amount of stool. He or she may pass small amounts of watery stool and experience severe stomach pain, discomfort, and bloating. Loss of appetite is a common complaint. Frail older adults may exhibit changes in cognition and develop a fever.

If a large impaction is present and enemas have been ineffective in removing the impaction, the feces must be broken up manually. Nurses tend to use enemas initially, followed up by laxatives to remove the impaction, using manual removal only as a last resort (Poulton & Thomas, 1999). The clinician must use caution with manual removal because stimulation of the vagus nerve in the rectal wall can slow the client's heart rate. For individuals with chronic illness who develop fecal impaction frequently, the nurse may need to teach the caregiver how to remove the impaction. The nurse should slowly insert a lubricated, gloved index finger approximately 5 cm into the rectum. The index finger should be inserted into the rectum using a rotating motion to stimulate relaxation of the internal anal sphincter and peristaltic contractions in the left colon. If the stool is hard and solid, an attempt should be made to break up the hard stool and remove it. This can be accomplished by pushing a finger into the center, splitting the stool and breaking it up into small sections.

Another method that may be successful is mixing 50 ml of water and 50 ml of hydrogen peroxide in a piston syringe, attaching a red rubber catheter to the tip of the syringe, and injecting this solution directly into the hard fecal mass. This mixture will cause foaming of the stool and will successfully break the mass into small pieces. Encourage the person to assist by bearing down using the Valsalva maneuver. It is recommended that an enema be used to remove stool that remains. Appendix A: Tips for Bowel Regularity discusses the use of a milk and molasses enema. If phosphate-containing Fleet enemas are used, only one enema at a time should be given because the colon may absorb some of the phosphate, which may lead to electrolyte imbalance.

DIARRHEA

Diarrhea is defined as the passage of frequent, watery bowel movements that can be seen in people with decreased anal sphincter pressures. The symptoms usually disappear quickly and are more an inconvenience than an illness. In certain cases, however, diarrhea may persist for days, weeks, and even months. If this occurs, the person may have viral or bacterial diarrhea resulting from exposure to the flu, a virus, or food poisoning or, in some cases, a parasite. Diarrhea caused by an infectious process raises particular concern in the institutional setting, such as hospitals or nursing facilities, where an infection may spread among the resident population. Usually the *Clostridium difficile* bacterium, which causes diarrhea, is treated effectively with medications. A stool culture will determine the presence of bacteria or parasites.

Another cause of diarrhea, especially in the older adult, is laxative abuse. Regular, frequent use of laxatives disrupts the nerves to the colon, dulling the sensation of the need for bowel elimination. Natural emptying mechanisms fail to work as the body becomes dependent on laxatives and enemas. Symptoms such as abdominal cramping; frequent passage of thin, watery stool; change in color and odor of stool; nausea and vomiting; and even fever may occur.

Prolonged diarrhea can cause skin irritation and breakdown around the anal, gluteal, and perineal area. After each bowel movement, the entire perineum should be cleaned with mild soap and water and thoroughly dried. Barrier skin products should be considered if any skin irritation or redness occurs. Antidiarrheal medications such as loperamide and diphenoxylate with atropine (Lomotil) should be used to treat acute diarrheal attacks.

FACTORS THAT CONTRIBUTE TO BOWEL DYSFUNCTION

Several risk factors have been identified as contributing to bowel disorders. This section discusses the most common contributing factors.

Insufficient Dietary Fiber

Dietary fiber is important for the successful long-term management of constipation. Soluble fiber sources such as oatmeal and peeled fruit can add bulk to liquid stool, absorb excess water in the colon, and increase the ability to form solid stool in people with fecal incontinence and diarrhea. A diet high in animal fats and refined sugars tends to be low in fiber. Fat delays gastric emptying and slows intestinal motility, which promotes constipation. High-fiber diets result in larger stools, more frequent bowel movements, and less constipation. Oral calcium supplements can also decrease the incidence of diarrhea by improving stool consistency

Hemorrhoids

Hemorrhoids can be internal, inside the rectum, or external, outside the anal opening. The presence of hemorrhoids causes pain, itching, and discomfort during defecation. Spasms can occur in the anal sphincters, causing the person to delay bowel movements.

Rectal Surgery

Any surgery in the area of the rectum that involves the anal sphincters can contribute to bowel dysfunction, especially if it results in disorders that in-

terfere with defecation. Hemorrhoidectomy may lead to a "keyhole" defor-
mity, which allows the passive seepage of liquid stool. Another common
anorectal procedure is a sphincterotomy, in which the lower third of the anal
sphincter is divided to relieve an anal fissure. It can inadvertently cause
sphincter damage in women.

Poor Fluid Intake

Drinking plenty of fluids, preferably water, helps stimulate intestinal activity.
Water and other fluids add bulk to stools, making bowel movements softer,
more frequent, and easier to pass.

Ignoring the Defecation Urge

People with chronic illness who have decreased functional mobility or a mental illness may ignore or inhibit the urge to defecate (the "call to stool"). Repeated inhibition of defecation can lead to constipation, fecal incontinence,
and impaction. This is believed to be one of the main causes of bowel disorders, especially fecal incontinence, in older people who are dependent on
caregivers or live in nursing facilities.

Pregnancy

Damage to one or both anal sphincters during delivery is the most common
cause of fecal incontinence in women. This is particularly the case in women
with third-degree tears that extend from the vagina through the anal sphincter. Women whose first delivery was assisted with forceps are the most likely
to develop incontinence. Women who are pregnant often have problems with
constipation, possibly as a result of increased pressure from the fetus on the
intestines, or hormonal changes.

Medications

Most of the medications commonly prescribed for older adults cause constipation. This is especially true with the following types of medications:

- Analgesics and opiates—inhibit gastrointestinal motility, particularly in
  the colon, by prolonging intestinal transit time. Orally administered opiates are more constipating than parentally administered agents.

- Anticholinergics (antihistamines, antiparkinsonian drugs, tricyclic antidepressants, and phenothiazines)—inhibit bowel function, particularly in
  the colon and rectum

- Antacids that contain aluminum and calcium; antibiotics—may cause diarrhea and constipation

- Calcium channel blockers—slow intestinal transit time by affecting autonomic nervous system function or smooth muscle contractility

- Iron supplements; calcium supplements—can slow colonic transit time, leading to constipation

Chronic Diseases

Underlying medical conditions, especially neurological diseases that affect nerves leading to the intestines or rectum and anus, can cause bowel dysfunction. *Irritable bowel syndrome* may cause refractory constipation. Parkinson's disease causes an abnormal response of the rectoanal inhibitory reflex, causing the anal sphincter to contract during defecation. Multiple sclerosis is associated with bowel dysfunction in more than two thirds of people who have this disease. The presence of fecal incontinence is correlated with the degree of disability, duration of disease, and bladder symptoms. People with multiple sclerosis also develop constipation as a result of slow colonic transit time and the inability to relax the pelvic floor muscles at the time of defecation. People with diabetes mellitus may suffer chronic diarrhea secondary to internal sphincter neuropathy and impaired sensation, which can also lead to fecal incontinence. Hypothyroidism may cause hypomotility and slow bowel transit time. Psychological factors such as depression and cognitive impairment, as seen in people with Alzheimer's disease or other dementias, predispose the older adult to constipation, fecal impaction, and fecal incontinence. The cause is believed to be neurological impairment that results in

- Inability to recognize or respond to an urge to have a bowel movement

- Inability to control the defecation

- Denial or avoidance of the urge to defecate

- Loss of social awareness of the need for continence

- Inability to identify toilet facilities appropriately

- In some cases, physical inability to cope with bowel function

Lack of Physical Activity

A decrease in mobility or prolonged bed rest as a result of an accident or illness may contribute to constipation and fecal incontinence. Decreased physical activity reduces both self-reported and objectively measured constipation in older adults. People are more apt to have fecal incontinence if they cannot get to the bathroom on sensing an urge to defecate. This is even more significant in the individual who has loose stools or diarrhea.

Laxative Abuse

Individuals who habitually take laxatives become dependent on them and may require increasing dosages, until the intestine ultimately becomes accustomed to the laxatives and does not respond to them.

Travel

When traveling, individuals often experience constipation, especially during long-distance trips and trips to other countries. This may be due to changes in drinking water, schedule, diet, and lifestyle.

EVALUATION OF BOWEL FUNCTION

The evaluation of a person with bowel dysfunction should include a focused history and physical examination. The checklist in Figure 5.2 can be used for this purpose. A detailed history can give important clues to the cause of the bowel dysfunction. Urgency and urge incontinence suggest an external sphincter defect. Passive soiling is likely to be caused by an internal sphincter problem, but the two can overlap, and it is impossible to be certain of the cause without further tests. Many commonly used medications, including calcium- and aluminum-containing antacids, beta-blockers, calcium channel blockers, anticholinergic agents, antidepressants, and opiates also cause constipation. Systemic diseases such as thyroid disease, diabetes mellitus, and neuromuscular diseases are yet other potential etiologies. Defecatory dysfunction is often a result of functional obstruction occurring because of pelvic floor muscle weakness with subsequent prolapse, including *rectocele* and *enterocele* (Jensen, 1997). Bowel function can also be affected by psychiatric disorders, including depression, dementia, and anorexia.

Another important part of the evaluation is asking the client to complete a bowel record or diary (Figure 5.3). The person should be asked to discuss the bowel problem in his or her own words (Jensen, 2000b). Using a pictorial scale such as the Bristol Stool Form Scale (see Figure 5.4) may aid the clinician in understanding stool consistency. Stool consistency can vary from hard lumps to very loose or pasty stool; the consistency often depends on how long the stools have been in the colon and how much water has been absorbed. Ideally stool should be formed into a smooth sausage shape, soft and comfortable to pass.

History

Elicit the client's definition of constipation and of bowel disorder.
Describe stool form (see Figure 5.4 for Bristol Stool Form Scale).
Determine onset, frequency, and duration of fecal leakage, constipation, and
   other bowel problems.
Determine current bowel management program.
Indicate any associated syptoms of fecal incontinence:
   O Abdominal pain and cramping
   O Abdominal bloating
   O Gas incontinence
Indicate associated symptoms of constipation:
   O Decreased stool frequency
   O Sense of incomplete evacuation
   O Pain and discomfort with defecation
   O Abdominal pain and cramping
   O Rectal pain
   O Straining on defecation
   O Digital help with defecation
   O Frequent laxative use
   O Change in mental status
Indicate associated symptoms of fecal impaction:
   O Anorexia
   O Nausea and vomiting
   O Abdominal pain
   O Acute states of confusion
   O Fecal incontinence
Determine the effect bowel dysfunction has had on quality of life.
Identify all primary and secondary medical problems to determine impact on
   gastrointestinal tract.
Specify type, frequency, and results of laxatives, stool softeners, mini-enemas,
   suppositories, and enemas used in the past.
Ask if the patient has had a previous problem with fecal impaction and
   intervention.
Identify current medication use: Any agents with side effects profiles that may
   contribute to bowel disorder?
Check diet and fluid intake:
   O Is dehydration present?
   O What is the total fluid intake in a 24-hour period?
   O How much caffeinated beverages and food are ingested?
Check past medical history:
   O Pelvic or urological disorders (e.g., urinary incontinence)
   O Previous gastrointestinal or pelvic surgery
   O Neurological disease (e.g., Parkinson's disease, multiple sclerosis)

Physical examination—the following may be noted on exam:

Abdomen:
   O Listen for presence of hyperactive or no bowel sounds.
   O Check for presence of abdominal cramping, bloating or discomfort,
      masses or bulges.

Figure 5.2.   Bowel function evaluation checklist.

○ Percuss to determine presence of gas.
○ Check for dullness that may indicate fecal mass.

Genitalia:
○ Visually inspect perineal skin for lack of integrity, rashes, and other effects of chronic leakage of stool.

Pelvic examination (women):
○ Are structural abnormalities present, such as pelvic organ prolapse, particularly retrocele?
○ Can pelvic muscle strength be assessed?

Anorectal examination:
○ Note color and characteristics of anal mucosa; note any gaping of the anus, which indicates an abnormal external sphincter tone.
○ Note presence and consistency of stool in rectal vault; note presence of fecal impaction.
○ Note anal wink, anal sphincter tone, impaired rectal sensation, and size and condition of rectum.
○ Note presence of external or internal hemorrhoids and rectal prolapse.
○ Perform hemoccult test to determine presence of occult blood.

Functional, environmental, and mental assessment

Mobility and ability to self-toilet:
○ Restraints (physical or chemical) used?

Environment:
○ Are toilet facilities accessible?
○ Are chairs desined for ease of rising?
○ Are grab bars available and within the resident's reach when toileting?

Mental:
○ Is a mini-mental exam needed?
○ Assess mood, affect, and comprehension.

Bowel record
Has resident's voiding and defecation pattern been assessed through collection of a 3-day record or some other method?

Other record
Anorectal manometry to provide baseline information on sphincter function and measurement of the rectal inhibility reflux.
Flexible sigmoidoscopy, especially in clients with hemoccult-positive stool, in clients who recently became constipated without obvious cause, and in clients with fecal incontinence.
Plain abdominal x-rays may be indicated for clients with constipation.
Barium enema if colonic obstruction is suspected.
Colonic transit time and motility testing in those clients with severe constipation that is not amenable to lifestyle modification treatments, such as fluids, diet, and exercise.
Defecography to determine aspects of anorectal and pelvic floor function.

1. Please descibe your stool:
    (Using the Bristol Stool Form Scale, circle the picture that most resembles your stool.)
2. Do you pass any blood or mucus when you move your bowels? ___Yes ___No
3. Do you have pain when you move your bowels? ___Yes ___No
4. If you do have pain, when does it occur:
    Before moving your bowels? ___Yes ___No
    When you are moving your bowels? ___Yes ___No
    After having a bowel movement? ___Yes ___No
5. When you move your bowels, do you have a strong urge and need to rush to the bathroom? ___Yes ___No
6. Do you ever not get to the toilet in time and have a "bowel accident"? ___Yes ___No
7. Do you have difficulty moving your bowels? ___Yes ___No
8. Do you need to strain or bear down to move your bowels? ___Yes ___No
9. Do you ever need to insert a finger to help get stool out? ___Yes ___No
10. Do you need to push on the area where your bowels move to help the stool come out? ___Yes ___No
11. Do you feel that you have not completely emptied your bowels? ___Yes ___No
12. Do you lose any stool when you do not want to or are unaware of it? ___Yes ___No
13. Can you control your gas (farts)? ___Yes ___No
14. Do you wear a pad for protection of leakage of stool? ___Yes ___No
15. Do you use laxatives or enemas to help move your bowels? ___Yes ___No
    What do you use? _____

Figure 5.3. Bowel record.

The physical examination should include a thorough abdominal, anorectal, and pelvic examination. Visual inspection of the perineal skin and anus should be performed. The anus is normally closed circumferentially. The examiner should stroke the perianal skin with a finger in the 9 and 3 o'clock positions. This normally elicits the anal wink, or visible contraction of the anal sphincter—the anus will pucker. The anorectal exam should include an inspection for soiling and an assessment of rectal contents. After inspection, a digital anorectal examination should be performed to determine the presence of a rectal tumor or mass, presence of fecal material, and strength of the anal sphincter. In order to determine overall anal sphincter tone, the strength and symmetry of the sphincter contraction, defects in the sphincter mechanism,

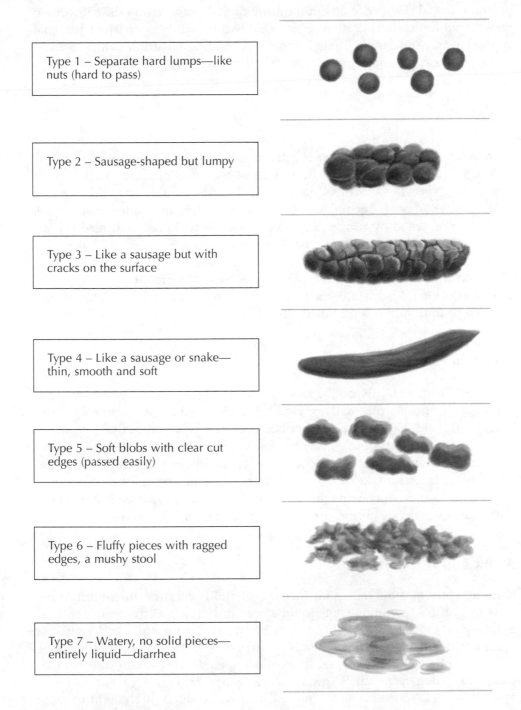

Figure 5.4. Bristol Stool Form Scale. (From Heaton, K.W., Radvan, J., Cripps, H., Mountford, R.A., Braddon, F.E.M., & Hughes, A.O. [1992]. Defaecation frequency, timing, and stool form in the general population: A prospective study. *Gut, 33,* 818–824.)

and the dynamic changes of the pelvic floor during a Valsalva maneuver, the person is asked to squeeze or strain during digital examination. Bearing down may reveal a rectal prolapse or enterocele. An inability to contract the anal sphincter may indicate neurological deficits. Additional studies such as anoscopy, proctoscopy, and barium enema radiography may be necessary.

TREATMENT

Management of bowel disorders is influenced by many factors, including tradition, culture, and people's expectations of what is "normal." Many bowel disorders, especially constipation and fecal incontinence, that are seen in older people who are dependent on caregivers or live in residential facilities could be prevented by proper attention to mobility, fluids, diet, medication, and establishment of good bowel habits. In residential facilities, staff attitudes are crucial: staff should not simply accept a situation as inevitable but rather approach it in an individualized manner (Benton, O'Harra, Chen, Harper, & Johnston, 1997). The strategies discussed in this section should be recommended to individuals with bowel disorders.

Maintain Adequate Fluid Intake

Daily fluid intake should not be less than six to eight 8-ounce glasses. Drinking a glass of prune juice daily or eating prunes may help with bowel regulation. Prune juice has almost no fiber but does have a laxative effect, probably because of its content of magnesium salts. There are creative ways to increase fluid intake. Setting the table or tray with two types of liquid at each meal helps increase total intake. If a person is averse to drinking additional amounts of juice and water, encourage the intake of foods that have a high water content, such as fruits (watermelon), soups, ice cream, and flavored ices.

Avoid Bowel Irritants

Caffeine consumption causes an increase of fluid secretion in the intestine, thus increasing the amount of liquid stool, and may contribute to fecal incontinence. Caffeine is presumed to stimulate the parasympathetic nervous system, thus increasing bowel motility. Avoiding foods that contain caffeine (i.e., tea, coffee, chocolate) is recommended. Some foods contain starches that escape digestion in the small bowel and may cause flatulence (gas) in the colon and lead to "gas" incontinence. Some of the foods commonly thought to cause flatulence include apricots, bananas, beans, Brussels sprouts, cabbage, carrots, celery, dried beans, eggs, lentils, milk and milk products, onions, peas, pretzels, prunes, raisins, salad ingredients (especially cucumber), and wheat germ.

Hot, spicy foods can increase the speed with which food travels along the bowel and increase gas production. People with incontinence of flatus can experiment to see if certain foods are affecting them and whether avoiding the offending food helps their condition.

Increase Fiber Intake

Fiber-Rich Foods   Increasing intake of dietary fiber is widely advocated as first-line treatment for clients complaining of constipation as it will increase bowel frequency (Hinrichs & Huseboe, 2001). Dietary fiber includes insoluble and soluble fiber. Insoluble fiber is found in wheat bran, vegetables, and whole grains. This type of fiber, especially wheat bran, is most helpful in preventing constipation. Soluble fiber is found in oat bran, barley, some beans, and certain fruits and vegetables. Soluble fiber has minimal benefit in preventing or treating constipation. The most beneficial means to prevent constipation is a combination of insoluble and soluble fiber by increasing dietary intake of bran, fruits, and vegetables. Fiber acts as a bulk-forming agent and is metabolized by colonic bacteria to nonabsorbable, volatile fatty acids, which act as an osmotic cathartic. As fiber passes through the colon it acts as a sponge by absorbing water. Fiber may bind with fecal bile salts and thus increase transit of stool through the intestine. While adding bulk, fiber also promotes retention of water in the stool thus decreasing the amount and frequency of watery liquid. High fiber foods include:

- Whole-grain breads and cereals (e.g., All-Bran). Whole-grain bread contains 8%–10% dietary fiber, but some fiber-rich breakfast cereals contain 25%.

- Raw vegetables, especially green leafy ones, and fresh fruits with skins (e.g., apples). Vegetables contain cellulose, hemicellulose, and lignin. Lignin is not digested in the human intestine and, therefore, adds to stool weight.

- Fresh fruit and raisins

Addition of Raw Bran   One solution to bowel dysfunction, especially if the person is not allergic to wheat products, is the use of whole, unprocessed wheat bran, often called miller's bran. Raw (unprocessed) bran has 40% fiber content and is the most concentrated form of fiber available. Wheat bran is a natural substance that is harmless to the body. Bran mixes with food residue in the colon, diluting the gut contents, facilitating evacuation, and speeding up colon transit time. Bran can also add bulk to stools that are too liquid.

The goal in using bran is to produce one bowel movement daily of soft, well-formed stool. Clinical trials on the efficacy of bran specifically using a "special bran recipe" have been performed on people with chronic constipation (Badiali et al., 1995; Behm, 1985; Smith & Newman, 1989). These studies used the combination of bran with applesauce and prune juice to regulate bowel function in nursing facility residents. Howard, West, and Ossip Klein (2000) reported an 80% reduction in total bowel medication use (laxative, suppository, or enema) in men living in nursing facilities who were placed on 4–5 tablespoons per day of a bran mixture. Unprocessed wheat bran is not the same as the commercial bran cereals that are widely advertised. Unprocessed wheat bran can be purchased very inexpensively at health food stores and local grocery stores. Bran may be added to cereal in the morning, mashed with bananas, or added to applesauce. Bran may also be added to soups, cottage cheese, ice cream, and puddings. Bran will not cause diarrhea, but, if bowel movements become too frequent, the individual should be instructed to decrease the amount (Behm, 1985).

Appendix A: Tips for Bowel Regularity can be used to explain to the individuals and caregivers how bran helps to promote bowel regularity. People should be instructed to begin using bran in small amounts, such as 1 tablespoon, and to gradually increase the amount over time. Use of bran can have side effects—flatulence, abdominal bloating, and cramps. However, by starting with small amounts and only gradually increasing the intake, the person can usually avoid any side effects. In any case, if side effects do occur, the adverse effects disappear in a few weeks. In nursing facilities, it is a good idea to team with the facility's dietary department to determine a "creative culinary solution" to getting residents to eat bran (Beverley & Travis, 1992). Some nursing facilities find it helpful to place the amount and administration time of the bran directly on the resident's medication card to ensure administration.

Promote Physical Activity

Physical activity in any form enhances colon peristalsis and motility. Walking for 15–20 minutes once or twice a day has been recommended as an aid to bowel motility, but even a small increase in physical activity has been shown to stimulate the bowel. Exercise together with abdominal massage can result in reduced fecal incontinence and a significant increase in the number of bowel movements. Chair or bed exercises, such as pelvic tilt, also help.

Establish a Routine Defecation Schedule

Improved bowel function can also be achieved by determining a timetable for bowel evacuation so that the person can take advantage of the "call to stool," or the urge to defecate. The schedule should be determined by the individual's bowel elimination pattern and previous timing of defecation. The person should be taught never to ignore the feeling that the bowel needs to be emptied. Also, the person must have adequate time to toilet.

Because the bowel is relatively quiet at night, the optimal time to schedule defecation is in the morning and after a meal, preferably breakfast. The gastrocolic reflex, or the mass propulsion of material through the large intestine, that occurs after a meal is strongest in the morning and on an empty stomach. The peristalsis created by this reflex propels feces to the descending colon and rectum. Normal defecation requires relaxation of the pelvic floor muscles, particularly the anal sphincter; adequate rectal tone; and sensation of rectal filling (Doughty, 1996). Normal sensation of rectal filling is key to providing motivation (a learned response), and underlines the cognitive component of normal defecatory function. This cognitive or behavioral component suggests that in some cases constipation may be a learned or conditioned response.

Heeding the urge to have a bowel movement and allowing sufficient time for undisturbed visits to the bathroom is especially important for residents in a nursing facility who need assistance to toilet. If a regular toileting time is not set aside for residents to empty their bowels, they will have fecal incontinence "accidents." Attention should be paid to body alignment; placing the feet on a footstool and thrusting the body slightly forward will promote complete evacuation and decrease straining. Massaging the abdomen can induce an increase in peristalsis and stimulate the gastrocolic reflex (Resende, Brocklehurst, & O'Neill, 1993). A bedridden person, whether living at home or in a nursing facility, may need to use a bedpan. If the resident is unable to sit, he or she should be positioned on the left side. However, attempting to defecate in a bedpan is very difficult for most people because this position causes undue strain. It forces the extension of legs, pushes the stomach (abdomen) out, and does not allow the pelvic muscles to aid in defecation. The caregiver should try to avoid using a bedpan if at all possible.

External Stimulation

If the individual is unable to defecate, some form of external stimulation should be considered because some people may need stimulation to initiate defecation. There are two types of external stimulation: use of a suppository and digital stimulation. *Suppositories* can be used to stimulate defecation until a pattern of regular defecation of soft, formed stools is established (Venn, Taft, Carpentier, & Applebaugh, 1992). The two most commonly used are glycerine and bisacodyl. To be successful, the suppository must be placed against the rectal wall and not into the actual stool.

Digital stimulation is commonly used in rehabilitation centers. Digital stimulation involves inserting a gloved, lubricated finger just inside the anus. Movement of the finger in a circular motion for 1–2 minutes will stimulate the rectum to contract. When the internal anal sphincter relaxes, the stimulation is stopped. Digital stimulation of the rectum can be performed as long as it does not cause the person pain and discomfort, or is not contraindicated by his or her condition. However, digital stimulation may not be acceptable to the caregiver and the individual.

Pelvic Muscle Rehabilitation Using Biofeedback Therapy

Pelvic muscle exercises, which involve tightening the pelvic floor muscles, are also very useful for learning to tighten the anal sphincter. This treatment modality is an established means of treating people with UI and other types of pelvic floor dysfunction. Biofeedback has been shown to be an effective treatment for fecal incontinence, with overall efficacy of 92% and, in individuals with constipation, an efficacy of 80% (Ko et al., 1997; Patankar, Ferrara, Levy, Williamson, & Perozo, 1997). The goals of biofeedback therapy are to improve the strength of the anal sphincter, improve the coordination between the rectum and the anal sphincter, and improve the sensory awareness for stool perception. A biofeedback-directed pelvic floor muscle rehabilitation program consists of instruction to the person regarding retraining of the pelvic floor muscles. In those individuals with constipation, "constipation exercises" (i.e., learning the "bearing down" maneuver) are taught. Usually a program consists of a biofeedback session displaying electromyographic activity of the pelvic floor muscles; education as to proper bowel diet, elimination regimen, and pelvic floor physiological function; and instruction in techniques to retrain these functions.

Use of Medications

In many cases, medications are prescribed to complement other strategies such as increased fluid and physical activity, addition of bran, and behavioral strategies. Bulk-forming laxatives have few side effects and minimal systemic effects. Bulk-forming agents have properties similar to those of dietary fiber. Table 5.2 lists common medications used to treat constipation.

Devices for Stool Collection

Figure 5.5 shows a fecal containment device that can be used with individuals with high-volume liquid diarrhea and fecal incontinence. This may be the best management option for people with incontinence resulting from prolonged immobility or other chronic neurological causes. When properly applied, these devices can reduce the risk of skin breakdown secondary to *Escherichia coli*. The least invasive product is the external perianal pouch. This is a drainable pouch that is attached to the skin using a synthetic, adhesive skin barrier. Application of the perianal pouch is similar to application of an ostomy pouch. The skin should be clean and dry. To prevent skin breakdown, a pectin-based powder (Stomahesive) is applied, followed by a plasticizing agent (skin prep). Once the opening to the pouch is sized relative to the anal opening, the pouch is pressed into place. The pouch spout can be clamped or connected to a drainage bag. The pouch will usually need to be changed every 2 days.

Table 5.2.   Common medications used for constipation and fecal incontinence

Type of bowel product	Action	Side effects
Fiber or bulk-forming agents Bran, psyllium (Metamucil), calcium polycarbophil (FiberCon), methylcellulose (Citrucel)	Safest laxatives but can interfere with absorption of some drugs. Increase fecal bulk while increasing colon motility and transit time. Should be taken with water because these agents absorb water in the intestine to make stool softer. Take 12 hours to 3 days to achieve effect.	Gas, bloating, bowel obstruction if not taken with enough water
Stool softeners Docusate sodium (Colace), docusate calcium (Surfak)	Cause absorption of water and fat. Provide moisture to the stool and prevent excessive loss of water. Used primarily to prevent constipation. Effective within 12–72 hours to produce a firm, semisolid stool. Recommended for situation where straining should be avoided.	Nausea, bitter taste Do not use with mineral oil.
Osmolar agents Lactulose (Chronulac), sorbitol	Metabolized by colonic bacteria. Cause increased retention of fluid and increased peristalsis by the colon. Take 24–48 hours to achieve effect.	Electrolyte imbalances, excessive gas, diarrhea, dehydration, hypermagnesemia, hypocalcemia, and hypophosphatemia in people with chronic renal failure; may be unpalatably sweet for certain individuals
Lubricants Mineral oil	Lubricate or soften the stool, allowing it to slip through the intestine more easily. Effects usually noted within 6–8 hours.	Can decrease reabsorption of vitamins A, D, E, and K if used long term
Saline cathartics Magnesium hydroxide (Phillips' Milk of Magnesia), magnesium citrate	Cause water to remain in the intestine for easier movement of stool. Produce watery stool in 1–3 hours.	Prolonged use can cause electrolyte and fluid imbalance.
Stimulants or irritants (cathartics) Anthraquinones (Senakot/Pericolace), bisacodyl (Dulcolax), phenolphthalein (Correctol, Ex-Lax)	Cause rhythmic muscular contractions in the intestines and increase fluid secretions. Should not be used daily or long term because they can damage bowel and cause electrolyte imbalance with continual use. Effects are usually noted within 6–12 hours.	Dermatitis, electrolyte imbalance, diarrhea, dehydration Avoid concomitant administration of antacids and pH-lowering agents, causes discoloration of gas

(continued)

Table 5.2.   *(continued)*

Type of bowel product	Action	Side effects
Suppositories Oil, glycerine, bisacodyl (Dulcolax)	Stimulate the defecation reflex and assist the rectum to empty any stool contents. Bisacodyl stimulates peristalsis by activating parasympathetic pathways. Glycerine works through lubrication and local stimulant effects. Work within 15 minutes.	Dehydration, electrolyte imbalance
Enemas Soap and tap water, saline, sodium phosphate (FLEET), milk and molasses, mini-enemas (Thera-vac)	Fluid instilled into the rectum to soften stool and to aid in removal. Must be retained for 10 minutes to work.	Dehydration, hypocalcemia, and hypophosphatemia in people with chronic renal failure

Surgery

Surgical procedures are usually reserved for people with fecal incontinence and include anal sphincter repair or replacement and fecal diversion (Jensen,

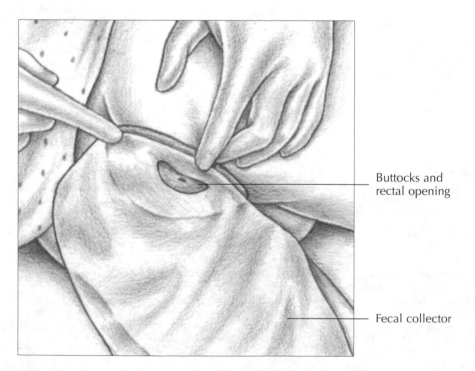

Buttocks and
rectal opening

Fecal collector

Figure 5.5.   Fecal collection device. (Courtesy of Hollister)

2000a). However, in older people, surgical intervention may worsen existing symptoms. In addition, surgery for constipation is not very successful.

REFERENCES

Badiali, D., Corazziari, E., Habib, F.I., Tomei, E., Bausano, G., Magrini, P., Anzini, F., & Torsoli, A. (1995). Effect of wheat bran in treatment of chronic nonorganic constipation—a double-blinded controlled trial. *Digestive Diseases and Sciences, 40*(2), 349–356.

Behm, R.M. (1985). A special recipe to banish constipation. *Geriatric Nursing, 6*(4), 216–217.

Benton, J.M., O'Harra, P.A., Chen, H., Harper, D.W., & Johnston, S.F. (1997). Changing bowel hygiene practice successfully: A program to reduce laxative use in a chronic care hospital. *Geriatric Nursing, 18*(1), 12–17.

Beverley, L., & Travis, I. (1992). Constipation—proposed natural laxative mixtures. *Journal of Gerontological Nursing, 18*(10), 5–12.

Chassagne, P., Landrin, I., Neveu, C., Czernichow, P., Bouaniche, M., Doucet, J., Denis, P., & Bercoff, E. (1999). Fecal incontinence in the institutionalized elderly: Incidence, risk factors, and prognosis. *American Journal of Medicine, 106*, 185–190.

Chiang L., Ouslander J., Schnelle J., & Reuben, D. (2000). Dually incontinent nursing home residents: Clinical characteristics and treatment differences. *Journal of the American Geriatrics Society, 48*(6), 673–676.

Doughty, D. (1996). Physiologic approach to bowel training. *Journal of Wound Ostomy Continence Nursing, 23*(1), 46–56.

Heaton, K.W., Radvan, J., Cripps, H., Mountford, R.A., Braddon, F.E.M., & Hughes, A.O. (1992). Defaecation frequency, timing, and stool form in the general population: A prospective study. *Gut, 33*, 818–824.

Hinrichs, M., & Huseboe, J. (2001, February). Research-based protocol: Management of constipation. *Journal of Gerontological Nursing*, 17–28.

Howard, L.V., West, D., & Ossip Klein, D.J. (2000). Chronic constipation management for institutionalized older adults. *Geriatric Nursing, 21*(2), 78–82.

Jackson, S., Weber, A., Hull, A.T., Mitchinson, A., & Walters, M. (1997). Fecal incontinence in women with urinary incontinence and pelvic organ prolapse. *Obstetrics and Gynecology, 89*(3), 423–427.

Jensen, L. (1997). Fecal incontinence: Evaluation and treatment. *Journal of Wound Ostomy Continence Nursing, 24*(5), 277–282.

Jensen, L.L. (2000a). Assessing and treating patients with complex fecal incontinence. *Ostomy/Wound Management, 46*(12), 56–60.

Jensen, L.L. (2000b). Assessment and management of patients with bowel dysfunction and fecal incontinence. In D. Doughty (Ed.), *Urinary and fecal incontinence: Nursing management* (pp. 325–383). St. Louis: C.V. Mosby.

Johanson, J.F. (1998). Geographic distribution of constipation in the United States. *American Journal of Gastroenterology, 93*(2), 188–191.

Johanson, J.F., Irizarry, F., & Doughty, A. (1997). Risk factors for fecal incontinence in a nursing home population. *Journal of Clinical Gastroenterology, 24*(3), 156–160.

Ko, C.Y., Tong, J., Lehman, R.E., Shelton, A.A., Schrock, T.R., & Welton, M.L. (1997). Biofeedback is effective therapy for fecal incontinence and constipation. *Archives of Surgery, 132*, 829–834.

Kumar, D., Bartolo, D.C.C., Devroede, G., Kamm, M.A., Keighley, M.R.B., Kuijpers, J.H., Lubowski, D.Z., Nicholls, R.J., Pemberton, J.H., & Read, N.W., et al. (1992). Symposium on constipation. *International Journal of Colorectal Disease, 7*, 47–67.

Nelson, R., Furner, S., & Jesudason, V. (1998). Fecal incontinence in Wisconsin nursing homes: Prevalence and associations. *Diseases of the Colon and Rectum, 41*(10), 1226–1229.

Nelson, R., Norton, N., Cautley, E., & Furner, S. (1995). Community-based prevalence of anal incontinence. *Journal of the American Medical Association, 274*(7), 559–561.

Patankar, S.K., Ferrara, A., Levy, J.R., Williamson, P.R., & Perozo, S.E. (1997). Biofeedback in colorectal practice: A multicenter statewide, three-year experience. *Diseases of the Colon and Rectum, 40,* 827–831.

Poulton, B., & Thomas, S. (1999). The nursing cost of constipation. *Primary Health Care, 9*(9), 17–20.

Resende, T.L., Brocklehurst, J.C., & O'Neill, P.A. (1993). A pilot study on the effect of exercise and abdominal massage on bowel habit in continuing care patients. *Clinical Rehabilitation, 7,* 204–209.

Resnick, B. (2001). Constipation. In A.M. Adelman, & M.P. Daly (Eds.), *20 Common Problems in Geriatrics* (pp. 311–335). New York: McGraw-Hill.

Sanburg, A.L., McGuire, T.M., & Lee, T. (1996). Stepping out of constipation: An educational campaign. *Australian Journal of Hospital Pharmacy, 26*(3), 350–355.

Smith, D.A., & Newman, D.K. (1989). The bran solution. *Contemporary Long Term Care, 12,* 66.

Venn, M.R., Taft, L., Carpentier, B., & Applebaugh, G. (1992). The influence of timing and suppository use on efficiency and effectiveness of bowel training after stroke. *Rehabilitation Nursing, 17*(3), 116–120.

6

Clinical Assessment and Evaluation

Careful assessment and identification of the cause(s) of urinary incontinence (UI) are essential first steps for appropriate and successful interventions. Despite a person's current age, age at onset of UI, length of time incontinent, and medical condition, he or she should receive an evaluation. Treatment decisions should be based on a diagnosis made after a reasonably thorough evaluation of genitourinary anatomy and physiology of bladder storage and emptying. Physical and mental status, expectations for treatment outcomes, motivation, and environmental barriers are important determinants of interventions. The basic evaluation of UI should incorporate recommendations outlined in the Agency for Healthcare Research and Quality (AHRQ; formerly the Agency for Health Care Policy and Research [AHCPR]) Clinical Practice Guidelines on Urinary Incontinence in Adults (Fantl et al., 1996).

The baseline evaluation of UI in nursing home residents is detailed in the Resident Assessment Program (RAP) and is supported by recommendations from the AHRQ and the American Medical Directors Association (1996) guidelines. Nursing facilities have a federal mandate to conduct a comprehensive assessment and screening of residents on admission and again quarterly during their stay. If the resident is incontinent or has an indwelling catheter, further assessment must be performed. Any change or decline in the resident's status also triggers an assessment. The RAP is considered to reflect the critical components of problem solving, care plan development, and treatment decisions in the provisions of comprehensive care and improvement of quality of life for the resident (Newman, 1998). The RAP includes evaluation for reversible/transient factors that may cause UI, such as a urinary tract infection (UTI), environmental factors, certain medical conditions, and medications, as outlined in Chapter 4. It focuses on people whose incontinence is persistent and chronic rather than transient. Nursing facility staff must uncover the cause and types of chronic UI and bladder dysfunction experienced by the resident. The components of the RAP for UI include situational factors, medical conditions, cause of transient incontinence, medications, abnormal laboratory values, cancer, and spinal cord lesions. A physician (e.g., primary care, internist, urologist, geriatrician, gynecologist) and nurse (nurse practitioner, clinical specialist, or registered nurse) can perform an evaluation for UI as part of an interdisciplinary team (Maloney & Cafiero, 1999). In the nursing facility and home care settings, the evaluation can be performed at the bedside.

CLINICAL ASSESSMENT

Incontinence can be the result of any dysfunction in the lower urinary tract or nervous system, or lack of coordination between the systems; cognitive and functional impairments; lack of motivation; or barriers in the environment. The assessment for identifying the problem or risk for incontinence problems should include a detailed history and physical examination, as well as mental, functional, and environmental components (Newman & Palmer, 1999). The checklist found in Figure 6.1 could be used when assessing the individual. Evaluation of bladder function begins with a good history. Generally, keeping a Bladder and Bowel Record (available in Appendix B) for 3 days of incontinence episodes and voiding times identifies the individual's pattern. If the person is able to perform this function, that is preferred; however, the caregiver or long-term care (LTC) staff may need to assist or complete the record.

Defining continence status can be helpful when performing an evaluation of the individual's UI. The following classification system (Fonda, 1990) was developed to understand the prevalence of incontinence in nursing facilities in Australia:

Independent continence—the person is able to maintain continence without assistance. He or she is aware of the urge sensation and can toilet independently, and is a candidate for retraining techniques to aid in self-toileting.

Dependent continence—the person has physical or mental impairment and is kept dry through the efforts of others. Caring for the person with dependent continence is a high labor cost for the LTC and home setting because staff or caregivers are needed to provide assistance with toileting.

Social continence—the person is incapable of maintaining continence independently or through assistance with regular toileting by caregivers and depends on absorbent products and other measures to contain urine leakage. This is probably the fastest growing group of people with UI—older, frailer, and more functionally and cognitively dependent. Currently, the use of absorbent products is the first choice for management of social continence in this population.

Palmer (1996) has added a new category to this classification system:

Partial continence—the person has the potential for improving or maintaining dryness levels but is unable to attain total continence. These individuals may use a combination of a scheduled toileting program and management of the urine leakage with devices or products.

History

Antecedents (e.g., observations by caregiver/long term care [LTC] staff)—when incontinence started, relationship to activities, what time of day incontinence occurs

Symptoms (e.g., urgency, frequency, nocturia, straining, hesitancy, dysuria, episodes of leakage)

Onset of the bladder dysfunction, length of time person has had problem with urinary incontinence (UI), urinary tract infection (UTI), or urinary retention

Awareness of need to urinate:
- ○ Is person aware of urge sensation?
- ○ When the bladder feels full or when there is an urge to go, how soon after the urge occurs does the urine start to flow?

Urine leakage:
- ○ When does the leakage occur: with standing (changing position), coughing, sneezing or laughing, or on the way to the bathroom?
- ○ How frequently does it occur: every time, sometimes, daily, once or twice a week?
- ○ How bad is it? Is the person using something to contain urine (tissues, pads, adult briefs)? How often do these products need to be changed per day?

Characteristics of the urinary stream:
Ask the person to describe or observe the following:
- ○ Character of the stream: when and how it starts once the person tries to initiate it
- ○ Whether the stream goes continuously or starts and stops
- ○ Strength of the stream
- ○ Whether straining (bearing down) is needed to get the urine out
- ○ If there is pain or discomfort (e.g., grimacing, wincing, moaning) with urination
- ○ Presence of postvoid dribbling

Initiation of urination:
- ○ Once on the toilet, can the person initiate the stream within one minute?
- ○ Does it take coaxing (e.g., running water or other triggers)?
- ○ What is the number of times that the individual actually urinates when on the toilet?

Emptying of the bladder:
- ○ Does the bladder feel completely empty once voiding is completed?

Characteristics of urine:
- ○ Color
- ○ Odor
- ○ Presence of sediment or mucus

Assessment of all acute/transient causes that can be reversed.

Identification of all primary and secondary medical problems to determine impact on lower urinary tract system.

Mental status:
- ○ Motivated to self-toilet and regain continence?
- ○ Cognition intact—alert enough to recognize bladder fullness (urge sensation)?
- ○ Can identify location of toileting facility (bathroom)?

Bowel history:
- ○ Systems of constipation, diarrhea, fecal incontinence, abdominal bloating
- ○ Type of laxatives used in the past—stool softeners, suppositories, enemas
- ○ Has the person had a previous problem with fecal incontinence and intervention?

(continued)

Figure 6.1. Genitourinary Assessment and Evaluation Form. (From Newman, D.K. [1998]. *Progress: Bladder and bowel rehabilitation program instructor's manual.* Eddystone, PA: SCA Hygiene Products; and Newman, D.K., & Palmer, M.H. [1999]. Incontinence and PPS: A new era. *Ostomy/Wound Management, 45(12),* 32–38, 40–44, 46, 48–49; adapted by permission.)

Figure 6.1.   *(continued)*

Observation of toileting process:
- ○ Is "toilet mapping" behavior present (person only frequents places where location of toilet is known in advance)?
- ○ Does the peson have the ability to suppress the urge long enough for caregiver/long term care staff to arrive and offer toileting?
- ○ What is the distance from the bed/chair to the bathroom/toilet?
- ○ Does the person have the ability to self-toilet with minimal assistance?
- ○ If caregiver/LTC staff offer and assist with toileting, does voiding occur (positive response to a prompt to void)?
- ○ Does the person use a device such as a bedside commode or urinal?
- ○ Does the person use an absorbant product, and is he or she able to remove the product to self-toilet?

Diet/fluid intake:
- ○ Are signs of dehydration present during physical examination (e.g., dry skin, poor skin turgor, dry mouth)?
- ○ What is the total fluid intake in a 24-hour period?
- ○ How much caffeinated beverages and food are ingested?

Relationship of incontinence to medical diagnoses:
- ○ History of bowel dysfunction?
- ○ Presense of diabetes, congestive heart failure, arthritis?
- ○ Neurological diseases (Pakinson's disease, multiple sclerosis [MS])?
- ○ Prostate problems in men (cancer or benign prostatic hyperplasia [BPH])?
- ○ History of chronic UTIs?
- ○ Psychiatric disorder?

Medications prescribed that may affect bladder function:
- ○ Psychotropic drugs—can accumulate in elderly people and cause sedation, confusion, and immobility resulting in functional incontinence?
- ○ Anticholingerics—cause urinary retention, urinary frequency, and overflow incontinence?
- ○ Calcium channel blockers—reduce smooth muscle contractility, causing urinary retention and overflow incontinence?
- ○ Rapidly acting diuretics (e.g., furosemide)—can overwhelm the bladder with rapidly produced urine, resulting in frequency and urgency?
- ○ Alpha-antagonists (common ingredient in cold preparations)—relax the sphincters to cause stress incontinence and urinary retention in men?
- ○ Neurological diseases (Parkinson's disease, MS)?

Physical examination

Abdominal examination:
- ○ Are bowel sounds present?
- ○ Are any masses present in abdomen?
- ○ Does the person complain of abdominal or suprapubic tenderness, discomfort, or fullness?

Genitalia examination:
- ○ Are dryness, redness, and thinning present on perineal and gluteal skin?
- ○ In men, what is the condition of foreskin, glans, scrotum, and testes?

Pelvic examination (women):
- ○ Are dryness, redness, and thinning present on mucosa (indicates atrophic vaginitis)?
- ○ Are structural abnormalities present, such as pelvic organ prolapse?
- ○ Can pelvic muscle strength be assessed?

Rectal examination:
- ○ Is fecal impaction present?
- ○ Assess the feel of rectal tone.
- ○ In men, determine size of prostate.

Neurological examination:
- ○ Difficulty walking?
- ○ Abnormal gait?
- ○ Presence or absence of reflexes?

Urinalysis results:
- ○ Are infection, red blood cells, bacteriuria, and glucose present?
- ○ Is there a need to send the urine for a culture?

Postvoid residual (PVR) urine:
- ○ Determine residual urine volume within 15–20 minutes after the person has voided.
- ○ Risk factors: suprapubic distention or tenderness, male sex, diabetes, anticholinergic drugs that interfere with bladder emptying, neurological disease
- ○ Method (straight catheterization or ultrasound [preferred])
- ○ Normal <50 ml
- ○ Abnormal >200 ml
- ○ If volume is between 50 and 200 ml, monitor PVR volumes on several occasions to determine clinical significance.
- ○ Does the person need a referral to a urologist?

Urdymanics tests:
- ○ Determine bladder capacity (may be done by having person drink water and scanning bladder at initial urge sensation).
- ○ Is the person a candidate for more bladder function tests? (should be considered for individuals with repeated UTIs that cannot be cleared and for continual urinary retention)

Bladder and bowel diary—objective information

Caregiver/LTC staff or individual keeps a diary for 3 days.
- ○ Determine the patterns during the day and during the night as well as frequency of urination.

Monitor intake and output for a minimum of 2 days. This can be accomplished using a bladder volume instrument such as BladderScan.

Functional and environmental assessment

Mobility:
- ○ How is toileting accomplished?
- ○ Would devices such as a bedside commode or urinal be helpful?
- ○ Can a person who uses a wheelchair propel the chair to the toilet in a timely fashion?
- ○ Are restraints, physical or chemical, being used that are causing UI? Physical restraints can include various straps and ties, as well as "geri-chairs." Sedating drugs can act as chemical restraints.
- ○ Is equipment that can enhance mobility (e.g., cane, walker, wheelchair) available?

Environment:
- ○ Can improved access to toilet lessen UI?
- ○ Is there poor color contrast in the bathroom, such as a white toilet and seat and light-colored floors and walls?
- ○ Are toilets at least 17 inches high with arms to assist the person in lowering or rising?
- ○ Does poor design of bathroom facilities interfere with use of walker or wheelchair and transfer to the toilet?
- ○ Are chairs designed for ease of rising?
- ○ Are grab bars available within the person's reach when toileting?

Functional Assessment

An assessment of the person's functional abilities should focus on self-care tasks or activities of daily living (ADLs), for example, the ability to ambulate, transfer to the toilet, disrobe, and use any necessary assistive devices (Jirovec,

1991). The individual should be assessed for the ability to perform more instrumental ADLs (e.g., cooking, shopping, driving, attending senior center activities). The person also should be rated on his or her level of dependence, according to the following classifications:

1.   Able to do the task without human assistance

2.   Able to perform the task with some assistance

3.   Unable to perform the task even with assistance

The use of chemical or physical restraints causes decreased mobility and contributes to UI. In nursing facilities, UI is partially iatrogenic in nature and is related to the atrophy of motor skills such as walking; therefore, nursing interventions need to enhance mobility skills. Difficulty ambulating increases the time required to reach the toilet, contributing to the severity of UI (Engberg et al., 1997). Slow ambulation has the potential to affect interventions such as prompted voiding and bladder retraining.

Direct observation of toileting will yield critical information that can direct interventions. Observing toileting skills can be accomplished using POTTI (performance on timed toileting instrument; Palmer, 1996). Ouslander et al. (1987) developed this instrument for use with residents in LTC. The instrument consists of five tasks that simulate toileting. They include ability to walk or move 15 feet, transfer to a toilet, unfasten hooks or snaps, unzip a zipper, and pull down a garment/pants.

Environmental Barriers

The following factors should be considered when performing an assessment of the individual's environment:

- *Change in living:* A change in continence status may occur if a person has changed rooms or has a new roommate.

- *Nighttime hours:* Nighttime UI can occur if the bed is too high, the bathroom is inaccessible, or the individual is fearful of falling. Falling while attempting to meet elimination needs is a serious problem in the older adult. People who have mobility or balance problems may be unable to suppress a strong urge to urinate until a caregiver arrives to help them with toileting. If they are independent, they may be unable to walk or propel themselves to the toilet in time when using a wheelchair or walker.

- *Clothing:* Clothing that is difficult to remove can contribute to the development of UI. Often sweatpants without underwear or the use of fabric that is fastened by Velcro rather than buttons and zippers can be very helpful in these cases.

- *Visual cues:* Inability to recognize the toilet (visual agnosia) is a frustrating situation for an individual. Visual cues such as a picture of a toilet on the bathroom door or of a man standing and voiding into a toilet might aid people with visual agnosia in identifying the proper location and use of the toilet. Also, painting the bathroom door a bright, eye-catching color that is different from the color of other doors may be helpful for some people with dementia.

- *Bathrooms:* Adequacy and availability of bathroom facilities and presence of toileting aids such as bedside commodes or urinals are important in promoting continence. In addition, the bathroom should be assessed for ease of toileting. The bathroom is considered the most hazardous room with respect to the chance of an older person falling. Size and layout of bathrooms are of paramount importance. Many older people who reside in metropolitan areas live in houses where the bathroom is on a different floor than where the person spends the majority of the day. Construction of a bathroom on the main living floor will promote continence. The bathroom should have good lighting. The bathroom mirror can be covered if individuals with cognitive impairment become confused and agitated when looking in the mirror.

- *Furniture:* Chairs with good back support, with a seat height of at least 19 inches, allow people to get to their feet more independently, quickly, and easily.

In the LTC setting, bathrooms may be adequate but residents may spend a large part of the day in public areas such as the dining room or in activities where access to and assistance in the bathroom is limited.

EVALUATION

The AHRQ clinical practice guideline recommends a history, physical examination, urinalysis, and determination of postvoid residual as part of the baseline evaluation to be performed before treatment can be instituted. Appendix B includes samples of medical record forms that have been used when completing a history and physical examination. These forms employ cue words because such a format results in higher levels of documentation than open-format forms (Palmer, McCormick, Langford, Langlois, & Alvaran, 1992).

Obtaining a History

The history should determine the characteristics of UI, noting the onset, duration, frequency, severity, and progression of incontinence and should assist in the differentiation of the cause and type of UI. It is important to include family members and caregivers when taking a history because they can add depth to the impact UI is having on the person's daily routine. Determining the symptom(s) most bothersome to the individual is especially important in guiding intervention and determining response. Precipitants of incontinence (e.g., situational antecedents, cough, previous pelvic surgery, injury, previous pelvic radiation therapy, trauma, new onset of diseases, new medications) and other lower urinary tract symptoms (e.g., nocturia, dysuria, hesitancy, poor or interrupted stream, straining, hematuria, suprapubic or perineal pain) are also an integral part of the history. The distinction among symptoms is important because this will determine treatment modalities.

Initially, the clinician should determine if the UI is of recent onset and may be caused by acute medical problems. These are discussed in Chapter 4 as transient causes of UI. If one of these problems is identified, treatment to correct the problem should be instituted. A current drug review will identify drug-related causes of UI. Medications that affect the lower urinary tract include diuretics, sedatives, hypnotics, analgesics, and antidepressants. Over-the-counter (OTC) drugs such as cold remedies can cause or contribute to UI.

The history should include a review of bowel function, fluid intake, and consumption of known bladder irritants. Chronic constipation can contribute to UI, and instituting a bowel regimen can improve incontinence (see Chapter 5). Determination of adequate fluid intake is an important component of the review of diet. It is also important to ask the person questions regarding sexual practices (e.g., urine leakage during intercourse, erectile dysfunction in men).

Bladder Record

Asking the person or caregiver to complete a Bladder Record, or a Bladder Diary, for 3–5 days is an essential component of the evaluation of UI. Often eliciting examples of incontinence episodes helps to objectively diagnose the type of incontinence. The recording of this information by the person can itself be an important intervention. A person may recognize the cause by the pattern of urinary accidents. These written records track the frequency, timing, and number of incontinence episodes. Data are usually collected in 24-hour intervals, with these periods further segmented into smaller time blocks to determine the frequency of diurnal and nocturnal voiding. Assessment of the person's voiding pattern and frequency of UI is a way of pinpointing antecedents and behaviors associated with urinary symptoms. If more than six episodes of voiding per day are noted, teaching the individual bladder training will improve this situation. The person, the caregiver, or both will need to estimate the volume of leakage during incontinence episodes. The following description of urine leakage can be used:

- Small volume: less than 30 milliliters (ml)—or enough to make underwear wet if no protective pad is worn

- Moderate volume: 31–60 ml—enough to wet or soak underwear and leak down the legs if no protective pad is worn

- Large volume: 61 ml or greater—soaks through clothing and onto floor or furniture and usually is the entire bladder volume

Because fluid intake and type of liquid consumed can be contributing factors to incontinence, most bladder records request that the person list daily intake, noting type and amount. Some records include measurement of voided volume (using a Frequency Volume Chart, see Appendix B) to determine an approximation of bladder capacity. The volume of voided urine is an important measure to determine functional and maximal bladder capacity, and daily and nocturnal urine volumes. By documenting each episode of incontinence, this bladder record can be used later to measure effectiveness of interventions.

In the LTC setting, the determination of a resident's voiding pattern and frequency of incontinence can assist staff in identifying interventions (e.g., identifying a voiding pattern for prompting voiding). In most facilities, this is accomplished through the use of a Bladder and Bowel Record (see Appendix B). To complete this record accurately, staff must check the resident hourly to determine wet or dry status. However, this method is cumbersome, has many inaccuracies, and usually lacks staff compliance. New technology that includes moisture detection devices and bladder volume instruments may prove to be more accurate in reporting, documenting, and tracking incontinence and voiding status automatically (Colling, Ouslander, Hadley, Eisch, & Campbell, 1992; Woolridge, 2000).

General Physical Examination

A general examination should be performed to detect conditions such as lower extremity edema that may contribute to increased renal perfusion in recumbent individuals, causing nocturia and enuresis; to detect neurological abnormalities that may suggest multiple sclerosis, stroke, spinal cord compression, or other neurological conditions; and to assess mobility, cognition, and manual dexterity related to toileting skills among frail older adults and those with functional impairments.

Abdominal Examination

The abdominal exam is best carried out with the person in the supine position. The exam is performed to detect the presence of bowel sounds, ascites (accumulation of fluid in the membrane lining of the abdomen), organomegaly (abnormal enlargement of organs), and the presence of surgical incisions, lower abdominal masses, and suprapubic bladder fullness or tenderness, which can influence intra-abdominal pressure and urinary tract function. It is generally possible to palpate or percuss the bladder above the level of the symphysis pubis if it contains 150 ml or more of urine. The finding of a palpable bladder may indicate incomplete bladder emptying or urinary retention.

Genitalia—Women

Pelvic Examination   All women who present with UI or related conditions should have a pelvic examination (with or without a speculum). Women should empty their bladders prior to the pelvic examination. A comprehensive examination is performed to determine the presence of atrophic tissue changes; pelvic organ prolapse; and perineal skin condition, color, and structural abnormalities. The examiner may use a mirror to demonstrate the findings to the woman. A pelvic exam is often deferred in older women, especially those who reside in a nursing facility. Reasons for not performing the exam include discomfort associated with atrophic vaginitis, patient and physician embarrassment with the examination, procedural difficulty because of the need for assistance with confused individuals, and time constraints of the physician. A bimanual, speculum exam is optimal, but, in older frail women, a digital exam may be more feasible. The urinary meatus should be identified, and its position and size should be noted. An erythematous, tender lesion arising from the meatus may represent a benign urethral *caruncle* or possible urethral carcinoma.

Inspection of the vagina and perineum can determine if the tissues are atrophic and estrogen deficient. Because the urethra and trigone are estrogen-dependent tissues, estrogen deficiency can contribute to UI and OAB (Batra & Losif, 1983). This assessment may reveal a pale, thin, shining, and poorly vascularized vaginal mucosa, indicating atrophy (atrophic vaginitis and urogenital atrophy). Atrophic vaginitis affects up to 40% of postmenopausal women. Symptoms of urogenital atrophy include both vaginal symptoms (burning/soreness, malodorous discharge, dryness, dyspareunia, itching) and urinary symptoms (frequency, urgency, dysuria, UI, nocturia, recurrent UTIs). Vaginal mucosa has a high density of estrogen receptors that respond to estrogen stimulation. The vaginal introitus (entrance to the vagina) will become less pliable and narrower (called vaginal stenosis) with estrogen deficiency. The presence of a urethral caruncle, which appears as an erythematous mass within the external urethral meatus, may also signify estrogen deficiency. The appearance of vaginal secretions may suggest a vaginal infection; urine within the vagina suggests a genitourinary fistula.

Testing of the vaginal pH serves as an accurate indicator of the state of the vaginal mucosa (Maloney & Oliver, 2001). A vaginal pH of 7 is considered neutral—an unrelated change. An alkaline environment (pH > 7) correlates with atrophic symptoms and hypoestrogenism. An acidic environment is a pH < 7. Vaginal pH can be tested using an indicator tape (Baxter diagnostic tape), which is placed inside the vagina past the *introitus*. In women with recurrent UTIs the vaginal pH is considerably higher (pH > 7) and warrants the use of topical estrogen cream. If the pH can be reduced through the use of estrogen, clinical improvement can be seen. For women who cannot use topical estrogen, OTC products (e.g., Replens, other intravaginal gels) can gradually reduce the symptoms of urogenital atrophy.

Pelvic Floor Muscle Evaluation   A very important part of the physical examination in women is determination of the strength of the pelvic floor muscles. The pelvic floor muscles are made up of the levator ani group and include the pubococcygeus, puborectalis, and iliococcygeus muscles. The levator ani can be palpated just superior to the hymeneal ring. The external urethral and anal sphincters are in continuity with these muscles, and both receive pudendal nerve innervation. The pelvic floor muscles provide support to all pelvic organs. The loss of pelvic muscle tone and strength can lead to both stress and urge UI.

Pelvic floor muscle function can be qualitatively defined by the tone at rest and the strength of a voluntary or reflex contraction as strong, weak, or absent or by a grading system. A pelvic muscle contraction may be assessed by visual inspection, by palpation, electromyography (EMG), or perineometry. Factors to be assessed include strength, duration, and repeatability (Abrams et al., 2002). Pelvic floor muscle function can be qualitatively defined during rectal examination by the muscle tone at rest and the strength of a muscle's voluntary contraction as strong, weak, or absent.

Functional testing of pelvic floor muscle strength by digital examination is a reliable assessment (Brink et al., 1994; Kerschan-Schindl et al., 2002). The woman should be placed in the semi-supine position with the hips flexed at about 45 degrees and the knees flexed at about 120 degrees. The legs should be abducted with the soles of the feet in contact with each other. This will prevent adductor muscle contractor. Digital measurement of pelvic muscle strength can be done by inserting the index finger into the vagina to the level of the first knuckle. The woman is asked to contract the pelvic muscles around the examiner's fingers with as much force and for as long as she is able. The muscle should be palpated bilaterally at the 5 and 7 o'clock positions. It is important to realize that, when asked to contract the pelvic muscle, many women will either use the wrong muscle, strain down, perform a Valsalva maneuver, or fail to activate all layers of the pelvic musculature. Most women are largely unaware that the pelvic floor muscles exist, and simple instruction in technique may not be adequate preparation. The examiner should confirm through observation that the woman is not contracting accessory muscles such as gluteal, abdominal, and thigh muscles.

When the woman is contracting the pelvic muscles, three criteria of muscle strength should be noted: pressure, duration, and alteration in position (Brink et al., 1994). The amount of pressure or strength of the muscle contraction can range from imperceptible to a firm squeeze. Duration involves the number of seconds that the examiner feels the muscle contraction. The woman should be asked to prolong the duration of the contraction to better assess the slow twitch fibers because the external urethral sphincter is solely, and the levator ani muscle mainly, composed of these fibers. In women with a well-supported pelvic muscle group, the muscle contraction can lift the base of the examiner's fingers. The use of an assessment tool for documentation is advised; Figure 6.2 presents a scale for grading digital evaluation of pelvic mus-

Check one: Vaginal exam ☐   Rectal exam ☐

Circle one: 0/5   No contractions
              1/5   Trace contractions: less than 1 second
              2/5   Weak contraction: with or without posterior elevation of fingers,
                        held for greater than 1 second but less than or equal to 3 seconds
              3/5   Moderate contraction: with or without posterior elevation of fingers,
                        held at least 4–6 seconds, repeated 3 times
              4/5   Strong contraction: with posterior elevation of fingers, held for at least
                        7–9 seconds, repeated 4–5 times
              5/5   Unmistakably strong contraction: with posterior elevation of fingers,
                        held at least 10 seconds, repeated 4–5 times

Use of accessory muscle groups
            Abdominal   ☐ Yes   ☐ No
            Gluteal   ☐ Yes   ☐ No
            Thigh/abductor   ☐ Yes   ☐ No

Evaluation—muscle hypertonus/spasm

Circle one: 0   No pressure or pain associated with exam
              1   Comfortable pressure associated with exam
              2   Uncomfortable pressure associated with exam
              3   Moderate pain associated with exam, intensifies with contraction
              4   Severe pain associated with exam; patient unable to perform muscle
                     contraction because of pain

EMG evaluation   ☐ Yes   ☐ No

Results: _____

_____

_____

Figure 6.2.   Scale for grading digital evaluation of pelvic muscle strength.

cle strength. When using the scale, the examiner should note the type of exam performed. When the woman contracts the pelvic muscles around the examiner's finger; the pressure, duration of contraction; and whether contraction causes the finger to change position should be noted, as well as whether the woman made use of accessory muscles. If the woman has pelvic muscle spasms, the examiner should note the degree of spasm.

Assessment for Pelvic Organ Prolapse   The presence and extent of pelvic organ prolapse (POP) should be noted. POP is a condition unique to women, in which the pelvic organs (bladder, uterus, rectum) descend within the pelvis, destroy the vaginal wall, and in some cases pass outside the vagina, bulging through the introitus (Rovner, 2000). At least 50% of women who have had children will develop prolapse in their lifetimes. The prolapse is considered a type of hernia. Certain factors may increase the risk of prolapse:

- Childbirth

- Effects of menopause (a decrease in the hormone estrogen)

- Radical pelvic surgery or trauma

- Chronic increases in intra-abdominal pressure resulting from chronic cough, chronic constipation and straining for stool evacuation, obesity, or chronic lifting

- Intrinsic factors such as race (white women have a higher prevalence), anatomy, connective tissue, and neurological conditions

Mechanical breakdown in the system of pelvic supports and organs can lead to UI and overactive bladder (OAB). Prolapse is categorized as urethrocele, cystocele, uterine prolapse, vaginal vault prolapse, rectocele, and enterocele (Brubaker & Saclarides, 1996). These types of prolapse are defined as follows:

- Urethrocele—descent of the lower part of the urethra into the vagina

- Cystocele—descent or prolapse of the anterior vaginal wall with the bladder behind it

- Uterine prolapse—descent of the uterus and cervix into the vagina. Women with a cystocele or uterine prolapse may complain of urinary urgency and frequency, UI, urinary retention with grade 3 or 4 prolapse, vaginal dryness or irritation, pressure or a bulging feeling in the vagina or perineum, or feeling as though they are sitting on a tennis ball.

- Vaginal vault prolapse—in women who have had a hysterectomy, the walls of the vagina can fall in on themselves and out of the vagina. Complaints include pelvic and vaginal pressure, low back pain, bleeding, and irritation from prolapsed mucosa rubbing on clothes or absorbent perineal products.

- Rectocele—protrusion of the posterior vaginal wall with the rectum behind it. Complaints include pelvic and vaginal pressure, vaginal bulge or mass, laxity with intercourse, difficulty with bowel movements (digital evacuation), constipation, and fecal incontinence.

- Enterocele—bulging herniation of the top of the vagina and small bowel into the vagina

Assessment of the extent of prolapse should be made during a Valsalva maneuver (having the women cough or bear down as though she is having a bowel movement). Grades (or stages) of prolapse are as follows:

Grade 1—the prolapse bulges halfway down the opening of the vagina (see Figure 6.3)

Grade 2—the prolapse is at the opening of the vagina (see Figure 6.4)

Grade 3—the prolapse protrudes or falls out of the vagina (see Figure 6.5)

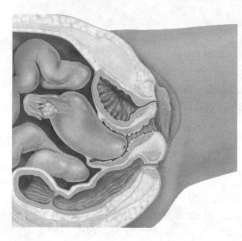

Figure 6.3.   Grade 1 uterine prolapse.
(Courtesy of Milex)

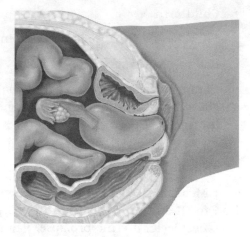

Figure 6.4.   Grade 2 uterine prolapse.
(Courtesy of Milex)

Grade 4—the vagina, with the vaginal vault and uterus, protrudes completely outside the body without a Valsalva maneuver (procidentia, the most severe form of prolapse; see Figure 6.6)

Childbirth, heavy lifting, chronic straining during bowel movements, and loss of estrogen may contribute to pelvic prolapse. As the population of American women ages, the prevalence of prolapse will rise. In prolapse cases, women may find that they have to empty their bladders more often or they may have unwanted urine leakage.

Genitalia—Men   Inspection of the penis will reveal obvious lesions of the skin and will define whether the man has been circumcised. The normal mea-

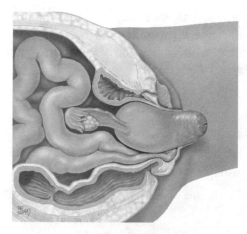

Figure 6.5.   Grade 3 uterine prolapse.
(Courtesy of Milex)

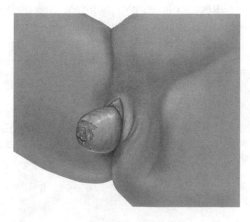

Figure 6.6.   Grade 4 uterine prolapse.
(Courtesy of Milex)

tus should be located at the top of the glans. In the uncircumcised man, the foreskin should be retracted and the glans and meatus should be assessed. Retracting the foreskin is a very important component of personal hygiene in the uncircumcised man. Once the foreskin is cleaned and dried, it should be replaced back over the glans to prevent *phimosis*. The normal meatus should be located at the tip of the glans. The scrotum should be assessed for lesions and size. The presence of an abnormal mass within the testes is best defined by careful palpation. The contents of each scrotal sac should be palpated in an orderly fashion. First, the testes should be examined; then, the epididymides. Next, the cord structures should be examined, and finally the area of the external inguinal ring should be checked for the presence of an inguinal hernia.

Anorectal Examination   A digital rectal examination (DRE) is performed in both men and women to assess for fecal impaction, to evaluate anal sphincter tone, and to rule out the presence of a tumor or mass. In men, assessment of the size, consistency, and contour of the prostate gland is determined. The normal prostate gland is walnut sized, with a flattened, heart-shaped configuration. A man with an abnormal or enlarged prostate is referred to a urologist. In men, assessment of the pelvic floor muscle can be performed by evaluating the anal sphincter contraction and tone. The individual should be instructed to perform a voluntary sphincter contraction by first relaxing and then contracting the anal sphincter and "bearing down" as if having a bowel movement. This will allow the clinician to assess the overall sphincter tone and the strength and symmetry of the sphincter and identify defects in the sphincter mechanism. The clinician should note any weakness in the pelvic floor, such as the presence of a rectocele or enterocele in women.

Neurological Examination

A focused neurological examination is divided into four parts: 1) mental status, 2) sensory function, 3) motor function, and 4) reflex integrity. Cognition is assessed by response to questions or through the use of a mental status exam. The Folstein Mini-Mental State examination is often used (Folstein, Folstein, & McHugh, 1975). Mental status examination should include assessment of mood, affect, orientation, speech pattern, memory, and comprehension. Cognitive status will determine if the person is a candidate for an educational retraining program (Jirovec & Wells, 1990).

A sensory function examination includes testing specific dermatomes (areas of the skin that are supplied by certain spinal nerves) for response to position, vibration, pinprick, light touch, and temperature. Relevant dermatomes include lumbosacral nerve roots L1 (innervates base of penis, upper scrotum, labia majora) and L1–2 (innervate midscrotum, labia minora) and sacral nerve roots S3–5 (innervate perineum and perianal skin) and S2–4 (innervate the striated muscles of the bladder and pelvic floor [external urethral and anal sphincter]). Tests used to evaluate the sacral nerve root reflexes include deep tendon reflexes, lower extremity strength, sharp/dull sensation, stimulation of the anal reflex (S2–5) and bulbocavernosus reflex (BCR). The test for the anal reflex involves lightly stroking the anus while observing for anal contraction—the anus should pucker or "wink." Absence of the anal wink in an older person is not pathological. The BCR refers specifically to the contraction of the bulbocavernosus muscle but is also used to test the innervation (S2–4) of all perineal striated muscles. To test the BCR, the examiner gently squeezes the glans penis in men or lightly taps the clitoris in women while observing for anal contraction. This should produce a reflex contraction of the external anal sphincter muscle. The BCR may be absent in up to 20% of neurologically normal women.

Because physical impairments have an impact on continence and UI treatments, the neurological exam should include an assessment of mobility. The person should be observed rising from a chair and walking. Watching the person manipulate clothing can assess fine motor skills and manual dexterity.

Urological Testing

The AHQR clinical practice guideline recommends basic tests that should be completed to identify bladder dysfunction. They include a urinalysis and determination of bladder emptying.

Urinalysis   A urinalysis is necessary to determine the presence of microorganisms, red blood cells, and glucose in the urine. Frequency, urgency, dysuria, lower abdominal or pelvic pain, nocturia, pyuria, UI, and low back pain are common symptoms suggestive of bacterial involvement of the lower urinary tract. In the nursing facility resident, symptoms of UI are often nonspecific and may include low-grade fever or change in temperature, increased confusion or delirium, worsening of incontinence, anorexia, and functional decline (Ouslander, Shapira, Schnelle, & Fingold, 1996).

Bacteriuria is common in nursing facility residents; its prevalence is 30%–50% among female residents. The accuracy of a rapid, enzyme-based screening test using a dipstick test for nitrate and leukocyte esterase has been demonstrated in nursing facility residents with UI (Ouslander, Schapira, Fingold, & Schnelle, 1995). This test can be performed easily by nursing facility staff. A urinalysis positive for leukocytes does not always require antibiotic treatment in older women. Gross, microscopic, and culture examinations of the urine may help distinguish between a noninfectious condition and an infectious agent. Colonization with more than 100,000 bacteria and symptoms of infection are the criteria for diagnosing a UTI. The infection should be treated before beginning UI therapy. The client with asymptomatic hematuria needs further tests to rule out the possibility of bladder cancer.

Specimens for testing are usually collected by a clean-catch midstream void. Ouslander, Shapira, and Schnelle (1995) found that having residents use a careful clean-catch technique yielded a comparable degree of accuracy compared with cultures obtained by catheterization from frail, incontinent female nursing facility residents. Therefore, most clinicians believe that nursing facility residents do not need to be catheterized to obtain a urine specimen for culture.

Postvoid Residual Urine Volume   Postvoid residual urine volume (PVR) determination should be performed on all clients to eliminate the possibility of urinary retention. Specific PVR measurement can be accomplished either by catheterization or by ultrasound within a few minutes of voiding (Newman & Smith, 1991). Portable ultrasound scanners are quick, easy to use, reasonable, sensitive, and very specific for determining elevated PVRs. Goode, Locher, Bryant, Roth, and Borgio (2000) compared portable ultrasound with catheterization in ambulatory women. They found the scanner to have a sensitivity of 66.7% and a specificity of 96.5% in detecting PVR ≥ 100ml. In acute care, LTC, and home care settings, the use of a BladderScan (Diagnostic Ultrasound Corporation, Bothell, WA) is the preferred method of obtaining a PVR (Colling, 1996; Ouslander et al., 1994; Wagner & Schmid, 1997). An ultrasound of the bladder with this instrument can be used as part of the evaluation of UI to determine PVR and as part of a bladder management program in residents with urinary retention (Newman, 2000).

It remains a point of contention whether all individuals presenting with symptoms of OAB require a PVR measurement prior to the initiation of treatment. It is desirable to measure the PVR in some individuals, particularly in older people with voiding symptoms, recurrent or persistent UTIs, or both; in those with neurological disease and voiding dysfunction; and in those with symptoms that suggest poor bladder emptying. There is also controversy regarding the amount of postvoid urine volume that should be considered abnormal. The normal range of residual urine is 50–60 ml; in people 65 years or older, a PVR of greater than 150–200 ml on at least two occasions is probably abnormal. Individuals who have abnormal volumes should be referred for further studies.

Pad Test   In certain cases, a client may be asked to save used perineal pads to be weighed to quantify urine loss. Appendix A: Pad Test contains an educational tool for clients.

Other Urological Tests   A cough test is a provocative test for stress UI. While standing, the person is asked to cough forcefully while the clinician observes for urine loss from the urethra. This test should be performed when the person's bladder is full, but not if the urge to void is present. If an instantaneous leakage occurs with cough, then stress UI is likely. If the leakage is not instantaneous, then other types of UI may be present. A cough test is very difficult to perform in people with cognitive and functional disabilities, and its usefulness in this population is questionable.

Individuals requiring further evaluation include those who meet the following criteria:

1. Uncertain diagnosis and inability to develop a reasonable management plan

2. Failure to respond to an adequate therapeutic trial

3. Hematuria without infection

4. The presence of comorbid conditions such as recurrent UTIs, difficult bladder emptying, severe POP, prostate nodule, and abnormal PVR

5. Consideration of surgical intervention

When diagnosis is uncertain or one of the above criteria is met, a series of tests called urodynamics may be indicated. *Urodynamics* are one or more of a series of tests that are designed to diagnose the cause of the person's symptom. Urodynamic tests are designed to determine the anatomic and functional status of the urinary bladder and urethra and are performed by qualified professional specialists. Numerous specialized diagnostic tests are available, and the evaluation must be tailored to the specific problem. These tests include cystoscopy, cystometrogram, uroflow, urethral pressure profile, voiding pressures, and electromygram.

MANAGEMENT OF PELVIC ORGAN PROLAPSE

Surgery can correct POP, especially a cystocele or uterine prolapse. However, standard treatment for prolapse is the use of a mechanical device called a pessary (device placed in the vagina to support the uterus). The word *pessary* can be found in both Greek and Latin literature. Some types of mechanical devices have been reported since the time of Hippocrates, who mentioned the use of fruit (a pomegranate) placed in the vagina to support a prolapse. Women report improved continence and ambulation with the use of a pessary; in addition, personal care is made easier and hygiene is improved. In the last few years, pessaries have become more widely used among older women. The use of pessaries may represent an alternative for frail older women who are not candidates for other therapies. Because this population frequently represents unlikely surgical candidates, a well-fitting pessary is often the preferred alternative.

Types of Pessaries

A pessary is a device made of silicone that looks like a contraceptive diaphragm, but the outside rim is hard (see Figure 6.7). The pessary rim's outside diameter is measured in inches. Current silicone pessaries are quite pliable and comfortable and come in a variety of sizes and shapes—round, cube, or "U" shaped:

*   *Ring (with and without support)*—useful in cases of grade 1 and 2 uterine prolapse and designed especially for uterine prolapse associated with a mild cystocele (see Figure 6.8). One of the most commonly and simplest to

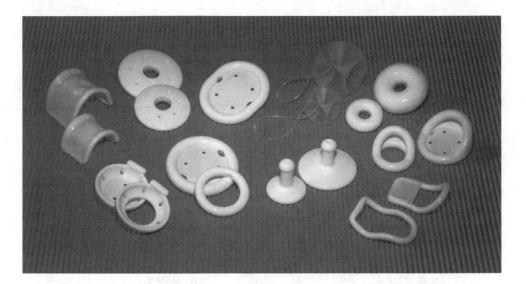

Figure 6.7.   A variety of pessaries. (Courtesy of Mentor)

use and fit, the ring mimics that of a contraceptive diaphragm. This pessary is easily managed by the patient.

- *Doughnut*—thicker than the ring, it is useful for third to fourth degree prolapse and/or vaginal vault prolapse (see Figure 6.9). Adequate integrity of the introital opening is necessary for this pessary to remain in place.

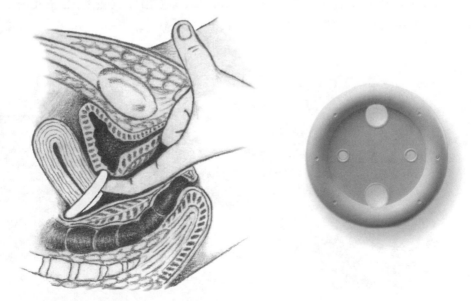

Figure 6.8.   Silicone incontinence ring. (Courtesy of Milex)

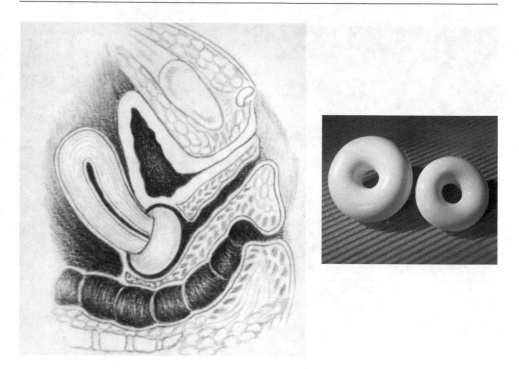

Figure 6.9.   Silicone doughnut pessary. (Courtesy of Mentor and Milex)

- *Gehrung*—an arch-like "U" shaped pessary, which is designed to support the anterior vaginal wall, raise the bladder floor, and thin out a rectocele (see Figure 6.10). The base of the arch should rest on the posterior vaginal wall and the curve supports the anterior wall. It is used with grades 2–4 cystocele and rectocele.

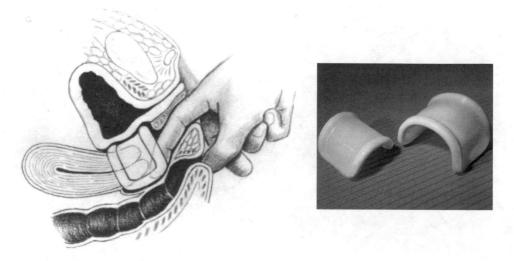

Figure 6.10.   Gehrung pessary. (Courtesy of Mentor and Milex)

- *Gellhorn*—supplied in a rigid, acrylic form and a flexible form, this is one of the most common pessaries used for grade 3 and 4 prolapse. This pessary relies on the integrity of the pelvic muscle for its retention. The Gellhorn pessary is placed with the wide, flat surface toward the anterior vaginal wall with the knob handle resting on the posterior vaginal wall. It must be removed for intercourse.

- *Cube and inflato-ball*—effective in some older patients where there is markedly decreased vaginal tone (rarely used). As the cube fills the entire vaginal vault there is no area for drainage, which can lead to vaginal discharge and infection. The inflato-ball provides general support to prolapsing vaginal structures. It has a filling port that allows for inflation and deflation. It is made of latex rubber. Both should be removed daily and need special care and removal.

- *Shaatz*—used for mild cystocele and uterine prolapse; was the original hard black rubber pessary

- *Incontinence dish and ring (with or without support)*—These are new types of pessaries (see Figure 6.11). These devices are occlusive as a bump or extra material at one part on the pessary rest against the base of the bladder to help press the bladder neck closed. As opposed to a regular pessary which is placed against the cervix in the posterior fornix, the incontinence pessary is placed at the base of the bladder to occlude the urethra and support the bladder neck. (Dierich & Froe, 2000). If properly fitted this type of pessary prevents urine loss during coughing, laughing and other physical exertion activities when standing. (Culligan & Heit, 2000).

The pessaries that are available are very effective for premenopausal women with grades 1–3 prolapse. Older women with large vaginal vaults and

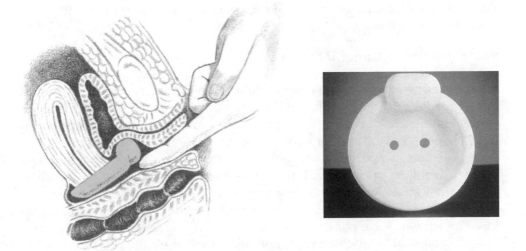

Figure 6.11. Incontinence dish with support. (Courtesy of Mentor)

grade 4 prolapse usually have a difficult time retaining the pessaries currently on the market. As stated previously, this population often represents unlikely surgical candidates and a well-fitting pessary is a preferred alternative.

Fitting a Pessary

Proper pessary fit is essential for effectiveness. It takes time and patience to fit pessaries, particularly in older woman. The use of local or topical estrogen replacement therapy aids in the success of pessary fitting (Schulz, 2001). The manufacturer usually recommends a certain pessary for different types and degrees of prolapse. The pessary should be fitted for comfort and support. Like a diaphragm, it is put into the vagina and rests against the cervix, lifting or supporting the prolapsed pelvic organs. A pelvic exam should always be performed before the introduction and fitting of a pessary because it helps to determine the appropriate pessary diameter. Manufacturers of pessaries will provide a fitting set, which may be a valuable aid in selecting the correct pessary.

To simplify insertion and removal, the pessary is folded so that the leading edge points in a downward direction. The folded pessary is then inserted past the cervix and into the posterior fornix. Once the pessary has passed the introitus, it is allowed to expand to its normal shape. It is recommended that the clinician rotate the pessary a quarter turn to prevent it from folding or being pushed out. To avoid risk of pressure necrosis, the clinician should be able to insert a finger between the rim of the pessary and the vaginal wall. Urinary retention can result if the pessary compresses the urethra into the pubic bone. Once in place, the pessary should not dislodge when standing, sitting, squatting, or bearing down. Unfortunately, many doctors are not familiar with pessary use (Cundiff, Weidner, Visco, Bump, & Addison, 2000; Palumbo, 2000). However, nurse practitioners have had success using pessaries in carefully selected women (Fritzinger, Newman, & Dinkin, 1997).

Pessary-Related Complications

When wearing a pessary, a woman should call her doctor or nurse if there is any vaginal discharge; itching; foul odor; localized pain; inability to urinate, empty the bladder, or have bowel movements; or back pain. Chronic irritation, erosion, and ulceration of the vagina, as well as vaginal fistulas, can occur in women who do not properly care for their pessary or who do not go for regular follow-up visits with their doctor or nurse. If ulceration and abrasion of the vaginal wall occur, the pessary should be changed to a smaller size. Adverse effects include back pain, foul-smelling vaginal discharge, and bleeding. Women who have not experienced UI should be warned that they have a risk of "potential" UI, which was previously masked by the prolapse. Leukorrhea (white watery discharge from the vagina) is related to the presence of a device in the vagina and is probably the most common problem associated with pessary use. This discharge should not be confused with an infection unless other symptoms are present (e.g., itching, burning, foul odor). Pessaries left in place for prolonged periods of time may be difficult to remove.

Pessary Care

The optimum method of care and the frequency of pessary removal differ from one type of pessary to another. For helpful information, see Appendix A: Taking Care of Your Pessary. Many patients prefer to remove the pessary at night in anticipation of sexual activity. Pessary care should occur at a minimum of every 6–8 weeks. Lubrication of either the pessary or the vagina is usually necessary prior to pessary insertion. The woman should be advised not to douche. Trimo-san, an OTC vaginal jelly with a pH of 4, helps restore and maintain normal vaginal acidity. This jelly coats the walls of the vagina with a lubricating film that helps prevent the growth of odor-causing bacteria. Trimo-san is inserted into the vagina using an applicator with the pessary in place.

REFERENCES

Abrams, P., Cardoza, L., Fall, M., Griffiths, D., Rosier, P., Ulmsten, U., van Kerrebroeck, P., Victor, A., & Wein, A. (2002). The standardization of terminology in lower urinary tract function: Report from the Standardisation Sub-committee of the Internationional Continence Society. *Neurourology and Urodynamics, 2.*

American Medical Directors Association. (1996). *Urinary incontinence clinical practice guideline.* Columbia, MD: Author.

Batra, S.C., & Losif, C.S. (1983). Female urethra: Target for estrogen action. *Journal of Urology, 129,* 418–420.

Brink, C., Wells, T.J., Sampselle, C.M., Tallie, E.R., & Mayer, R. (1994). A digital test for pelvic muscle strength in women with urinary incontinence. *Nursing Research, 43,* 352–356.

Brubaker, L.T., & Saclarides, T.J. (1996). *The female pelvic floor—Disorders of function and support.* Philadelphia: F.A. Davis.

Colling, J. (1996). Noninvasive techniques to manage urinary incontinence among care-dependent persons. *Journal of Wound Ostomy Continence Nursing, 23*(6), 302–308.

Colling, J., Ouslander, J., Hadley, B.J., Eisch, J., & Campbell, E. (1992). The effects of patterned urge response toileting (PURT) on urinary incontinence among nursing home residents. *Journal of the American Geriatrics Society, 40,* 135–141.

Culligan, P.J., & Heit, M., (2000). Urinary incontinence in women: Evaluation and management. *American Family Physician, 62,* 2433–44, 2447, 2452.

Cundiff, G.W., Weidner, A.C., Visco, A.G., Bump, R.C., & Addison, W.A. (2000). A survey of pessary use by members of the American Urogynecologic Society. *Obstetrics and Gynecology, 95*(6), 931–935.

Dierich, M., & Froe, F. (2000). *Overcoming incontinence.* New York: John Wiley & Sons.

Engberg, S.J., McDowell, B.J., Weber, E., Brodak, I., Donovan, N., & Engberg, R. (1997). Assessment and management of urinary incontinence among homebound older adults: A clinical trial protocol. *Advanced Practice Nursing Quarterly, 3*(2), 48–56.

Fantl, J.A., Newman, D.K., Colling, J., et al., for the Urinary Incontinence in Adults Guideline Update Panel. (1996). *Urinary incontinence in adults: Acute and chronic management. Clinical practice guideline* (No. 2. Update; AHCPR Publication No. 96-0682). Rockville, MD: Agency for Health Care Policy and Research.

Folstein, M.F., Folstein, S.E., & McHugh, P.R. (1975). "Mini-Mental State": A practical method for grading the cognitive state of patients for the clinician. *Journal of Psychiatric Research, 12,* 189–198.

Fonda, A. (1990). Improving management of urinary incontinence in geriatric centers and nursing homes. Victorian Geriatrician Peer Review Group. *Australian Clinical Review (Sydney), 10*(2), 66–71.

Fritzinger, K., C.M., Newman, D.K., & Dinkin, E. (1997). Use of a pessary for the management of pelvic organ prolapse. *Lippincott's Primary Care Practice, 1*(4), 431–436.

Goode, P.S., Locher, J.L., Bryant, R.L., Roth, D.L., & Burgio, K.L. (2000). Measurement of postvoid urine with portable transabdominal bladder ultrasound scanner and urethral catheterization. *International Urogynecology Journal and Pelvic Floor Dysfunction, 11*(5), 296–300.

Jirovec, M.M. (1991). The impact of daily exercise on the mobility, balance and urine control of cognitively impaired nursing home residents. *International Journal of Nursing Studies, 28*(2), 145–151.

Jirovec, M.M., & Wells, T.J. (1990). Urinary incontinence in nursing home residents with dementia: The mobility-cognition paradigm. *Applied Nursing Research, 3*(3), 112–117.

Kerschan-Schindl, K., Uher, E., Wiesinger, G., Kaider, A., Ebenbichler, G., Nicolakis, P., Kollmitzer, J., Preisinger, E., & Fialka-Moser, V. (2002). Reliability of pelvic floor muscle strength measurements in elderly incontinent women. *Neurourology and Urodynamics, 21*(1), 42–47.

Maloney, C., & Cafiero, M. (1999). Implementing an incontinence program in long-term care settings. *Journal of Gerontological Nursing, 25*(6), 47–52.

Maloney, C., & Oliver, M.L. (2001). Effect of local conjugated estrogens on vaginal pH in elderly women. *Journal of the American Medical Directors Association, 2*(2), 51–55.

Newman, D.K. (1998). *Progress: Bladder and bowel rehabilitation program instructor's manual.* Eddystone, PA: SCA Hygiene Products.

Newman, D.K. (2000). *Program of excellence in extended care.* Bothell, WA: Diagnostic Ultrasound Corporation.

Newman, D.K., & Palmer, M.H. (1999). Incontinence and PPS: A new era. *Ostomy/Wound Management, 45*(12), 32–49.

Newman, D.K., & Smith, D.A. (1991). A portable bladder scanner. *Nurse Practitioner Forum, 2*(4), 243–245.

Ouslander, J.G., Morshita, L., Blaustein, J., Orzeck, S., Dunn, S., & Sayre, J. (1987). Clinical, functional, and psychological characteristics of an incontinent nursing home population. *Journal of Gerontology, 42,* 631–637.

Ouslander, J.G., Schapira, M., Fingold, S., & Schnelle, J. (1995). Accuracy of rapid urine screening tests among incontinent nursing home residents with asymptomatic bacteriuria *Journal of the American Geriatrics Society, 43,* 772–775.

Ouslander, J.G., Schapira, M., & Schnelle, J.F. (1995). Urine specimen collection from incontinent female nursing home residents. *Journal of the American Geriatrics Society, 43,* 279–281.

Ouslander, J.G., Schapira, M., Schnelle, J., & Fingold, S. (1996). Pyuria among chronically incontinent but otherwise asymptomatic nursing home residents. *Journal of the American Geriatrics Society, 44,* 420–423

Ouslander, J.G., Simmons, S., Tuico, E., Nigam, J.G., Fingold, S., Bates-Jensen, B., & Schnelle, J.F. (1994). Use of portable ultrasound device to measure post-void residual volume among incontinent nursing home residents. *Journal of the American Geriatrics Society, 42,* 1189–1192.

Palmer, M.H. (1996). A new framework for urinary continence outcomes in long-term care. *Urologic Nursing, 16*(4), 146–151.

Palmer, M.H., McCormick, K.A., Langford, A., Langlois, J., & Alvaran, M. (1992). Continence outcomes: Documentation on medical records in the nursing home environment. *Journal of Nursing Care Quality, 6*(3), 36–43.

Palumbo, M.V. (2000). Pessary placement and management. *Ostomy/Wound Management, 46*(12), 40–45.

Rovner, E. (2000). Pelvic organ prolapse: A review. *Ostomy/Wound Management, 46*(12), 24–37.

Schulz, J.A. (2001). Assessing and treating pelvic organ prolapse. *Ostomy/Wound Management, 47*(5), 54–59.

Wagner, M., & Schmid, M. (1997). Exploring the research base and outcome measures for portable bladder ultrasound technology. *MEDSURG Nursing, 6*(5), 304–314.

Woolridge, L. (2000, June). Ultrasound technology and bladder dysfunction. *American Journal of Nursing* (Suppl.), 3–14.

7

Self-Care Practices to Reduce Urinary Symptoms

Very little information is available relevant to incontinence prevention and continence promotion. Self-care practices such as regular toileting, increased fluid intake, exercise, and weight reduction are thought to be ways to prevent or reduce urinary incontinence (UI) but are not actively promoted. Research has shown that there is incontinence prevention potential in community-dwelling older women (Association of Women's Health, Obstetric and Neonatal Nurses [AWHONN], 2000a, 2000b). It was estimated that, by increasing the number of women who discussed UI with their doctors from 41% to 71% and by assuming that they all performed effective bladder training, incontinence could be reduced by 50,000 cases annually (Fantl et al., 1996). Risk factors have been identified for incontinence, and interventions have been successful in modifying these risk factors. Thus, the potential for designing preventive interventions or promoting self-care practices is enhanced.

This author has been involved in promoting "bladder health" to seniors in the Philadelphia metropolitan area (Newman, Wallace, Blackwood, & Spencer 1996). Older consumers are taught about UI and overactive bladder (OAB) and given ways to prevent or reduce the problem, including good bowel habits, diet changes, and bladder retraining. The program uses self-care practices to improve quality of life for people experiencing bladder problems. The behavioral methods include diet modification, daily self-monitoring of voiding habits, bladder training techniques, bowel management, and the use of absorbent products. The goal of the program has been to educate older adults about behaviors that may precipitate bladder symptoms, to outline self-care practices, and to decrease bladder symptoms.

Modification of factors such as type and amount of fluid intake, constipation, use of bladder irritants, and techniques to facilitate complete bladder emptying can decrease symptoms of UI and OAB. Clients can take control of UI and OAB by identifying daily practices that have a detrimental effect on the urinary system. If clients learn to alter certain lifestyle habits through self-care practices, further treatments may not be necessary. This chapter targets those behaviors that, if altered, will have a positive impact on bladder function. Providers in all settings can easily teach the methods described in this chapter.

DIETARY RESTRICTIONS AND MODIFICATIONS

People can decrease urine leakage, urgency, and frequency through modification of certain diet habits; see Appendix A: Diet Habits that Can Affect Your Bladder.

Fluid Intake

It is important to teach the person that adequate fluid intake is necessary to prevent UI. The recommended daily fluid intake is 1,500 milliliters (ml), but many authorities believe that a more appropriate intake is 1,800–2,400 ml/day. It is thought that older adults must consume at least 1,500–2,000 ml of liquids per day to be adequately hydrated (Kayser-Jones, Schell, Porter, Barbaccia, & Shaw, 1999). Many people who have bladder control problems reduce the amount of liquids they drink because they fear incontinence and urinary urgency. Although drinking less liquid does result in less urine in the bladder, the smaller amount of urine may be more highly concentrated and irritate the bladder lining. Highly concentrated (dark yellow, strong smelling) urine may cause urgency and frequency. It can also encourage bacteria to grow, which can lead to a bladder infection (Dowd, Campbell, & Jones, 1996). In contrast, many people, especially women who are dieting, may drink excessive amounts of fluids that total 4,000 ml per day. If they are experiencing UI, they should be encouraged to decrease the amount.

Contrary to popular belief, maintaining adequate fluid intake is important, especially for older adults who already have a decrease in total body water and are at risk for dehydration. Nursing facility residents are chronically dehydrated because most require assistance from staff to eat and drink (Colling, McCreedy, & Owen 1994; Gaspar, 1999). Also, as nursing facilities attempt to limit the number of times medication is dispensed, there are fewer times that residents are offered liquids. In nursing facilities, the majority of fluids tend to be given between 6:00 A.M. and 6:00 P.M. Another belief is that staff may restrict fluids in order to reduce urinary output and thus decrease UI. Approaches that have been successful in increasing hydration in nursing facility residents include offering more between-meal snacks, supervision of residents at mealtimes to ensure adequate ingestion of liquids, and designating a certified nurse assistant who is responsible for offering fluids every 2 hours from a "water cart."

Bladder Irritants

Certain dietary factors that are considered common bladder irritants, such as caffeine, artificial sweeteners, spicy foods, and citrus fruits may influence continence status (Wyman, 2000). Caffeine, a central nervous system stimulant that is found in many beverages, foods, medications, and dietary supplements, reaches peak blood concentrations within 30–60 minutes after ingestion. Caffeine has been shown to have an excitatory effect on detrusor muscle contraction (Lee, Wein, & Levin, 1993). This can cause a significant rise in detrusor pressure and subsequent urinary urgency and frequency following caffeine ingestion (Creighton & Stanton, 1990). Caffeine is also believed to have a diuretic effect.

More than 80% of the U.S. adult population consumes caffeine in the form of coffee, tea, or soft drinks on a daily basis. Caffeine occurs naturally in coffee beans, tea leaves, and cocoa beans. Caffeine is found in liquids such as sodas (e.g., Mountain Dew, Pepsi, Coca-Cola) and foods and candy that contain milk chocolate. In addition, many over-the-counter drugs (e.g., Excedrin, Anacin) and prescription medications (e.g., Darvon compound, Fiorinal) contain caffeine (Newman, 1999). Nutritional supplements, puddings, and cakes that contain cocoa are favorite foods and daily staples in nursing homes. However, cocoa is also a source of caffeine. Table A.1 (see Appendix A: Avoiding Foods and Liquids with Caffeine) lists the caffeine content of many drinks, foods, and medications.

Research has shown that UI decreased (63% decrease in urine leakage) when caffeine consumption was reduced from 23 to 14 grams (g) (Tomlinson et al., 1999). Arya, Myers, and Jackson (2000) found that women with detrusor instability had a higher caffeine intake than women without detrusor instability. Even though current research is not conclusive, people with UI and OAB should be assessed for amount of caffeine intake. It is recommended that an individual drink no more than 2 cups of caffeinated drinks per day. People should be advised about the possible adverse effects caffeine may have on the detrusor muscle and the possible benefits of reduction of caffeine intake (Gray, 2001). Switching to caffeine-free beverages and foods or eliminating those with caffeine may cause urgency and frequency to decrease. The individual should be taught to restrict caffeine through behavior modification. Instructions should include encouraging the person to gradually replace caffeinated beverages or foods with noncaffeinated ones. Because caffeine crosses the blood–brain barrier and can reduce blood flow to the brain, a sudden withdrawal from caffeine can cause headaches, nervousness, nausea, and muscular tension.

Constipation

Dietary changes should also be recommended to people who have constipation because chronic constipation can contribute to incontinence. The use of bran and other approaches to improve constipation are outlined in Chapter 5.

MANAGEMENT OF NOCTURIA

Nighttime voiding and incontinence are major problems for many people. The largest amount of urine production occurs at rest and usually between the hours of midnight and 8:00 A.M. (Colling et al., 1994). During the night, there is a lower level of physical activity and fluid moves more quickly from one part of the body to another, causing an increase in the amount of urine in the bladder. The loss of urine during sleep is called nocturnal enuresis (nighttime incontinence). Because greater quantities of potassium, sodium, and solute are excreted into the urine at night, nighttime incontinence may also lead to skin irritation in older people. The following preventive measures can be employed to decrease nighttime UI:

- Some people may benefit from fluid restriction in the evening, usually after dinner. These individuals should maintain adequate fluid intake by drinking the bulk of their liquids before dinner.

- Individuals who develop edema of the lower extremities during the day should be advised to elevate their lower extremities for several hours during the afternoon. This will help to stimulate a natural diuresis and limit the amount of edema present at bedtime.

- The use of diuretics has been associated with lower nighttime urine volumes; altering the timing of the administration of diuretics may decrease nocturia (Ouslander, Schnelle, Simmons, Bates-Jensen, & Zeitlin, 1993).

- Some individuals may also benefit from elimination of caffeine-containing beverages and foods in the evening.

- Residents in nursing facilities who are put to bed after dinner, usually around 7:00 P.M., will need to toilet before midnight. This may be a task for the night nursing staff.

   The issues surrounding continence care during the night are complex and will require coordination of the efforts of all nursing staff. Staff who are responsible for the purchase of care products must be aware of improved absorbent products and the correct use of skin cleansers, protection creams, and powders.

TECHNIQUES TO FACILITATE VOIDING AND BLADDER EMPTYING

Manual techniques are available that will assist the bladder in complete emptying. These techniques are helpful for the individual with urinary retention and overflow incontinence. The following maneuvers can be used to teach the person how to completely empty the bladder manually:

- The *Credé maneuver* is a means of direct manual compression to empty the bladder. The person presses firmly with one hand (or both hands) directly into the abdomen over the bladder during voiding.

- A program of double voiding may be effective in cases of mild to moderate urinary retention. The individual is taught to void twice during each trip to the bathroom to reduce residual urine volumes. The person is instructed to void, to remain on the toilet, and to void again after a rest period of 2–10 minutes. Another method of double voiding is to have the person void, then stand up, sit back down, and attempt to void again.

- People without a spinal cord injury may be able to identify a "trigger" to initiate a bladder contraction. One common method is called "suprapubic tapping," which involves drumming the abdomen overlying the bladder. Other trigger mechanisms include pulling on pubic hairs, stroking the abdomen or inner thigh, digital anal stimulation, running water in the sink, placing the hands in a basin of warm water, drinking warm fluids, and pouring warm water on the perineal area. Staff may want to have residents experiment to discover which technique works best and easiest for them.

REFERENCES

Arya, L.A., Myers, D.L., & Jackson, N.D. (2000). Dietary caffeine intake and the risk for detrusor instability: A case-control study. *Obstetrics and Gynecology, 96*(1), 85–89.

Association of Women's Health, Obstetric and Neonatal Nurses. (2000a). *Evidence-based clinical practice guideline: Continence for women*. Washington, DC: Author.

Association of Women's Health, Obstetric and Neonatal Nurses. (2000b). *Quick care guide: Continence for women*. Washington, DC: Author.

Colling, J., McCreedy, M., & Owen, T. (1994). Urinary tract infection rates among incontinent nursing home and community dwelling elderly. *Urologic Nursing, 14,* 117–119.

Creighton, S.M., & Stanton, S.L. (1990). Caffeine: Does it affect your bladder? *British Journal of Urology, 66,* 613–614.

Dowd, T.T., Campbell, J.M., & Jones, J.A. (1996). Fluid intake and urinary incontinence in older community-dwelling women. *Journal of Community Health Nursing, 13*(3), 179–186.

Fantl, J., Newman, D., Colling, J., et al., for the Urinary Incontinence in Adults Guideline Update Panel. (1996). *Urinary incontinence in adults: Acute and chronic management. Clinical practice guideline* (No. 2. Update; ACHCPR Publication No. 96-0692). Rockville, MD: Agency for Health Care and Policy Research.

Gaspar, P.M. (1999). Water intake of nursing home residents. *Journal of Gerontological Nursing, 25*(4), 22–29.

Gray, M. (2001). Caffeine and urinary continence. *Journal of Wound Ostomy and Continence Nursing, 28,* 66–69.

Kayser-Jones, J., Schell, E.S., Porter, C., Barbaccia, J.C., & Shaw, H. (1999). Factors contributing to dehydration in nursing homes: Inadequate staffing and lack of professional supervision. *Journal of the American Geriatrics Society, 47,* 1187–1194.

Lee, J.G., Wein, A.J., & Levin. R.M. (1993). The effect of caffeine on the contractile response of the rabbit urinary bladder to field stimulation. *General Pharmacology, 24*(4), 1007–1011.

Newman, D.K. (1999). *The urinary incontinence sourcebook* (2nd ed.). Los Angeles: Lowell House.

Newman, D.K., Wallace, J., Blackwood, N., & Spencer, C. (1996). Promoting healthy bladder habits for seniors. *Ostomy/Wound Management, 42(10),* 18–28.

Ouslander, J., Schnelle, J., Simmons, S., Bates-Jenson, B., & Zeitlin, M. (1993). The dark side of incontinence in nursing home residents. *Journal of the American Geriatrics Society, 41,* 371–376.

Tomlinson, B.U., Dougherty, M.C., Pendergast, J.F., Boyington, A.R., Coffman, M.A., & Pickens, S.M. (1999). Dietary caffeine, fluid intake and urinary incontinence in older rural women. *International Urogynecology, 10,* 22–28.

Wyman, J.F. (2000). Management of urinary incontinence in adult ambulatory care populations. In J.F. Fitzpatrick (Series Ed.) & J. Geoppinger (Vol. Ed.), *Annual review of nursing research: Vol. 18. Chronic illness* (pp. 171–195). New York: Springer-Verlag.

8

Implementing Toileting
and Retraining Programs

Toileting and bladder retraining programs are part of behavioral methods that target restoration or maintenance of bladder function with the goal of returning an individual to continence. These interventions, called behavioral therapies, include adjusting the intake of fluids and eliminating bladder irritants (discussed in Chapter 7), scheduled or timed toileting, prompted voiding, and bladder retraining with pelvic muscle rehabilitation (Newman, 2000). Behavioral therapies are now recommended as the first line treatment for urinary incontinence (UI) and overactive bladder (OAB, Fantl, Newman, & Colling, 1996; Wilson et al., 1999). Most ambulatory, cognitively intact adults can learn or can relearn to regulate bladder or bowel performance sufficiently to achieve and to maintain clinically significant, improved function.

The best way to learn new behavior or to relearn old behavior is by identifying the desired or optimal behavior and outlining the steps to be taken to gradually achieve it. This shaping of desired behavior is achieved through goal setting and positive reinforcement or reward. For example, toilet training toddlers involves providing rewards as a motivating factor for the child to void appropriately—in the toilet. An additional component of any behavioral treatment program for UI is monitoring voiding patterns and specified behavior, accomplished through the use of a Bladder Record (discussed in Chapter 6). A critical part of any behavioral program is the feedback from the clinician or caregiver in settings such as long-term or in-home care. Feedback should be provided about compliance, progress with the program, and positive reinforcement for success.

In the long-term care (LTC) setting, behavioral interventions such as timed/scheduled toileting use a caregiver delivery system to achieve the goal of continence. In the home care setting, the need for a caregiver to provide teaching, assistance, and feedback is a problem unless a family member is available throughout the day or a hired paraprofessional is in place. However, the following tips can be used by home caregivers to promote safe and independent toileting:

- Try to give the person his or her own private bathroom so someone else is never using it. If a bathroom is inaccessible, use a bedside commode, urinal, or bedpan.

- Ensure that bed height is sufficient so that when the person sits on the edge of the bed, his or her feet are flat and he or she can easily accomplish going from sitting to standing.

- Keep a clear, unobstructed, direct walking path to the bathroom and place night-lights along the path.

- Make sure the person can easily use the toilet (e.g., raised toilet seat, grab bars).

- Make sure the person's clothing is easy to remove. Encourage the use of underwear whenever possible. Underwear serves as a reminder to stay dry and as a stimulus to use the toilet and not to wet oneself if it can be avoided.

- Encourage the person to void before going to bed.

- Locate bathroom facilities when traveling, or bring a portable urinal. Choose seats in restaurants, theaters, and other such locations that are near a bathroom.

- Use underpads (reusable or disposable) under bedsheets, on chairs, and in the car. Avoid use of garbage bags, rubber pads, or shower curtain liners because these may be too slippery or may irritate skin.

- Open windows or use deodorizers to cut down on odors. (A cut-up onion will absorb odors in a room without leaving its own smell. Also, an open box of baking soda will reduce odors.)

TOILETING PROGRAMS

The initial treatment approach to someone with incontinence depends on the overall condition of the person and his or her ability to participate in a toileting program. People who can benefit from such programs may have mobility or cognitive impairment or may need assistance (e.g., one-person assist) but are able to cooperate with toileting. A caregiver–dependent program that provides toileting on a scheduled time basis may be the simplest initial approach. If residents in LTC facilities or people living at home have an available and willing caregiver, a timed toileting program should be established. At least 60% of care-dependent individuals with incontinence can benefit from a toileting assistance program. The premise of these programs is that if the person is taught to void frequently, incontinence will not occur. The programs most commonly used are routine or scheduled toileting, habit training, and prompted voiding.

Prior to determining which program is the most appropriate, assessment, determination of the underlying pathophysiology, and identification of the expected outcomes must be done. Also, the assessment should determine which individuals would not benefit from a scheduled toileting or retraining program and should be just "checked and changed." With the recent implementation of a prospective payment system (PPS) in nursing facilities that includes a classification system based on amount of resources needed to care for residents, assessment becomes all the more critical. One classification, special rehabilitation, identifies two specific toileting programs, scheduled toileting and bladder retraining, both programs that staff can implement. Therefore, nursing facility staff, especially the direct caregivers, such as certified nurse assistants, must be aware of the key components of these programs and how to determine which residents can be successfully retrained to obtain optimal bladder function.

Habit Training/Scheduled Voiding

Habit training establishes timed toileting on a rigid, fixed schedule. Toileting takes place regardless of whether a sensation to void is present. This pattern may or may not be followed during sleep hours. The goal is to keep the person dry, and no effort is made to motivate the person to resist the urge to urinate and delay urination. The schedule for toileting is based on the Bladder Record or on data collected using a bladder volume recording instrument or from an electronic device used to monitor and record incontinence episodes, providing a more accurate record. In nursing facilities, preestablished toileting times are usually used, or the schedule may be related to certain events such as lunch or bedtime. A schedule is usually determined by administrative staff for those people who cannot toilet themselves. If the person self-toilets independently, then scheduled times are readjusted.

The following are components of a toileting program:

- Identify specific times the person is likely to void by recording the voiding pattern for at least 3 days. Based on the pattern/times observed using a Bladder and Bowel Record (see Appendix B), efforts are made to schedule toileting opportunities around these times. If the person is taking a diuretic, the toileting schedule may need to be altered because the urine volume will be increased at the diuretic's peak action time. A common toileting interval used is every 3–4 hours. An example is to toilet

    After breakfast

    After lunch

    After dinner

    Before bedtime

    In settings such as nursing facilities, the person should toilet on last incontinence rounds or on awakening.

- Negotiate the voiding interval and toileting times with people who are cognitively intact to increase compliance.

- Observe body language for cues about need to use the toilet. Look for fidgeting, nervousness, and pacing or increased anxiety.

- Ensure complete bladder emptying by having the person toilet upright in a bathroom commode or a bedside commode rather than a bedpan.

- Institute visual cues to indicate the location of the bathroom (e.g., put the word "toilet" on the outside of the bathroom door; show a picture of a man using a toilet).

- Facilitate voiding by

    Using a raised toilet seat or bedside commode to avoid having the person sitting too low.

    Having the person slowly back up to the toilet until he or she can feel the back of his or her knees touching it. After placing both hands on the commode armrests or the grab bar and edge of seat, the person lowers him- or herself slowly by bending at the knee and hip.

    Reversing the procedure by having the person stand up by using the grab bars and seat or commode armrests with one hand and perhaps a walker with the other. Instruct the person to keep knees bent and feet firmly on the floor when attempting to stand.

This type of toileting program is helpful for residents in nursing facilities who are not incontinent more often than every 2 hours and in homebound people living with a caregiver, usually a family member, who can assist with toileting. Research has shown that, with nursing facility residents, a timed, scheduled toileting program can be successful in decreasing the number of incontinence episodes. This is probably also true in people being cared for in their homes.

Prompted Voiding

Prompted voiding is a scheduled toileting program that employs behavior modification to reinforce both appropriate toileting behaviors and the individual's desire to stay dry (Pinkowski, 1996). Prompted voiding is used with people who are able to recognize urine leakage and are able to respond (will void) when prompted. Prompted voiding stresses active communication and interaction between a caregiver and the individual, allowing the person to take an active part in his or her incontinence and toileting behavior. This type of toileting program is most successful if the individual

- Has a bladder capacity of at least 100 milliliters

- Has a low number of incontinent episodes per day

- Responds to caregivers if prompted (asked and taken to the toilet) to void

- Can control urination until the toilet is reached

A prompted voiding program tries to increase the person's awareness of the need to void and to ask for assistance to toilet. Like habit training, this program is used with more frail, ill people who require assistance from family members, professional caregivers, or both. The person should be given a therapeutic trial of prompted voiding (Schnelle, 1990). Research in LTC facilities has shown that at least 25%–40% of incontinent residents respond well to toileting assistance, while approximately 38% cannot successfully toilet even when provided assistance by research assistants (Ouslander et al., 1995; Schnelle, 1990). A decrease in UI rates can be seen within 3 days, but maximal response may not be realized until after several weeks of treatment (Ouslander et al., 1995; Palmer, Bennett, Marks, McCormick, & Engel, 1994).

Steps of a Prompted Voiding Program   There are five major steps in a prompted voiding program as used in a LTC facility.

1. Check   The caregiver should give the resident a chance to request to toilet. Clothes, linens, and absorbent products are checked by the caregiver on a regular, scheduled basis. It is important that both the inside and outside of clothes and absorbent products are checked. The caregiver should inform the resident of what is being done and why.

2. Talk   The resident is encouraged to discuss the bladder/incontinence problem. The caregiver should ask the resident if he or she knows whether he or she is wet or dry (to determine accuracy and to see if the resident is in denial). The caregiver should verbally verify the accuracy of the resident's response. These efforts will increase the resident's awareness about his or her condition. If the resident is dry, the caregiver should indicate approval or praise the resident. If resident is wet, the caregiver should provide corrective verbal feedback such as disappointment.

Examples: "That's right, Mrs. Ryan, you are dry. That is good." (praise)
             "Oh, dear, Mrs. Ryan, you are wet." (corrective feedback)

The caregiver should inquire as to the resident's need to void prior to going anywhere new (e.g., before physical therapy). In addition, the caregiver should make sure the resident knows how to communicate with staff regarding the need to toilet if he or she is in a new room or place in the facility and should show the resident the location of and how to access the toilet in that area.

3. Prompt   Because the goal is to have the resident take an active part in the voiding process, he or she is asked (prompted) to try to use the toilet regardless of continence status. The caregiver should be very persuasive to get the resident to void by offering assistance and providing privacy during toileting. Residents should not be rushed, but rather allowed 15 minutes to relax and void. Relaxation is needed to allow the external urethral sphincter to open. However, if the resident does not want to void, the caregiver should not attempt to toilet him or her because more than likely voiding will not occur.

Example: "Mrs. Ryan, would you like to use the bathroom?"
"Mrs. Ryan, maybe you'd better try because I won't be back for 3 hours."
If client is still not sure:
"Mrs. Ryan, please give it a try, okay?"

4. Praise   The caregiver should praise the resident for 1) being dry (continence) or 2) making an effort to use the toilet. The resident should be informed of the terms of the next scheduled prompted voiding time.

Example: "Very good, Mrs. Ryan. You tried to use the bathroom."
"Mrs. Ryan, it has been 3 hours, and you have remained dry. I will be back in 3 hours. Please try to be dry again."

5. Correct   If the resident is wet, the caregiver should indicate to him or her that the expectation is that he or she will stay dry.

Example: "Mrs. Ryan, you were incontinent this time. Please ask me (push on your call bell) before you have to go to the bathroom the next time."

Outcomes of Prompted Voiding Programs   Research supports the value of prompted voiding programs because most residents can become continent within 3 days when they are given prompts and assistance with toileting (Fantl et al., 1996). The outcomes of prompted voiding have been identified through clinical trials and include

- Identification of individual patterns of UI
- Decrease in average urine volume of incontinent episodes
- Increased recognition of urge to void
- Increase in daily average number of dry checks and nonwet (continent) episodes

However, key elements must be in place if these practices are to be transferred effectively to a clinical setting and residential population. Elements identified (Ouslander et al., 1995) include

1. Assessment to determine if the person is a candidate for a toileting program. Residents in LTC facilities with high baseline incontinence rates (usually incontinent more than every 2 hours), who have small voided urine volumes, and who were unsuccessful at reported toileting regimens using prompted voiding techniques are usually not responsive to toileting programs (Lekan-Rutledge, 2000).

2. Ability of the individual to ambulate independently or with the assistance of one person

3. Ability of the individual to void into a toileting receptacle when prompted at least 50% of the time

A more successful program may involve toileting residents and other care-dependent individuals at times when they are most likely need to void, which is determined by tracking voiding and UI and determining patterns using such techniques as computerized recordings of wetness (Colling, Ouslander, Hadley, Eisch, & Campbell, 1992). Another use of technology would be to toilet residents based on actual bladder volume. Some LTC facilities have instituted the use of an ultrasound scanner to determine bladder volume when attempting to toilet a resident. The following is an example of one facility's approach to prompted voiding using a bladder volume scanning instrument:

1. Anticipate the needs of the resident related to voiding.

2. Listen to the resident for complaints of pain, discomfort, and need to urinate.

3. When the resident requests toileting, determine bladder volume using the BladderScan device. Inform the resident of the scan results, explaining what the volume means.

4. If the amount is more than 200–250 ml, toilet the resident using prompted voiding techniques.

5. If the amount is 150 ml or less, explain to the resident that the volume is not sufficient to necessitate voiding. If amounts are consistently low (<150 ml) for a given resident and the resident does not appear to be voiding adequate amounts, or at least four to five times per day, consider increasing fluid intake.

Despite the availability of such new technologies, however, LTC facilities have not seemed to embrace their use. Unfortunately, with regard to toileting programs, there is a wide gap between what is known and what is actually used. Despite documented research of positive outcomes, prompted voiding interventions largely have not been adopted in LTC settings. Improvement in continence on the part of residents can only be maintained if the prompting continues, because the residents do not achieve complete independence from staff (Schnelle, Newman, & Fogarty, 1990; Schnelle et al., 1993). Research has documented the success of a staff training program called the behavioral supervision model, which defines responsibilities of staff members for the prompted voiding intervention, gives staff feedback regarding performance, and establishes consequences based on staff performance evaluation (Burgio & Burgio, 1990).

Providers should consider combining treatments to maximize the effects in residents in LTC. In female residents diagnosed with atrophic vaginitis, topical estrogen cream may improve urogenital atrophy. In residents clinically diagnosed with urge UI and other symptoms of OAB, a combination of an anticholinergic (e.g., Tolterodine, ditropan) and a toileting program may maximize the benefit. Ouslander, Maloney, Gravel, Rogers, and Salamander (2001) placed 50 clinically stable residents on a toileting program and the increase in dryness was 16%. When residents ($n = 31$) were given the combination treatment of toileting and Tolterodine, an increase in dryness was noted to be 29%.

If instituted correctly, nursing facility residents and families should benefit from improvement in incontinence rates, a lowered incidence of complications secondary to UI, less absorbent product (e.g., adult briefs) use, and greater dignity. Nursing facility chains or consortiums should consider using a central data collection process and a program coordinator to produce graphs of outcomes and to provide ongoing feedback to faculties and staff. For a toileting program to be successful, facilities must be motivated, have in place an efficient training process, provide good oversight, continuously monitor the process, and identify "program champions" who will take ownership of the program (Ouslander et al., 2001). Figure 8.1 is an example of a treatment pathway for UI in a LTC environment.

Bladder Retraining

A bladder retraining program requires people to resist the sensation of urgency, to postpone voiding, and to urinate by the clock rather than in response to an urge. The goals of a bladder retraining program are to

- Improve ability to control bladder urgency

- Decrease urinary frequency

- Increase bladder capacity

- Reduce incontinence episodes

Mechanisms of action are not well understood, but it is believed that bladder retraining improves cortical inhibition over detrusor contractions, facilitates cortical control over urethral closure during bladder filling, strengthens pelvic striated muscles, and alters behaviors that affect continence (e.g., frequent response to urgency).

Initially, bladder retraining was prescribed for functional disorders of the bladder for which surgical intervention was not expected to be successful. It was a technique used in hospitals and with those people who were thought to have bladder dysfunction secondary to psychological disorders. The management regimen included education followed by a strict schedule of voluntary voiding with specific instructions to avoid responding prematurely to urinary urgency. This type of bladder retraining was the basis of a large randomized, controlled clinical trial of 123 women with detrusor instability, stress UI, and mixed UI. Results from the group taught bladder retraining showed that more than 50% experienced a reduction in UI ranging from 50% to 75%. On average, fewer than 15% of women had complete resolution of UI and associated symptoms (Fantl et al., 1991).

Bladder retraining helps to promote continence by gradually increasing the intervals between voiding in an attempt to correct the habit of frequent

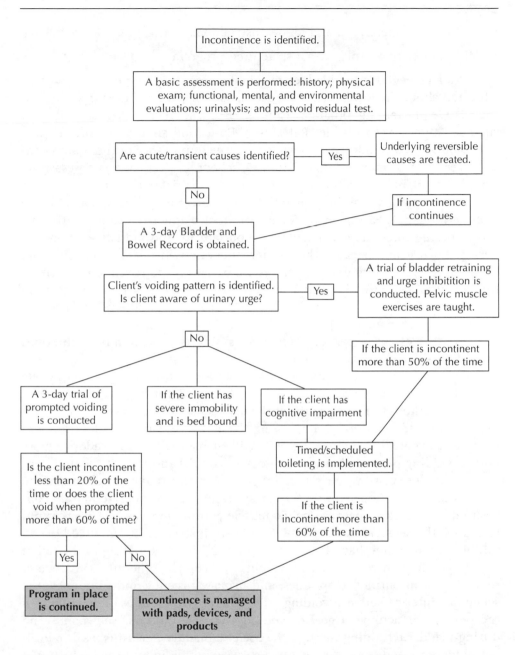

Figure 8.1   Treatment pathway for urinary incontinence in a long-term care setting.

voiding, to suppress bladder instability, and eventually to diminish urgency. This type of therapy is most appropriate for individuals with

- Stress, urge, or mixed incontinence
- Intact cognition
- Ability to sense the urinary urge sensation

- Ability to comprehend and follow instructions
- Willingness to comply with a structured program

Prior to beginning a bladder retraining program, the person should be educated about the lower urinary tract, causes of urinary incontinence, and the bladder retraining program using easy-to-understand educational aids, such as Appendix A: Bladder Retraining. Education should include the fact that "continence" is a learned behavior and the importance of the brain's control over lower urinary tract function. A scheduling regimen is an essential component of bladder retraining. The clinician initiates the program by assigning a voluntary voiding schedule, which includes voiding every 30–60 minutes (Tobani & Fantl, 1999). The initiation of bladder retraining with very short voiding intervals is particularly important for individuals who are experiencing urgency because the shorter intervals will decrease or eliminate these symptoms. The voiding intervals are based on the baseline micturition frequency as determined by the Bladder Record. The use of timers such as an electronic pill timer or stopwatch can be beneficial to help the person keep on a schedule (Newman, 1999).

Another essential part of bladder retraining is education on techniques to achieve the cortical ability to delay voiding and strategies for distraction. Concentration on a task requiring close attention is useful in distracting the individual from the sensation of urgency (Wyman & Fantl, 1991). The person is taught methods to resist or inhibit the urge sensation so an expanded voiding interval can be adopted. Improving the ability to suppress the urge sensation and eventually diminish urgency will enable the person to adopt a more normal voiding pattern. A useful strategy to control and inhibit the urge sensation is the use of slow, deep breathing to relax and reduce or eliminate the urge. Another method is to do five or six rapid, intense pelvic muscle contractions, or "flicks," because pelvic muscle contraction has also been found to reduce the sensation of urgency. People are instructed to practice learned inhibition when they have an urge to void or before ambulating to the toilet.

Depending on the individual's ability to keep the schedule, evidence of reduction of incontinence episodes, and urinary urgency and frequency, the scheduled interval between voiding is increased by 30 minutes each week until the person can achieve a goal of voiding every 3–4 hours. Self-monitoring during bladder retraining through the use of a Bladder Record is used to evaluate adherence and to determine the next weekly voiding interval. The use of a signed agreement or "contract" with the individual stating personal outcome goals can be helpful in motivating him or her to adhere to the program, and it also outlines expectations. It has been shown that incontinent women have diverse goals for incontinence treatment; in some cases they may desire an improvement in urine leakage and not continence (Sale & Wyman, 1994). The relationship between the clinician and client is very important to the success of the retraining. The clinician must monitor the client's progress and provide praise and encouragement where appropriate.

Bladder retraining can be very successful in the LTC setting if the appropriate resident is identified. A bladder retraining program in a LTC facility must be flexible enough to be modified to the resident's needs. The following are the components of a LTC bladder retraining program:

- When usual voiding times have been established, arrange for the resident to be toileted one half-hour prior to the next expected time. If there is no observable voiding pattern, toilet the resident at 1-hour intervals, beginning at 7:00 A.M. or 8:00 A.M. and continuing hourly until bedtime. The resident should be awakened to void at less frequent intervals during the night.

- Timing is crucial to success. Teach the resident to control the urge to void by teaching the following:

  Explain to the resident that the urinary urge, called urgency, is that uncomfortable feeling that occurs when the bladder needs to be emptied. It can lead to sudden urine leakage or urge incontinence. Urgency follows a wave pattern: it starts, grows, peaks, and then subsides until it stops.

  The key to controlling urinary urge is not to respond by rushing to the bathroom. Rushing may precipitate a bladder contraction, which in turn increases urgency, so teach the resident never to rush or run to the bathroom or toilet. Substitute walking slowly. The ultimate goal of bladder retraining is to have the resident go to the bathroom every 3–4 hours.

- Staff must give the resident consistent encouragement and positive feedback. If UI continues, focus the resident's attention on successes that are achieved each day.

- When the resident has remained dry most of the time for 1 week, the toileting interval should be increased to 2 hours, and finally to 3 hours. Some residents will never be able to retain urine longer than 2–3 hours, but others will regain more extended control.

- Institute the self-care strategies discussed in Chapter 7.

- Continue to record intake and voiding times on the Bladder and Bowel Record. Progress can be monitored, and adjustments can be made to the voiding schedule and fluid intake as necessary.

Decreasing Obsessive Toileting

Some individuals request toileting as frequently as every 20 or 30 minutes. These people fear that, if they do not void, they will be incontinent. It is thought that at least 5% of LTC residents exhibit obsessive toileting behavior. This includes residents who

- Have been diagnosed with neurogenic bladder

- Frequently request toileting assistance (every 20 minutes, 30 minutes, 1 hour)

- Frequently self-toilet (every 20 minutes, 30 minutes, 1 hour)

The goals for such residents are

- To stop obsessive toileting behavior

- To educate the resident about normal bladder volumes through the use of a bladder volume recording instrument

- To expand and increase intervals between voiding

- To decrease the time the staff spend with frequent toileting of the same resident

The resident is taught to reduce the number of incontinence episodes through combining "dependent" continence and "independent" continence. In "dependent" continence, the staff toilet the resident based on an adequate bladder volume as determined by ultrasound scanning. In "independent" continence, the resident takes a more active role in developing awareness of the need to void based on adequate bladder volume and is able to delay voiding through urge inhibition techniques. The ultrasound bladder scanner may be a helpful tool with the resident who has an obsession with toileting. Knowledge about bladder volume at any given time helps eliminate unnecessary toileting and allows for accurate assessment of the resident's hydration state (Woolridge, 2000). With the resident who repeatedly asks to be toileted before the scheduled time (or before an adequate volume of urine is present in the bladder), the following techniques can be used:

1. Scan the bladder; if under 100–150 ml, show the resident the results. Usually these individuals will have 50- to 75-ml volumes. Include the resident in the scanning process by encouraging the resident to look at the bladder scanner screen and explain what the numbers indicate. Show the resident the printout of the bladder volume.

2. Ask the resident if he or she understands that there is actually very little urine in the bladder and encourage the resident to extend toileting times. If the resident is cognitively intact, teach him or her urge inhibition techniques to delay voiding (see previous section on Bladder Retraining). Ask the resident to delay voiding for 15–30 minutes.

3. Monitor fluid intake because these residents often intentionally decrease fluid intake for fear of becoming incontinent or having to use the bathroom too often. Education and demonstration with the bladder scanner help residents realize that increasing fluid intake actually improves bladder function.

An 84-year-old female resident, continent of bowel and bladder, put on her call light every 15 minutes requesting assistance to the toilet. When taken to the bathroom, she was unable to void. The resident reported to the staff that she was not drinking liquids because she feared being incontinent and not being able to make it to the bathroom on time. The staff were able to convince the resident to let them scan her bladder before toileting to show her the amount of urine that was in her bladder and whether she needed to void. The resident was reluctant at first and stated, "When I've gotta go, I've gotta go. There ain't no contraption that's gonna tell me when to go to the bathroom."

Through much persuasion and visual education regarding the bladder scanner, the staff were able to get her to agree to allow them to scan her bladder to measure volume. The resident slowly increased her fluid intake and was able to use the toilet on a more regular schedule. The staff used the scanner to show the resident her increasing bladder volumes and when those volumes necessitated voiding. Within a couple of weeks, the resident was more comfortable, and the staff did not have to answer the resident's call bell every 15 minutes. The resident's fear of incontinence decreased, incontinence products were eliminated, and the voiding interval improved to every 3–4 hours.

PELVIC MUSCLE REHABILITATION

In the late 1940s, Dr. Arnold Kegel implemented a comprehensive program of progressive contractions of the pelvic floor muscles (PFMs)—specifically the levator ani muscle, which is under voluntary control—conducted under direct supervision by a trained nurse and incorporating biofeedback technology. These Kegel exercises, or pelvic muscle exercises (PMEs), also known as pelvic floor muscle training, were shown to decrease urine leakage in women with stress UI (Fantl et al., 1996). PMEs consist of repeated, high-intensity contractions of the muscles of the pelvic floor. A strong and fast pelvic muscle contraction will cause closure of the urethra and increase urethral pressure to prevent leakage during sudden increases in intra-abdominal pressure. PMEs will also press the urethra against the pubic symphysis to create a mechanical pressure rise and will prevent urethral descent during increases in intra-abdominal pressure. The pelvic muscle "reflex" contraction will precede increases in bladder pressure and may inhibit bladder contraction.

As part of a rehabilitation program, PMEs increase support to the urethral sphincter and detrusor muscle, thereby preventing stress, urge, and mixed UI. They are most appropriate in people who

- Do not have cognitive impairments
- Are motivated to comply with the program
- Have a pelvic floor that is neurologically intact

The goal of pelvic muscle training is to isolate the PFMs, specifically the levator ani. The PFMs are a striated, skeletal muscle group that is under voluntary control and are important to maintaining urinary and fecal continence and to providing urogenital support (see Figures 8.2 and 8.3). The functional demands on the fibers of the PFMs include sustaining force over time, especially during increases in intra-abdominal pressure; developing force quickly; and contracting and relaxing voluntarily. During voiding, the person must relax the PFMs to open the external urethral sphincter to allow voiding. When these muscles do not function properly, women in particular may develop stress UI, fecal incontinence, and pelvic organ prolapse.

The PFMs consist of two types of muscle fibers: Type I, or slow-twitch muscle fibers, and Type II, or fast-twitch muscle fibers. At least 65% of the levator ani muscle consists of Type I muscle fibers. These fibers produce less force on contraction and assist in improving muscle endurance by generating a slower, more sustained, but less intense contraction. Over time, the continuous though lower intensity contraction of these muscle fibers maintains a general level of support and urethral closure pressure. Type I muscle fibers are also fatigue resistant. Type II, or fast-twitch fibers, aid in strong and forceful contractions. These fibers come into play during sudden increases in intra-abdominal pressure by contributing to urethral closure. These fibers are like the leg muscles used during a sprint; they are powerful and explosive. Muscle inactivity, aging, and innervation damage can contribute to a decrease in the proportion of Type II fibers. Because these Type II fibers fatigue easily, people with UI are taught to perform a small number of PMEs. By exercising these fibers, pelvic muscle strength will increase.

Dr. Kegel described four phases in the performance of the exercises:

1. Awareness of the function and coordination of the PFM muscles. For older adults and people whose pelvic muscles are severely relaxed, this may take several weeks.

2. Gains over muscle identification, control, and strength. Muscle strength is the maximal force that can be generated by the PFMs. Because the PFMs must adapt to different or changing requirements, they must have contractibility and build force quickly when contracting.

3. Firmness, thickening, broadening, and bulking of the muscles to increase muscle endurance. Muscle endurance is a performance characteristic that indicates the ability of the PFMs to execute repeated contractions to an initial level of strength often called a "submaximum" contraction.

4. Improvements of the symptoms indicating that the muscles are strengthening. At this point, some people believe that their incontinence is so improved that regular exercising is no longer needed; however, persons need to incorporate exercises in routine daily activities.

Instruction on the correct technique of PMEs is important. Many people may have a difficult time identifying and isolating these muscles. Inability to

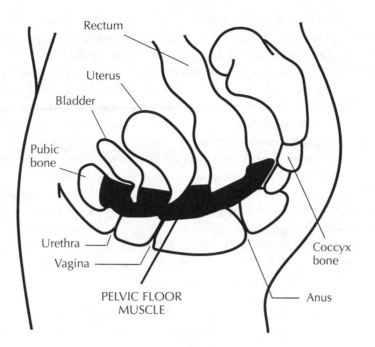

Figure 8.2. Location of pelvic floor muscles in women.

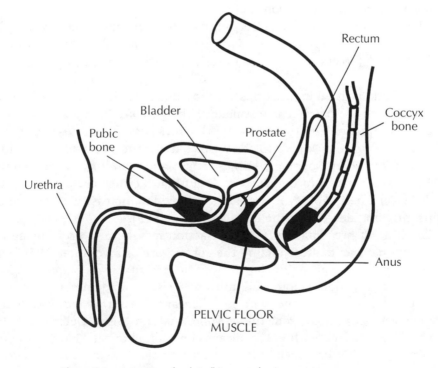

Figure 8.3. Location of pelvic floor muscles in men.

isolate and identify the pelvic muscle will usually cause contraction of accessory muscles, primarily the gluteal and abdominal muscles. The gluteal muscles attach to the posterior aspect of the pelvis as well as the femur. Because they are a large muscle group, they can overpower the pelvic muscles. For this reason, the gluteal muscles should be relaxed. The abdominal muscles attach to the pubic bone. If contracted, they will increase pressure on the bladder, pelvic, and urogenital muscles, which will make pelvic muscle contraction more difficult. In addition to contracting the pelvic muscles, some clients may benefit by combining contraction of both pelvic muscles and the internal obturator muscle. This can be accomplished by having the client stand with feet turned outward and slightly more than hip width. Instruct the client to do a plié by bending the knees 2 inches to 3 inches as they pull up and in with the pelvic muscles. They should hold this position for 10 seconds then return to upright position and relax for 10 seconds.

This may be a difficult exercise for older, unsteady women. Without sufficient information, the person may mistakenly bear down or exercise ineffectively. Specifically, women are told to "draw in" and "lift up" the perivaginal and anal sphincter muscles (see Appendix A: How to Do Pelvic Muscle Exercises). Once the person is able to identify the correct muscles, he or she is instructed to perform a series of "quick flicks," or 2-second contractions, followed by sustained contractions of 5 seconds or longer (endurance contractions) as part of a daily exercise regimen. At least 10 seconds of relaxation is recommended between each contraction. The individual is encouraged to aim for a high level of concentrated effort with each pelvic muscle contraction because greater contraction intensity is associated with improvement in pelvic muscle strength (Bo et al., 1990; Bo, Talseth, & Holme, 1999; Dougherty et al., 1993).

Verbal and written instructions are provided for a daily exercise program that is based on the baseline assessment of the person's PFM strength, as assessed by contraction endurance during the initial assessment session. People are instructed to exercise two to three times daily and optimally to perform the exercises in three positions: lying, sitting, and standing. A minimum of 30–45 PMEs per day is recommended. A gradual increase in number of contractions over a period of PME practice is believed to increase muscle strength significantly and decrease urine loss (Newman, 1999).

Teaching of preventative PFM contraction may help to avoid urine loss with exertional events. Recognizing the correct use of a voluntary PFM contraction to prevent leakage during a stressful activity is an acquired motor skill. PFM contraction before and during a rise in abdominal pressure is termed the Knack because the word *knack* means a task that requires dexterity or a clever way of doing something (Miller, Ashton-Miller, DeLancey, 1998). The Knack, when used with PMEs, means contraction of the PFMs just before and throughout the time of the physical activity that increases intra-abdominal pressure and causes urine leakage. The individual should be instructed to contract the PFMs at the time of a UI episode (e.g., when coughing, on the way to the bathroom; Miller, Ashton-Miller, & Delancey, 1996). In addition, contracting them before such activities as sneezing, coughing, lifting, standing up, or swinging a golf club can prevent stress UI from occurring (see Appendix A: Pelvic Muscle Exercises During Activities of Daily Living).

The PFMs also can be contracted when the individual feels a strong urge to void. Results may not occur until after 6–8 weeks of exercise, and optimal results usually take longer. Self-monitoring through the use of a calendar record and audio- and videotaped material that reviews the exercises can improve protocol compliance.

A large body of research has demonstrated the efficacy of behavioral intervention that includes PMEs. The majority of PME research has used biofeedback therapy to teach the exercises (see Use of Biofeedback Therapy later in this chapter). The 1996 clinical guideline on urinary incontinence in adults (Fantl et al., 1996) outlined the research that demonstrated that PMEs are indicated for people with stress incontinence and can reduce urgency and prevent urge UI. PFM reeducation has proven to be effective in women with sphincter deficiency and detrusor instability (Association of Women's Health, Obstetric and Neonatal Nurses, 2000a, 2000b; Burgio et al., 1998; Holtedahl, Verelst, & Schieflow, 1998; Sampselle et al., 1998, 2000a, 2000b; Wyman, Fantl, McClish, & Bump, 1998). Burgio et al. (1998) reported a mean 80.7% reduction of incontinence in their research on older women with urge UI. A study of older women living in rural counties in Florida employed a sequenced use of behavioral interventions (prevention/lifestyle changes, bladder retraining, and biofeedback PMEs) based on the woman's personal goals (Dougherty et al., 2002). At 2 years, the UI severity had decreased by 61%. Self-monitoring (fluid volume, elimination of caffeinated beverages, bowel regulation, and reduction of nocturia) and bladder retraining was felt to account for most of the improvement.

Long-term studies have demonstrated that improvement persists over time (Bo & Talseth, 1996). Practice of PMEs in women pregnant with their first child resulted in fewer UI symptoms during late pregnancy and postpartum (Sampselle et al., 1998). Behavioral modifications, pelvic muscle rehabilitation, and bladder retraining programs have successfully decreased UI in homebound older people (Flynn, Cell, & Luisi, 1994; McDowell et al., 1999; McDowell, Engberg, Weber, Brodak, & Engberg, 1994; Rose, Baigis-Smith, Smith, & Newman, 1990). A study of men with UI following radical prostate surgery showed that 88% of the treatment group achieved continence in 3 months using PMEs, compared to 56% of the control group (Van Kampen et al., 2000). Another study (Burgio, Locher, & Goode, 2000) examined the effects of combining behavioral treatment and drug treatment for urge UI in ambulatory women. The subjects' reduction of incontinence went from a mean of 57.5% with behavior therapy alone to a mean of 88.5% with combined behavior and drug (anticholinergic) treatment.

Use of Biofeedback Therapy

The goal in using biofeedback as a treatment for UI is to alter the responses of the detrusor and pelvic muscles, which control urine loss. Biofeedback teaches the person how to control the external sphincter by measuring the action of the PFMs and "feeding back" to the person information about how well the muscles are performing. The information is stored, processed, and fed back to the person in the form of sound, lights, or images (see Figure 8.4). Information about the status and condition of PFMs, pelvic nerves, and bladder function is immediately accessible and can be interpreted simultaneously by both the clinician and client. Biofeedback therapy is also used as treatment for muscle dysfunction (abnormality).

Motivation and active participation play a big part in the success of biofeedback therapy. Biofeedback therapy can be performed lying, standing, or sitting in a chair. For incontinence, biofeedback therapy uses computer graphs or lights as a teaching tool to help people identify and learn to control the correct muscles. Biofeedback helps the individual locate the pelvic muscles by changing the graph or light when the correct muscle is squeezed or tightened. Optimal biofeedback therapy includes visualization of both pelvic and abdominal muscle movement; therefore, a two-channel system is preferable.

Generally, visual, auditory, and verbal feedback techniques are used for neuromuscular conditioning. These methods help to reinforce a particular task being performed. For example, a monitor screen can be used to display the pressure of the anal sphincter as electromyographic changes, providing instant visual feedback to the individual regarding his or her performance. Similarly, during muscle contraction, the intensity (pitch of the electrical activity) of the sphincter muscle contraction provides corresponding auditory feedback to the person regarding performance. Throughout the training session, the clinician reinforces the client's behavior and provides compliments and other appropriate advice. This constitutes verbal feedback to the client. All three maneuvers are complimentary.

Several tests can be used to measure pelvic muscle activity. The electromyogram (EMG) measures activity through electrodes placed on the skin surface or sensors that are inserted into the vagina or rectum. EMG feedback uses electronic instrumentation to detect and feed back the myoelectric signals from the muscle to the client. Manometry, or pressure feedback, can only be done by inserting sensors into the vagina or rectum. By contracting the PFMs against the sensor, the EMG displays PFM contraction, allowing the client to identify and isolate the correct muscle group. To determine outcome of PMEs, two indices that can be recorded by electromyography or manometry are recommended—the peak muscle contraction value (strength) and the average muscle contraction (endurance)—in addition to other factors:

• Strength, recorded as the peak maximum pressure (the highest waveforms) and the ability to sustain or hold the contraction

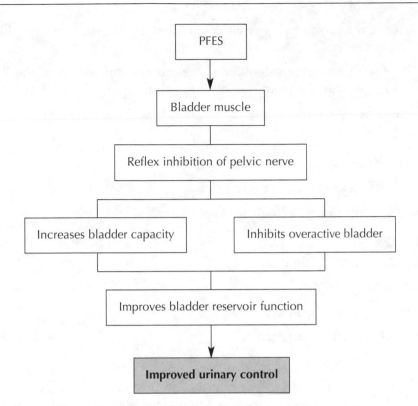

Figure 8.6. Pelvic floor electrical stimulation (PFES) for urge incontinence. (Courtesy of Empi)

pulses per second (PPS). The optimal frequency of electrical stimulation is determined by how quickly the impulses pass through the nerve being targeting (conduction velocity). The lower ranges (13 Hz) will inhibit the bladder, so they are used for people with urge UI; the higher ranges (50 Hz) are optimum for urethral closure. High frequency (50 PPS) builds strength (bulks up muscle, increases urethral closure). Low frequency (13 PPS) has a calming effect on the detrusor muscle, thus decreasing inhibited bladder contractions.

5. *"On" time* is the amount of time that the electrical current is delivered to the muscle. *"Off" time* is the amount of time when there is no electrical current to the muscle, allowing it to recover. The time needed to allow the muscle to recover is determined by the clinician using the following guidelines:

- At no time should the exposure to the electrical current be at more than a 1-to-1 ratio; in other words, the time when the current is off should never be less than the time when it is on.

- In many cases, a 1-to-2 ratio, with 1 representing on time and 2 representing off time, will be the most appropriate (e.g., 5 seconds on, 10 seconds off). This is especially true in the beginning stages of therapy when the person has very weak muscle strength, or when using higher frequencies.

There are no adverse side effects to electrical stimulation of the PFMs, but PFES is contraindicated in the following situations:

Complete denervation of the pelvic floor (PFMs will not respond)

Dementia

Demand cardiac pacemaker

Unstable or serious cardiac arrhythmia

Pregnancy or planning/attempting pregnancy

Rectal bleeding

Active infection (UTI/vaginal)

Unstable seizure disorder

Swollen, painful hemorrhoids

Presence of vaginal vault prolapse

Pelvic surgery in past 6 months

Electrical stimulation can be performed in the clinician's office or may be prescribed as a home program using a battery-operated home unit. The home program consists of using the stimulator for 15 minutes twice a day for several weeks to months. It is recommended that the person perform PFES initially in the lying (side) position until he or she becomes comfortable changing to the seated position.

REFERENCES

Association of Women's Health, Obstetric and Neonatal Nurses. (2000a). *Evidence-based clinical practice guideline: Continence for women*. Washington, DC: Author.

Association of Women's Health, Obstetric and Neonatal Nurses. (2000b). *Quick care guide: Continence for women*. Washington, DC: Author.

Bo, K., Hagen, R.M., Kvarstein, B., Jorgensen, J., & Larsen, S. (1990). Pelvic floor muscle exercises for the treatment of female stress urinary incontinence: III. Effects of two different degrees of pelvic floor muscle exercises. *Neurourology & Urodynamics, 9*(5), 489–502.

Bo, K., & Talseth, T. (1996). Long-term effect of pelvic floor muscle exercise 5 years after cessation of organized training. *Obstetrics and Gynecology, 87,* 261–265.

Bo, K., Talseth, T., & Holme, I. (1999). Single-blind, randomized controlled trial of pelvic floor exercises, electrical stimulation, vaginal cones and no treatment of genuine stress urinary incontinence in women. *British Medical Journal, 318,* 487–493.

Boyington, A.R., & Dougherty, M.C. (2000). Pelvic muscle exercise effect on pelvic muscle performance in women. *International Urogynecology Journal and Pelvic Floor Dysfunction, 11,* 212–218.

Burgio, K.L., Locher, J.L., & Goode, P.S. (2000). Combined behavioral and drug therapy for urge incontinence in older women. *Journal of the American Geriatrics Society, 48,* 370–374.

Burgio, K.L., Locher, J.L., Goode, P.S., Hardin, J.M., McDowell, B.J., Dombrowski, M., & Candib, D. (1998). Behavioral vs. drug treatment for urge urinary incontinence in older women: A randomized controlled trial. *Journal of the American Medical Association, 280*(23), 1995–2000.

Burgio, L.D., & Burgio, K. (1990). Institutional staff training and management: A review of the literature and a model for geriatric long-term care facilities. *International Journal of Aging and Human Development, 30,* 287–302.

Colling, J., Ouslander, J., Hadley, B.J., Eisch, J., & Campbell, E. (1992). The effects of patterned urge response toileting (PURT) on urinary incontinence among nursing home residents. *Journal of the American Geriatrics Society, 40,* 135–141.

Dougherty, M., Bishop, K., Mooney, R., Gimotty, P., & Williams, B. (1993) Graded pelvic muscle exercise. Effect on stress urinary incontinence. *Journal of Reproductive Medicine, 39*(9), 684–691.

Dougherty, M.C., Dwyer, J.W., Pendergast, J.F., Boyington, A.R., Tomlinson, B.U., Coward, R.T., Duncan, R.P., Vogel, B., & Rooks, L.G. (2002). A randomized trial of behavioral management for continence with older rural women. *Research in Nursing and Health, 25,* 3–13.

Dougherty, M.C., Dwyer, J.W., Pendergast, J.F., Tomlinson, B.U., Boyington, A.R., Vogel, W.B., Duncan, R.P., Coward, R.T., & Cox, C.L. (1998). Community-based nursing: Continence care for older rural women. *Nursing Outlook, 46*(5), 233–244.

Engberg, S.J., McDowell, B.J., Weber, E., Brodak, I., Donovan, N., & Engberg R. (1997). Assessment and management of urinary incontinence among homebound older adults: A clinical trial protocol. *Advanced Practice Nursing Quarterly, 3*(2), 48 56.

Fantl, J., Newman, D., Colling, J., et al., for the Urinary Incontinence in Adults Guideline Update Panel. (1996). *Urinary incontinence in adults: Acute and chronic management. Clinical practice guideline* (No. 2. Update; AHCPR Publication No. 96-0692). Rockville, MD: Agency for Health Care and Policy Research.

Fantl, J.A., Wyman, J.F., McClish, D.K., Harkins, S.W., Elswick, R.K., Taylor. J.R., & Hadley, E.C. (1991). Efficacy of bladder training in older women with urinary incontinence. *Journal of the American Medical Association, 265*(5), 609–613.

Flynn, L., Cell, P., & Luisi, E. (1994). Effectiveness of pelvic muscle in reducing urge incontinence among community residing elders. *Journal of Gerontological Nursing, 20*(5), 23–27.

Holtedahl, K., Verelst, M., & Schieflow, A. (1998). A population based, randomized, controlled trial of conservative treatment of urinary incontinence in women. *Acta Obstetricia et Gynecologica Scandinavica, 46,* 870–874.

Lekan-Rutledge, D. (2000). Diffusion of innovation. *Journal of Gerontological Nursing, 26(4),* 25–33.

McDowell, B.J., Engberg, S., Sereika, S., Donovan, N., Jubeck, M.E., Weber, E., & Engberg, R. (1999). Effectiveness of behavioral therapy to treat incontinence in homebound older adults. *Journal of the American Geriatrics Society, 47*(3), 309–318.

McDowell, B.J., Engberg, S., Weber, E., Brodak, I., & Engberg, R. (1994). Successful treatment using behavioral interventions of urinary incontinence in homebound older adults. *Geriatric Nursing, 15*(6), 303–307.

Miller, J., Ashton-Miller, J.A., & DeLancey, J.O.L. (1996). The Knack: Use of precisely timed pelvic muscle exercise contraction can reduce leakage in SUI. *Neurourology & Urodynamics, 15,* 302–393.

Miller, J.M., Ashton-Miller, J.A., & DeLancey, J.O.L. (1998). A pelvic muscle contraction can reduce cough-related urine loss in selected women with mild stress urinary incontinence. *Journal of the American Geriatrics Society, 46*(7), 870–874.

Newman, D.K. (1999). *The urinary incontinence sourcebook* (2nd ed.). Los Angeles: Lowell House.

Newman, D.K. (2000). *Continence for women: Research-based practice*. Washington DC: Association of Women's Health, Obstetric and Neonatal Nurses.

Ouslander, J.G., Maloney, C., Gravel, T.H., Rogers, L., & Salamaner, C.A. (2001). Implementation of a nursing home urinary incontinence management program with and without tolterodine. *Journal of the American Medical Directors Association, 2,* 207–214.

Ouslander, J.G., Schnelle, J.F., Uman, G., Fingold, S., Nigam, J.G., Tuico, E., & Bates-Jensen, B. (1995). Predictors of successful prompted voiding among incontinent nursing home residents. *Journal of the American Medical Association, 273*(17), 1366–1370.

Palmer, M.H., Bennett, R.G., Marks, J., McCormick, K.A., & Engel, B.T. (1994). Urinary incontinence: A program that works. *Journal of Long Term Care Administration, 22* (2), 19–25.

Pinkowski, P.S. (1996). Prompted voiding in the long-term care facility. *Journal of Wound Ostomy and Continence Nursing, 23*(2), 110–114.

Rose, M.A., Baigis-Smith, J., Smith, D., & Newman, D.K. (1990). Behavioral management of urinary incontinence in homebound older adults. *Home Health Nursing, 8,* 10–15.

Sale, P.G., & Wyman, J.F. (1994). Achievement of goals associated with bladder training by older incontinent women. *Research Briefs* (pp. 93–96). Philadelphia: W B Saunders.

Sampselle, C.M., Miller, J.M., Mims, B.L., Delancey, J.O.L., Ashton-Miller, J.A., & Antonakos, C.L. (1998). Effect of pelvic muscle exercise on transient incontinence during pregnancy and after birth. *Obstetrics and Gynecology, 91,* 406–412.

Sampselle, C.M., Wyman, J.F., Thomas, K.K., Newman, D.K., Gray, M., Dougherty, M., & Burns, P.A. (2000a). Continence for women: A test of AWHONN's evidence-based protocol in clinical practice. *Journal of Obstetric, Gynecologic, and Neonatal Nursing, 29*(1), 18–26.

Sampselle, C.M., Wyman, J.F., Thomas, K.K., Newman, D.K., Gray, M., Dougherty, M., & Burns, P.A. (2000b). Continence for women: Evaluation of AWHONN's third research utilization project. *Journal of Obstetric, Gynecologic, and Neonatal Nursing, 29*(1), 9–17.

Schnelle, J.F. (1990). Treatment of urinary incontinence in nursing home patients by prompted voiding. *Journal of the American Geriatrics Society, 38,* 356–360.

Schnelle, J.F., Newman, D.R., & Fogarty, T. (1990). Management of patient continence in long-term care nursing facilities. *Gerontologist, 30,* 373–376.

Schnelle, J.F., Newman, D.R., White, M., Abbey, J., Wallston, K.A., Fogarty, T., & Ory, M.G. (1993). Maintaining continence in NH clients through the application of industrial quality control. *Gerontologist, 33,* 114–121.

Tobani, L., & Fantl, J.A. (1999, March/April). Urinary incontinence in women and the use of bladder training for its management. *Mature Medicine,* 90–93.

Van Kampen, M., De Weerdt, W., Van Poppel, H., DeRidder, D., Feys, H., & Baert, L. (2000). Effect of pelvic-floor re-education on duration and degree of incontinence after radical prostatectomy: A randomised controlled trial. *Lancet, 355*(8), 98–102.

Wilson, P.D., Bo, K., Bourcier, A., Hay-Smith, J., Staskin, D., Nygaard, I., Wyman, J., & Shepard, A. (1999). Conservative management in women. In P. Abrams, S. Khoury, & A. Wein (Eds.), *Incontinence proceedings from the First International Consultation on Incontinence* (pp. 579–636.). Plymouth, UK: Health Publications.

Woolridge, L. (2000, June). Ultrasound technology and bladder dysfunction. *American Journal of Nursing,*(Suppl.), 3–14.

Wyman, J.F., & Fantl, J.A. (1991). Bladder training in ambulatory care management of urinary incontinence. *Urologic Nursing, 11,* 11–17.

Wyman, J.F., Fantl, J.A., McClish, D.K., & Bump, R.C. (1998). Comparative efficacy of behavioral interventions in the management of female urinary incontinence. *American Journal of Obstetrics and Gynecology, 179*(4), 999–1007.

9

Urinary Collection and Management Products

Each year, millions of Americans, primarily older adults in acute care hospitals, extended care facilities, and their homes, use urinary collection (often referred to as containment) devices (Warren, 1997). Catheters, devices, and absorbent products used to contain or collect urine are a part of the management of bladder dysfunction. The objective for using these products is for the person to remain as dry as possible while preserving dignity and quality of life. The role of urinary collection devices in managing urinary incontinence (UI) is viewed by clinicians and caregivers as an essential adjunct of treatment for most people with UI. Brink (1996) stated that the products used for incontinence are effective as primary management in those individuals who 1) are unable to achieve any effects from interventions, 2) have advanced dementia and are cognitively unable to respond to standard treatment, and 3) are bed bound or frail and are not candidates for other treatments. These products also relieve caregiver burden and act as a supplement to bladder retraining programs in those individuals undergoing treatment. People who use containment devices are classified as being "socially" continent and are managed by the most appropriate product technology.

Even though these products are an integral part of the nursing care of people with urinary dysfunction, there is little to no research on their long-term use. In Great Britain, government-funded, multicenter evaluations of urinary collection devices provided research-based evidence for product selection (Fader, Cottenden, & Brooks, 2001). This chapter reviews the use of these products.

CATHETERS

A catheter is used for two common medical problems: UI and urinary retention. To ease these conditions, the catheter is put into the bladder to drain the urine. It may stay in place for a short or long time depending on the type

of catheter and the reason for its use. Catheters are used in several different ways:

- They are put intermittently into the bladder (*intermittent catheterization*).

- They are placed in the bladder on a more permanent basis (*indwelling urethral catheterization*).

- They are inserted into the bladder through the abdomen (*suprapubic
catheterization*).

- They are used on the outside of the body for men (*external condom catheters*).

Most of the medical literature states that infection should be the factor when
deciding which type of catheter to use for people requiring urinary collection. Yet most professionals in clinical practice would agree that the use of
catheters is governed by caregiver/client preference and ease of urinary management. Figure 9.1 shows suprapubic and urethral catheters.

Indwelling Urethral (Foley) Catheters

An indwelling urethral (Foley) catheter is a closed sterile system inserted
through the urethra to allow for bladder drainage. In the 1930s, Frederick
Foley designed a rubber tube with a separate lumen used to inflate a balloon
to hold the catheter in place in the bladder (Newman & Blackwood, 1991).
Historically, indwelling catheters have been used in older adults with chronic
medical conditions. Indwelling urethral catheters are currently being used to
relieve urinary retention and to manage long-term UI, and are being supervised primarily by nurses. However, this type of "management" or drainage
system has several medical and nursing care problems. Long-term use of these
catheters, defined as greater than 30 days, provides access for bacteria from a
contaminated environment into a vulnerable body organ and system. As a result, catheter-associated urinary tract infections (UTIs) are the most common
type of infection acquired in hospitals and long-term care (LTC) facilities. Indwelling catheters are associated with multiple complications and side effects
as well as increased morbidity and mortality. Long-term catheterization should
only be used as a last resort in the person with UI.

Indications for Use   Indications for catheter use are based on guidelines developed by the Agency for Health Care Policy and Research (Fantl
et al., 1996). The use of an indwelling (Foley) catheter is allowed on a long-term
basis in people residing in skilled nursing facilities in the following instances:

1. Urethral obstruction or urinary retention is present with the following
   conditions:

   a. Persistent overflow incontinence, symptomatic infections, or kidney
      disease

   b. Surgical or pharmacological interventions have been unsuccessful or
      there are clinical reasons they would not be appropriate for the par-
      ticular resident

   c. Intermittent catheterization in a resident with retention is contraindicated

2. When irreversible medical conditions are present and bed, clothing, and
absorbent product changes may be painful or disruptive (e.g., metastatic
terminal disease, coma, end stages of other conditions such as congestive
heart failure or chronic obstructive pulmonary disease)

3. In residents who have incontinence and grade 3 or 4 pressure ulcers that
are not healing because of continual urine leakage

An additional indication has been applied to people who are being cared for
in their homes when the person or caregiver, or both, prefer the indwelling
catheter for management of UI or retention and do not want or cannot pursue
other management options. This may occur despite efforts to educate the per-

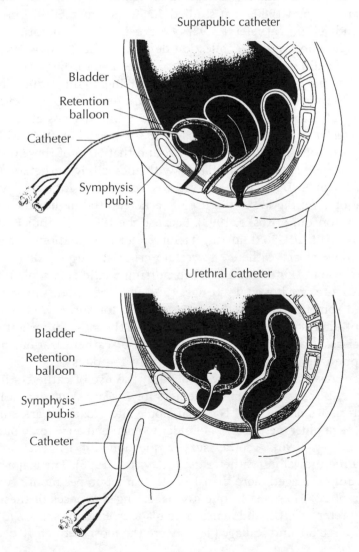

Figure 9.1. Suprapubic and urethral catheters. (Courtesy of Bard)

son and caregiver as to the risks associated with use of the catheter. In many cases, the person may live alone and a caregiver is unavailable to provide other management options.

In the medical literature, the short-term use of these catheters has been documented in hospitalized patients. However, the number of people who use a catheter indefinitely to manage UI or because of urinary retention has not been well documented in medical or nursing research. The settings where the prevalence of long-term indwelling catheter usage is the greatest are 1) skilled nursing facilities with residents with UI and 2) homes where the person requires skilled nursing visits. In the home care setting, the prevalence of indwelling catheters is increasing with the increasing numbers of older adults.

Prevalence of indwelling catheter use in skilled nursing facilities has been documented in three studies. Warren, Steinberg, Hebel, and Tenney (1989) completed a randomized certified sample of nine Maryland nursing facilities in the mid-1980s that studied 4,259 residents. Of 972 men, 6.4% were using indwelling catheters, 5.9% were using condom catheters, and 2.7% were using another urine collection device. In the 3,287 women, 9.4% were using indwelling catheters and 0.7% were using other urine collection devices. An analysis of Virginia Medicaid nursing facility admissions from 1984 to 1985 found that 15.2% of residents had urethral catheterizations, with the majority of indwelling catheters inserted 9 months postadmission (Moseley, 1994). Ouslander, Kane, and Abrass (1982) reported on 954 residents in seven nursing facilities in California. They found that 50% of these residents had UI and, of these, 28% were managed with indwelling catheters. Of that 28%, 43% developed UTIs. Catheter rates were used to indicate level of nursing quality of care: the lower the use of catheters, the higher the quality of care (Zinn, Aaronson, & Rosko, 1993). Because the 1990 Omnibus Budget Reconciliation Act (PL 101-508) nursing facility reform regulations limited the use of indwelling urinary catheters to certain criteria, the prevalence of indwelling catheter use in United States skilled nursing facilities has fallen to 7%.

In acute care hospital settings, 15%–25% of patients may have a catheter inserted sometime during their stay, usually for surgery, urine output measurement, urinary retention, and UI. Because the most important risk factor for catheter-associated bacteriuria is duration of catheterization, most catheters in hospitalized patients are placed for only 2–4 days.

Few research studies have looked at the use of catheters in homebound people. A publication from the Centers for Disease Control and Prevention on characteristics of the 1994 National Home and Hospice Care Survey reported that 12% of older men and 7% of older women had an ostomy or an indwelling catheter (Day, 1996). Another survey questioned 471 agencies from 45 states concerning indwelling catheter use (ConvaTec, 1996). The majority of agencies responding managed more than 16 Foley catheters per month, with a national average of 28. The most frequently occurring diagnoses of these clients were urinary retention, UI, and neurogenic bladder. Bladder spasms (37%), catheter blockage (48%), and leakage (48%) were the most frequently occurring problems, necessitating unscheduled client visits for almost half (46%) of these agencies. Chronic UTI was reported as a problem in most clients, with one to two episodes per year. It is thought that catheter use in clients requiring skilled nursing visits increases overall costs and number of nursing visits and contributes to nursing care problems. In fact, one visiting nurse agency noted that the presence of catheters in clients with UI meant the continuation of skilled nursing services, home health aide services, and Medicare-covered catheter supplies (Newman, Parente, & Yuan, 1997).

Catheter-Related Complications Clients with indwelling Foley catheters are at increased risk for catheter-related problems that range from simple obstruction (blockage) to serious infections, *sepsis,* and death (Fantl et al., 1996). Catheter-associated complications occur frequently. The most severe and common complication, which can lead to urosepsis and septicemia, involves nosocomial infections, which are common in acute and LTC settings.

Bacteriuria Bacteriuria usually occurs within 2–4 weeks after the catheter is inserted and is due to the presence of a foreign object, the catheter (Warren, 1997). There are three catheter-associated entry points for bacteria: the urethral meatus, the junction of the catheter–bag connection, and the drainage port of the collection bag. Microorganisms that are present on the meatus or distal urethra can be transferred directly into the bladder during the insertion of the catheter (Sedor & Muholland, 1999). Although insertion of an indwelling catheter is a sterile procedure, depending on the technique and setting, bacteria can enter the system at the time of insertion. In acute and long-term care, sterility is usually not a problem because additional skilled staff are available to assist the nurse doing the catheterization with positioning the person and maintaining the sterile field. However, in the home care environment, where sometimes the nurse is the only other individual in the home, it is hard to maintain sterility, especially in women, because of inadequate lighting and positioning. In women, it is important to clearly see the perineum and urethral meatus, so the woman should lie on her back with her legs bent at the knees. Catheters should be inserted aseptically using sterile equipment. Gloves should be worn, the person should be draped, and the urinary meatus should be cleansed using an antiseptic solution (e.g., povidone-iodine [Betadine]).

The second entry point for bacteria is the junction of the catheter tubing and drainage bag. If possible, the catheter should not be disconnected from the drainage tube for any purpose. Each time the system is disconnected, bacteria can enter the system. The third point of entry for bacteria is the drainage bag outlet port. All drainage bags should be kept off the floor and the outlet tube should not be dragged. Selecting a bag that prevents migration of bacteria through this port (antireflux chamber) would be preferable. Two catheter hygiene principles should be used to prevent bacteriuria: use a "closed" system and remove the catheter as soon as possible (Warren, 1997). The basic components of a closed system include the catheter, a preconnected collecting tube with an attached sampling port, and a vented drainage bag with a port for drainage. To maintain integrity of the sterile closed system, urine samples should be collected aseptically through the sampling port. When obtaining a urine specimen, the specimen port should be wiped with disinfectant (e.g., alcohol) before and after sampling. Catheter-associated bacteriuria is usually asymptomatic and uncomplicated and resolves after the catheter is removed.

Urinary Tract Infection   UTIs are the most common complication associated with long-term use of indwelling catheters and may occur at least twice a year, requiring hospitalization. The risk of infection is related to the length of time the catheter is in place, and in most clients UTI is inevitable. Infection is more common in women than men because of anatomical differences. The urethra in women is only 1.5 cm in length, and the proximity of the anus to the urethra causes migration of *Escherichia coli*, the organism most frequently seen in catheter-related infections.

A problem in hospitals and LTC facilities is infection with vancomycin-resistant *enterococci* (VRE) and methicillin-resistant *Staphylococcus aureus* (MRSA). Residents in LTC facilities are believed to be especially at risk because of their exposure to patients transferred from acute care hospitals, where VRE and MRSA prevalence rates are high. If individuals with VRE are identified and isolated at the time of admission to the LTC facility, the chance of spreading VRE is low (Silverblatt et al., 2000; Terpenning et al., 1994). In addition to identification and isolation of residents, staff should practice strict hand washing and standard precautions (single room, gowns and gloves, and additional cleansing) to prevent spread of the organism resulting from environmental contamination.

Despite common belief by LTC staff, an indwelling catheter does not carry infections. However, catheters are a good medium for bacterial growth because bacterial biofilms (layers of organisms) adhere to the many surfaces of the catheter system (Fiers, 1994; Morris, Stickler, & Mclean, 1999). Because bacteria migration occurs both inside and along the outside of the catheter, it is recommended that the drainage bag be emptied at least every 4 hours, if at all possible.

Catheter-related infections are difficult to eliminate by antibiotic therapy while the catheter remains in place. Standard practice is to treat with antibiotic therapy only those infected individuals whose symptoms suggest that the bloodstream or upper renal tracts (kidneys) have been infected (Warren, 1997). Cranberry juice or tablets are increasingly being recommended to prevent and treat UTIs (Avorn et al., 1994; Dignam et al., 1998; Kuzminski, 1996). Urine acidification also can be promoted with the use of ascorbic acid (1,000 mg daily).

Urosepsis   Urosepsis can result from frequent and repeated UTIs leading to sepsis, and death from severe UTIs has been reported. Mortality has been documented as more than three times higher in catheterized than in noncatheterized individuals. In the past, standard practice was catheter irrigation to "wash out" the bacteria; however, it has been shown that the use of such irrigation to prevent or eradicate bacteria in indwelling catheters is ineffective because more organisms will gain entry to the irrigated catheters through disconnection of the system. Also, research has proven that use of prophylactic antibiotics, antimicrobials, or both, is not of any benefit in preventing symptomatic UTI (Fantl et al., 1996; Nicolle, 2001; Warren, 1997).

Other Complications   *Bladder stones* occur in at least 8% of people with indwelling catheters. Therefore, people with these catheters should be seen by a urologist annually. The urologist will perform a cystoscopy to determine the environment within the bladder and the presence of stones or cancer.

Three primary types of urethral damage can result from use of an indwelling catheter:

1. *Urethritis*, or inflammation of the urethral meatus, is seen and may be due to frequent insertion of catheters.

2. *Erosion of the urethra* occurs in people, especially men, who have had indwelling catheters for a long period of time. This erosion is usually secondary to catheter tension on the distal urethra at the meatus.

3. *Creation of a false passage* can occur primarily in men with persisting urethral strictures. Men with enlargement of the prostate gland are most at risk.

Other complications include

Urethral fistulas can occur in people being managed long term with a urethral catheter. Fistula formation develops in women between the bladder and the anterior vaginal wall. Many times the woman who has developed a fistula will complain of leakage and drainage from the vagina. Fistula formation occurs in men between the prostate and urethra.

Epididymitis caused by urethral and bladder inflammation, and *scrotal abscess*, are seen in men.

Hematuria occurs in people who have long-term catheters and is a possible sign of bladder cancer or kidney stones. Some bleeding may occur during catheter insertion, but, if the bleeding persists, the physician should be notified.

Bladder cancer can occur in some people using catheters. Those most at risk for developing squamous cell carcinoma are long-term catheter users.

Types of Indwelling Catheters   Indwelling Foley catheters are soft, flexible tubes that have double lumens, one that allows for urine drainage and the other for inflation and deflation of the retention balloon. Once inflated, the balloon allows for retention of the catheter in the bladder. The tip of the catheter has two openings called *eyeholes* to allow the urine to drain. Catheter products have changed significantly in their composition, texture, and durability during the past 5 years. A wide range of catheter materials is available, and the material selected should be chosen for the following characteristics: comfort, presence of latex sensitivity in the intended user, ease of insertion and removal, and ability to reduce the likelihood of complications such as urethral and bladder tissue damage, colonization by microorganisms, and encrustation. It is important for the clinician to be aware of the results of research in the use of indwelling catheters. There are reported increases in allergies and reactions in people with indwelling latex catheters. If the person is latex sensitive, silicone catheters should be used. Avoiding latex catheters may also decrease the incidence of encrustation. Bonded catheters may be longer lasting than silicone catheters because their hydrogel coating prevents bacterial adherence and reduces mucosal friction.

Silicone-Coated Latex Catheters   These catheters have a latex core with a chemically bonded coating of silicone elastomer or Teflon. The coating helps prevent urethral contact with the latex. These catheters tend to be yellow or golden in color. The most commonly used catheter is a silicone-coated latex catheter.

All-Silicone Catheters   These are thin-walled catheters that have a larger diameter drainage lumen compared with silicone-coated catheters. Fewer problems seem to occur in long-term use because these catheters are compatible with the lining of the urethra and do not allow build-up of protein and mucus. In a study of encrustation of different catheter materials, although all catheters became blocked, the all-silicone catheters took longer to become blocked than other types (Morris, Stickler, & Winters, 1997). However, this may be because all-silicone catheters have a slightly wider lumen than other coated catheters. Silicone catheters are now popular because people are developing allergies to latex catheters. These catheters are clear or white in color.

Bonded Hydrogel-Coated Latex   Hydrogels are polymers that absorb water to produce a slippery outside surface. Catheters with hydrogel bonding are less likely to become encrusted and may be better tolerated and preferred by the person for long-term usage. Urine leakage may be less of a problem with the hydrogel-coated than the silicone catheters.

Other Coated Catheters   In an attempt to prevent bacterial colonization, catheters have been coated with *antibiotics*. Usually the outer wall and inner drainage lumen of these catheters are impregnated with an antibacterial agent (e.g., nitrofurazone), which elutes from the catheter over a period of days after insertion. It is unclear if these catheters, which are more expensive, have any effect on infection. *Silver-coated catheters* are thought to cause less inflammation and have a bacteriostatic effect (Verleyan, De Ridder, Von Poppel, & Baert, 1999). It may be reasonable to consider using a silver alloy–coated catheter in people who are at highest risk for developing consequences from UTI.

Catheter Size The golden rule is to use the smallest catheter size that allows for adequate drainage. The outer circumference of the catheter is measured in a unit called French (Fr). The use of 14, 16, or 18 Fr catheters is recommended because catheters with larger diameters can cause more erosion of the urethral mucosa, can cause stricture formation, and do not allow adequate drainage of periurethral gland secretions. A large catheter can cause pain and discomfort, as well as occlusion of periurethral glands, increasing the chances of infection. In men, a coudé-tipped catheter, which is angled upward at the tip to assist in negotiating the upward bend in the male urethra, may be indicated. This feature facilitates passage through a bladder neck that has a slightly enlarged prostate gland (e.g., benign prostatic hyperplasia).

Balloon Size The preferred balloon size is 5 ml, which is to be instilled with 10 ml of sterile water for inflation. If a 5-ml balloon is inflated with more than 10 ml of water, irritation may occur unilaterally on the bladder wall from increased pressure of the balloon. Underfilling or overfilling may interfere with the correct positioning of the catheter tip, which may lead to irritation and trauma of the bladder wall. The catheterized bladder is in a collapsed state as a result of constant urine drainage. A balloon size greater than 10 ml, such as a 30-ml balloon, will not allow for correct bladder drainage and can lead to bacterial overgrowth (see Figure 9.2). In addition, with a large balloon, there will be a greater chance of contact between the balloon or catheter tip and the bladder wall than with a smaller one (5 ml), leading to bladder spasms that may cause urinary leakage. The 30-ml balloons are used primarily to facilitate traction on the prostate gland to stop bleeding in men after prostate surgery or in women after pelvic surgery.

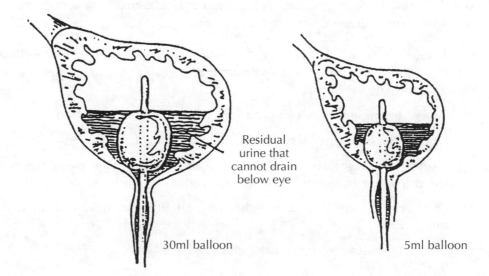

Residual urine that cannot drain below eye

30ml balloon   5ml balloon

Figure 9.2. Urine drainage with two different balloon sizes. (Courtesy of ConvaTec)

Drainage Bag   Indwelling catheters are attached to overnight or leg drainage bags. The manual dexterity of the person and caregiver determines which drainage system will be selected. An overnight or bedside bag is usually of 1,500- or 2,000-ml capacity, with a long tube that is used for overnight drainage. The bag should be hung over the side of the bed below the level of the catheter so that the urine will flow easily. Leg bags come in different sizes and shapes (horizontal or vertical) and are made from a variety of materials. More active people may prefer a leg bag for use at home or when away from home. These smaller bags are more discreet, so the person can attach the bag to the upper thigh or calf and conceal it under clothing. They are held in place with straps, mesh, elastic straps with Velcro closures, or knitted bag holders. Using these leg bags allows more freedom of movement.

When selecting a drainage bag for a catheter system, certain factors must be considered. Leg bag attachments that are too tight can restrict circulation. Attention should be paid to the selection of the drainage port, because some people may be able to manipulate a flip-flow valve but not a sliding type. Also, there is no research that shows the benefit of adding antibiotic or antimicrobial solutions to the bag to prevent the development of catheter-related infection.

Changing Schedule   Usual medical practice is to change indwelling catheters every month; however, this practice is based not on research but on insurance reimbursable allowances. Most experts believe that changing schedules should be arranged according to the user's needs. The catheter should be changed more often if obstruction occurs, if the person develops frequent infections, or if difficulty with removal of the catheter or deflation of the balloon occurs. To prevent the occurrence of catheter-related problems, clinicians should identify when problems occur and develop a changing schedule that helps to prevent their recurrence.

Management of Indwelling Catheters   Management of indwelling catheters varies according to the setting and the caregiver. The objectives of effective catheter care are to

- Prevent or minimize the complications related to catheterization

- Promote the independence, comfort, and dignity of the person

- Ensure that individuals and their caregivers are knowledgeable of and proficient in the management of long-term catheters

Problems arising from long-term indwelling catheters are described in Table 9.1 and include

- Unprescribed (inadvertent) dislodgment

- Leakage

- Obstruction or encrustation

Table 9.1. Common problems with long-term catheterization

Problem	Causes	Intervention
Inadvertent dislodgment (catheter falling out, usually with balloon inflated)	Occurs in 41% of clients with indwelling catheters. Causes: • Client pulling the catheter out because of confusion, discomfort; may occur in the client who doesn't like or want the catheter • Secondary to catheter tension, where increased pressure and weight on the catheter cause it to dislodge. • Detrusor overactivity or bladder spasms will cause expulsion of catheter with balloon intact	Consider alternative urinary collection device. Use an anchor strap. Consider changing catheter more frequently.
Leakage of urine around the catheter (referred to as catheter bypass)	Occurs 65% of the time with catheterized clients. Causes: • Bladder spasms • Infection • Obstruction • Catheter size too large • Secondary to an irritated bladder mucosa caused by long-term catheter use	If infection is suspected, consider acidification and dilution of urine. Consider changing catheter more frequently.
Obstruction or blockage of catheter	Occurs in more than 50% of clients with catheters. Cause: encrustation resulting from the collection of bacteria, crystallization of protein, or mucus plugs. Crystalline deposits can cover the balloon and obstruct the eyehole and lumen of the catheter (Morris, Stickler, & Winters, 1997). Formation of encrustation usually occurs around the tip of the catheter, around the balloon, or within the catheter lumen.	Make sure catheter is not kinking or looping. If encrustation causes occlusion of the catheter, the entire system needs to be changed.
Catheter/balloon malfunction	Failure of the balloon to deflate as a result of malfunction of inflation valve, obstruction of the inflation channel by external encrustation of the balloon	Cut balloon at the port distal to the junction. If this fails to deflate the balloon, push narrow-gauge guidewire through balloon port into the balloon to allow fluid to drain. Do not inject air, water, or any chemical into balloon port to rupture the balloon.
Pain and urethral discomfort	More than 50% of clients find catheters painful (Saint, Lipsky, Baker, McDonald, & Ossenkop, 1999). Discomfort may be secondary to catheter's size (too large) or occlusion of periurethral glans.	Decrease catheter size. Use large amounts of lubrication at time of insertion to decrease pain and discomfort. Lubricate the urethra, not just the catheter. Consider removal of catheter and alternative management of bladder disorder.

- Catheter or balloon malfunction
- Pain and urethral discomfort

The catheter management strategies outlined next (Newman, 1998) can prevent complications and nursing care problems.

1. Always insert the catheter using an aseptic (sterile) procedure. Difficulty passing the catheter may mean that the catheter is going in the wrong direction and the urethra is being damaged. Once the catheter enters the bladder, a good flow of urine confirms its location and the balloon can be inflated. If there is no urine return, it is because either there is no urine in the bladder or (the most common reason) the lubricating jelly is occluding the catheter port.

2. A smaller catheter (16 or 18 Fr) is preferred because it is likely to be better tolerated, cause less urethral irritation, and decrease occlusion of periurethral glands. Always use a 5-ml balloon (instill 10 ml of sterile water in a 5-ml balloon).

3. The catheter insertion site should be cleaned on a daily basis. Routine perianal and meatal care should exclude the use of antiseptics (e.g., Betadine solution or ointment). Wash the meatal areas with soap and water or a perineum wash and avoid frequent and vigorous cleansing of the area. *Wash hands immediately before and after manipulating the catheter site or apparatus.*

4. To avoid migration of bacteria up the lumen of the catheter, the urine in the drainage bag should be emptied at least every 4–6 hours. To avoid cross-contamination, do not empty catheter bags from a number of people into one container or using the same pair of gloves. When attaching the drainage bag to a bed or chair, make sure the bag is above the floor.

5. The catheter should be anchored or stabilized at all times to prevent urethral tension, which can lead to tears. The catheter should follow the natural curve of the urethra. The catheter should be anchored on the upper thigh in women and ideally to the abdomen in men. Avoid kinks or loops in the catheter and tubing that might decrease or impede the flow of urine. The catheter or drainage tube should never be clamped.

6. Current practice for changing catheters has been to change them every 4–8 weeks. However, catheters should be changed according to the individual's usual pattern of catheter wear rather than waiting until infection or encrustations occur. If an infection occurs frequently or obstruction is common, the catheter should be changed more often. Keep a record of when catheter-related problems occur so that a proactive changing schedule can be determined.

7. Maintaining a high fluid intake produces less concentrated urine, which impairs bacterial growth in the bladder and catheter system. The flush-

ing action of large quantities of dilute urine will reduce the likelihood of bacteria ascending the bag and catheter. Dilute urine may also reduce the concentration of substances that precipitate the development of encrustations that lead to catheter blockage. Forcing fluids is especially difficult in older people because aging causes a loss in the sense of thirst, so they do not know when they should be drinking. Foods that have a high liquid content may be substituted (e.g., Jell-O, Popsicles, soups).

8. Repeated use of antibiotics and antimicrobials to prevent symptomatic UTI should be avoided because they do not have a significant effect on urethral flora. In people with repeated infections, maintaining an acidic environment in the bladder may prevent recurrence. Check urine pH; if pH is greater than 5, consider acidification of urine by having the person drink 3–8 oz. of cranberry juice or take 1 g of ascorbic acid daily.

9. Catheters should not be irrigated with any type of solution (e.g., antimicrobials, antibiotics). Historically, bladder irrigations were used to minimize the likelihood of catheter-associated UTIs and to dissolve blockages from encrustations. The evidence to support this practice is not found in the medical literature. Bladder irrigation is not only ineffective in treating UTI, but may also further disrupt the already damaged bladder epithelium, leading to further infection.

10. Routine cultures in the absence of infection should be avoided because all individuals with long-term catheters will have bacteria in the bladder and the organisms change frequently, about once or twice per month. Urine cultures should only be obtained when there is suspected clinical sepsis based on objective signs or symptoms. If a symptomatic infection does occur, change the catheter before obtaining a specimen for cultures. Obtain a sample of the urine that drains through the new system because urine in the old system may reflect not bladder urine but "catheter" urine.

Research has shown that the majority of people know nothing about catheters before actually using one themselves, and only 43% of users stated that they received initial advice about how to care for the catheter (Roe, 1990). Those using catheters and their caregivers should be informed about the catheter's location, use, and subsequent management. Educating new and established catheter users about their catheters will improve their ability to cope with catheter use. Appendix A: Care and Use of a Urinary (Foley) Catheter and Appendix A: How to Care for Your Catheter Drainage Bag provide information on emptying, changing, and managing the entire system.

Alternatives to Indwelling Urethral Catheters   People with indwelling catheters must be reevaluated periodically to determine whether a voiding trial or bladder retraining program may be effective in eliminating the need for the indwelling catheter. Most urologists recommend that suprapubic catheters be used in people, especially men, who require chronic, long-term bladder drainage and for whom no other alternative therapy is possible. Intermittent catheterization is the safest bladder management method in terms of urological complications and should always be considered before the use of a urethral or suprapubic catheter (Weld & Dmochowski, 2000).

Bladder Retraining After Catheter Removal   People can successfully regain bladder function and undergo retraining following indwelling catheter use (Newman, 1998); however, it may take as long as 6 weeks after catheter removal to determine the success of a bladder retraining program. Prior to catheter removal, a thorough genitourinary history and examination must be obtained (see Chapter 6). The presence of medical conditions that may precipitate urinary retention must be ascertained prior to catheter removal. The catheter removal plan should be discussed with the person's physician to determine if there are contraindications to the catheter's removal. One of the most important assessments is the client's motivation to regain bladder function. Also, caregiver involvement and agreement is imperative because many caregivers feel the person is easier to manage with a catheter than without. The caregiver should be informed of the benefits of catheter removal. Once the catheter is removed, the person, no longer restricted by the indwelling catheter, is able to increase mobility and could become more independent and productive. Removing an indwelling catheter requires persistent nursing evaluation and intervention.

The following is a step-by-step approach to catheter removal:

Step 1: Obtain a urine culture. Regardless of the results of the urine culture, the person is usually treated with antibiotics for 3 days to eradicate any bacteriuria.

Step 2: Remove the catheter. Clamping the catheter before removal is not necessary; clamping routines have never been shown to be helpful.

Step 3: Place the person on a timed voiding schedule or on habit training. Usually the individual is instructed to void at 2-hour intervals except during the night. The person should always void on awakening and before going to bed.

Step 4: Monitor bowel function. Fecal impaction can cause compression of the urethra, leading to urinary retention. Implement a bowel regimen if necessary.

Step 5: Have the person/staff/caregiver monitor the voiding pattern. Keeping a record that notes frequency, time, and amount of continent voids, as well as incontinence episodes, allows the nurse to ascertain the success of the program and identifies areas that may require further instruction. The fluid intake pattern should be monitored as well. For the first few days after catheter removal, the person should be monitored for urinary retention. In people who have a history of urinary retention, it may take days or weeks for the bladder to regain normal function. If postvoid residuals remain elevated, the person should have a urological consultation before the indwelling catheter is reinserted (Resnick, 1993).

Step 6: Once the person is able to maintain a 2-hour voiding schedule, he or she is encouraged to delay voiding as long as possible. Bladder retraining techniques that inhibit the urge sensation are helpful. In addition, teaching the person pelvic muscle exercises to strengthen the muscles that support the bladder will decrease UI episodes.

Suprapubic Catheterization

Suprapubic catheterization is a technique used in people with urinary retention who have urethral damage from long-term catheterization. The catheter is introduced into the bladder via an incision through the anterior abdominal wall (above the pubic bone) into the bladder to permit drainage. The incision is usually placed 2 cm above the pubic bone (suprapubic). Suprapubic catheterization has been used mainly in clients who are undergoing urological or gynecological procedures. A suprapubic catheter may be the best choice for a person who needs to have a catheter in place for a long period of time because this type of catheter is more convenient for the person and caregiver.

A suprapubic catheter is preferable to an indwelling catheter in people who require chronic bladder drainage and for whom no other alternative therapy is possible because it decreases the risk of contamination with organisms from fecal material, decreases the risk of infection, and eliminates damage to the urethra. The anterior abdominal wall possesses a lower microbial load than the periurethal area and has a lower risk of infection (Sedor & Mulholland, 1999). Additional advantages are that the catheter is easier to change and clean (Fantl et al., 1996). In men who require long-term catheterization, suprapubic catheterization may also reduce the risk of local genitourinary complications such as meatal erosion, prostatitis, and epididymitis (Sheriff et al., 1998). Suprapubic catheters may be more comfortable for women using wheelchairs who find sitting on a urethral catheter uncomfortable. Despite these data, suprapubic catheters are not commonly used for long-term management of urinary dysfunction.

Although anatomical complications such as urethral erosion and fistula formation may be less with suprapubic catheters, potential problems include uncontrolled urine leakage, skin erosion, hematoma, and problems with catheter reinsertion. Suprapubic catheters have a higher rate of satisfaction and a lower risk of UTIs than indwelling urethral catheters. These catheters need to be changed, just like an indwelling catheter, at least every 4 weeks. Swelling at the site of insertion, bleeding, and bowel injury can occur at the time of inserting the catheter; however, these incidents are rare. A problem exists with long-term medical and nursing management of suprapubic catheterization because of lack of knowledge and expertise on the part of the health care clinician and because of the inability of the homebound person to access medical care quickly if a problem arises. Research is lacking in the area of long-term management because the medical literature has only documented postsurgical, short-term suprapubic catheter use. Prevention of complications and catheter management are similar to that used with indwelling urethral catheters.

Changing the Catheter   A new suprapubic tract usually takes between 10 days and 4 weeks to become established (McMahon-Parkes, 1998). After that, the catheter should be changed. Usually a regular 16–22 Fr Foley catheter is used to drain the urine. The following are some guidelines for changing a suprapubic catheter:

- Place the person in bed and remove the cystotomy dressing.

- Cleanse the abdomen around the cystostomy site with soap and water. Cleanse the cystotomy with vinegar and water to remove crusting and discharge, if necessary.

- Remove the existing catheter from the cystotomy opening. Gently rotate the catheter to release any growth and deflate the balloon.

- Open the new catheter package using aseptic technique. Test the balloon for leaks, then apply lubricant. Cleanse the cystotomy site with sterile cotton balls and antiseptic.

- Insert the new catheter immediately after removal of the old catheter because the passage can begin to close within a few minutes if insertion of a new catheter is delayed. If necessary, gentle pressure may be used. Insert the catheter gently downward toward the pelvic floor until urine flows. Inflate the balloon with sterile water.

- Attach the catheter to its closed drainage tubing and system, anchor the catheter by securing the tubing to the lateral abdominal wall with tape, and reapply a dressing.

- Teach the person, caregiver, or both to wash the skin area around the catheter with soap and water daily. Keep the area dry.

- Avoid the use of powder or creams around the catheter. The person can shower with this catheter in place and should not disconnect the catheter when showering.

- If the skin around the catheter gets red, swells, or opens, the person should contact the physician or nurse because this may be caused by an infection.

Intermittent Catheterization

Intermittent catheterization (IC) is the insertion and removal of a sterile or clean catheter several times a day to provide bladder emptying. Sterile (aseptic) technique implies genital disinfection and the use of sterile catheters, gloves, and other equipment. Clean technique implies ordinary washing techniques and the use of disposable or cleansed reusable catheters (Abrams et al., 2002). This form of catheterization has been used in the management of people with urinary retention and other voiding dysfunction for the past 20 years. Clean intermittent catheterization (CIC) has become the standard of care for performing self-catheterization (performed by the patient) in people with spinal cord injuries.

During urination, the bladder contracts and the pelvic floor muscles relax to allow urine to pass through the urethra. Normally, after the bladder empties, a small amount of urine (less than 90 ml) remains in the bladder, called the postvoid residual. If the person cannot urinate or empty the bladder completely, the residual urine volume increases and can cause UTIs, overflow UI, and permanent damage to the bladder and kidneys. By inserting the catheter several times during the day, episodes of bladder overdistention are avoided. Usually the person, caregiver, or both are taught to perform this type of catheterization. Long-term use of IC is preferable to indwelling urethral catheterization because of the low chance of infection and other problems.

Research has shown that regular bladder emptying reduces intravesical bladder pressure and improves blood circulation in the bladder wall, making the bladder mucous membrane more resistant to infectious bacteria. Older people and those with impaired immune systems (e.g., people with acquired immunodeficiency syndrome, those receiving chemotherapy) are at risk for developing urinary infections, and this sterile technique is best for them. Despite research indicating equivalent efficacy of CIC and sterile IC, sterile technique is used for IC in acute care facilities because of the high risk of nosocomial infections (Rainville, 1994). CIC has been used in people residing in the community; however, few data are available about the safest method in long-term facilities. A study in a Veterans Administration LTC facility found no difference in frequency of UTIs between clean and sterile IC in the male residents (Duffy et al., 1995). The long-term use of prophylactic antibiotics in most people regularly using CIC is not advisable because such long-term use is associated with the development of resistant bacterial strains. If an infection occurs in these individuals, it should be treated. In people with an internal prosthesis (pacemaker, heart valve), however, the use of prophylactic antibiotic therapy for bacteria in the urine is often recommended.

Common Complications   Common problems that can result from IC include bacteriuria. This is seen in 50% of CIC users, but rarely leads to urinary tract infections. The majority of individuals usually have no symptoms and therefore should not be treated with antibiotics.

Urinary tract infections occur in 10%–15% of people using IC and are more prevalent in those who have higher residual urine volumes at the time of catheterization. Chronic pyelonephritis rarely develops in people performing CIC.

Urethral damage from IC in men is similar to the problems seen with indwelling catheters:

1. *Urethritis*, or inflammation of the urethral meatus, may be due to frequent insertion of catheters.

2. *Urethral stricture* is the result of urethral inflammatory response to re-peated catheterization. The risk of a urethral stricture increases with the number of years using CIC. The use of hydrophilic catheters may decrease the incidence of strictures (Perrouin-Verbe et al., 1995). Difficulty with insertion is a sign of the presence of a urethral stricture.

3. *Creation of a false passage* can occur primarily in men with persisting ure-thral strictures. The false passage occurs because of trauma to the urethra and the site of the external sphincter. It is more common in men than women.

Epididymitis, caused by urethral and bladder inflammation, and scrotal abscess are seen in men. Bladder stones may occur in people who perform CIC over the long term. Stones have been shown to grow around introduced pubic hairs.

Types of Intermittent Catheters   There are several different types of in-termittent catheters. The clinician who instructs the person usually makes the catheter choice. The preferred catheters for CIC are clear and made of plastic material. Red rubber catheters are more flexible, and some clients find them more difficult to insert. Plastic catheters fall into two main groups (Easton, 2000):

1. Those that require lubrication to be applied before insertion

2. Those for which the coating provides the lubrication when water is applied

Straight catheters are plastic, silicone, or rubber catheters that have two eyeholes at the tip that allow for urine drainage. Length is either 5 inches (for women) or 12 inches (for men).

Coudé or *curved catheters* have a slight curve at the tip that aids in inser-tion. An olive-tip catheter may help a woman in identifying her urethra. Using a coudé or curved-tip catheter makes it easier for men to thread the catheter past the prostate gland. A clear, more rigid catheter makes insertion easier, but in some cases a red rubber catheter may be used.

Prelubricated hydrophilic-coated catheters have recently been introduced in the United States. The catheter is coated with a substance that absorbs water and binds it to the catheter surface. This extremely slippery layer of water stays on the catheter during insertion and withdrawal. These catheters are for one-time use only. They allow for easier insertion, minimize discom-fort, and protect the urethral mucosa from damage and irritation (Newman, 1998). They may be indicated for clients who experience particular discom-fort during catheterization or have difficulty with other types of catheters (Diokno, Mitchell, Nash, & Kimbrough, 1995).

Self-contained systems are closed systems that provide sterile catheteriza-tion. This system is 100% latex-free and uses a prelubricated catheter. The catheter passes through a special guide mechanism at the top of the pocket. This guide provides two main benefits: It keeps the catheter straight as it is advanced and, when squeezed, it prevents the catheter from slipping during insertion. Once the catheter is inserted, the urine drains into the bag. The use of this system may decrease chances of infection.

Coated catheters have a coating of an antibacterial agent (e.g., nitrofurazone) in the outer layer to produce local antibacterial activity.

Catheterization Schedule   The catheterization schedule should be based on the urine volume. As a general rule, bladder volume should not exceed 400 ml. When starting CIC, the person, caregiver, or both should record the amount of urine drained from the bladder. If the person voids, catheterization should always be performed after voiding. Based on a person's average output, catheterization is usually done four times during the day.

Before using CIC, it is important to consider the age of the person being catheterized, the physical ability of the person who will perform the catheterization, and the willingness and self-discipline of both. People who can feed themselves usually have the manual dexterity to self-catheterize. People and caregivers who are well motivated and cooperative and have adequate manual dexterity to manipulate the catheter can be taught to perform IC. Appendix A: Clean Intermittent Self-Catheterization (CIC) for Women and Appendix A: Clean Intermittent Self-Catheterization (CIC) for Men provide instruction for performing CIC. It should be noted that there is a lack of uniformity and standardization in nursing practice in terms of performing CIC.

External Catheter Systems

External catheter systems are condom-type sheaths that are placed over the penis for urine collection. External catheters are referred to as a condom catheter, penile sheath, or external male catheter. These catheters are made from latex rubber, polyvinyl, or silicone material. The catheters are secured to the penile shaft by a double-sided adhesive or a latex or foam strap that encircles the penis. They are connected to a urinary drainage bag by a collection tube. This system is suitable for men with moderate to severe UI and may also be used for men with urgency or frequency in circumstances in which it would be difficult to make frequent trips to restrooms. Men at one Veterans Administration medical center found the condom catheter more comfortable, less painful, and less restrictive on their activities. The only complaint was of urinary leakage (Saint et al., 1999). This study also indicated that nurses also preferred these catheters to indwelling catheters.

There are external collection devices for women that funnel the urine to tubing via a pouch (Figure 9.3). These devices are flexible or plastic pouches that are attached to the skin by adhesive or straps. The ideal device for women would be one that is easy to place and works well for women who transfer from beds to chairs or who use wheelchairs. Unfortunately, none of these devices have proven to be totally useful for women who use wheelchairs or those who are bedbound.

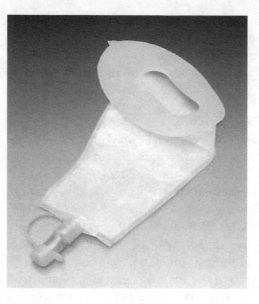

Figure 9.3.   External female pouch. (Courtesy of Hollister)

Common Complications   Once an external catheter is applied, careful attention must be given to avoid problems such as contact dermatitis, maceration of the tip of the penis, ischemia, penile edema, and penile obstruction. Most of these adverse effects are the result of improper and prolonged use of these devices. These effects go unreported in men with decreased penile and scrotal sensation.

1. Use of a condom catheter introduces the chance of *infection*, but the risk is less because it avoids instrumentation of the urethra.

2. *Maceration and irritation of the skin* can occur from the friction caused by an external catheter. In older men, the penis may have retracted (decreased in length and size) and it may be difficult to keep a condom catheter from falling off. *Retracted penis* pouches are available that can easily be applied by the man or his caregiver (see Figure 9.4).

3. *Phimosis* is present when the orifice of the foreskin is constricted, preventing retraction of the foreskin over the glans. This can occur as a result of overconstriction of the penis from a condom catheter.

4. Constriction or *strangulation of the penis* can occur when using a double-sided adhesive strap to secure the condom catheter. Two types of straps are available: adhesive-coated foam straps and adhesive barrier straps. Barrier straps stretch and have the capacity to return to original size and shape. These are the preferred type in men who retain erectile function. Foam straps are not elastic, so they will not stretch.

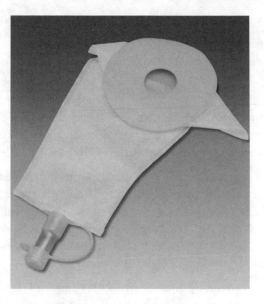

Figure 9.4.   External retracted penis pouch. (Courtesy of Hollister)

Considerations for Use   Before deciding that external catheterization is appropriate for an individual, the following assessment must be completed:

- *Dexterity*—If a client has difficulty with dexterity and manipulation of small objects, the ease of application and removal may be an issue. Identification of a caregiver or family member who will apply the catheter must be considered. In a LTC facility, staff can be taught to apply these catheters.

- *Size of the penis*—The penis length must be sufficient to support the catheter. With aging and prostate cancer treatments, penile size may decrease, causing the penis to *retract*. If this is the case, consideration should be given to a retracted penis pouch.

- *Condition of the skin*—The penis and scrotum must be assessed for redness, open areas, and rashes because external catheters should only be considered in men who have intact skin. If the client is at risk for possible skin breakdown, use of a barrier film product should be considered when applying the device.

As with most urinary collection devices, the clinician will make the decision about catheter type and size. The following should be considered when choosing the best product for the client:

- Penis size (width and length or circumference and length)
- Risk for infection

- Mechanical damage to the penis resulting from adhesives, tapes, or shape of condom

- Catheter material contributing to blockage of urine flow

- Wear time

Types of Condom Catheters   Several different external condom catheters made of latex rubber, polyvinyl, or silicone are available. They are attached to the shaft of the penis by one of five different methods:

1. *Self-adhesive external catheters* are very popular. These are rolled over the shaft of the penis and pressed to stick. Recent new technology includes all-silicone external catheters, which cause less irritation and fewer adverse reactions and are recommended for men who have an allergy to latex. Another attractive feature is that these catheters are made of clear material, allowing for monitoring of skin condition.

2. *Hydrocolloid strips* have adhesive on both sides and can be applied around the penile circumference. The catheter sheath is rolled up and over the strip and penis, and pressed against the penis to stick. Catheters with a circumferential band may be too restrictive for the shaft of the penis and should only be used by men who are cognitively intact and have penile sensation.

3. *Retracted penis pouches* are specific for men with retracted or short penises, who cannot use a regular condom catheter. Adhesive urinary pouches (one or two piece) are available; however, more preparation is needed for the application of these devices. Pubic hair should be removed from the base of the penis. The hair should be trimmed, not shaved, because shaving causes more irritation. The opening in the adhesive surface should be cut to the size of the base of the penis. The pouch can be connected to straight drainage or the man can empty the pouch as needed.

4. *Reusable external catheter systems* are available for men who experience UI after prostate surgery. Some men use no method of attachment and prefer a nonadhesive condom, using a foam-and-elastic reusable band fastened with Velcro to secure the catheter. There is no direct skin adhesion, and thus less chance of skin breakdown.

External Catheter Size and Application   Because there are several sizes of condom catheters, it is important to select the correct size. Measuring (sizing) guides are very helpful when fitting a man with a condom catheter. The clinician should take the time to find the size that fits the client's needs. When choosing a size, the clinician should allow for nocturnal erections in the sizing of the device. Nothing should ever be applied to the penile shaft circumferentially, because this may cause pressure and ulceration. The catheter should be examined for tightness; fit should be snug but not constrictive. A medical adhesive (commonly used when applying ostomy bags) can be applied around the circumference of the penis to ensure that the catheter "sticks" to the penis. The adhesive must be dry before rolling on the catheter. A skin barrier product can be applied to the penis to protect penile skin from breakdown secondary to repetitive application and removal of an adhesive device. Men need to be instructed on correct application of external catheters (see Appendix A: How to Use an External "Condom" Catheter).

PENILE CLAMP

A penile clamp or compression device is used by men with UI. These devices mechanically compress the soft tissue of the penis, thus preventing any flow or leakage via the urethra. Often these clamps are used by men after prostate cancer surgery to stop stress UI, or by men with continuous urine leakage. Usually the clamp is placed halfway down the shaft of the penis and then tightened to compress the urethra (see Figure 9.5). The inside of the clamp has a flexible portion made of soft foam that conforms to fit the penis. The outside is made of metal with several notches on the side to adjust the tightness. When closed, it should pinch off the urine flow without discomfort. Another type of compression device is adjustable, encircles the penis, and is inflated with air to stop the flow of urine. A penile clamp should be used with caution and is only appropriate in men who have penile sensation and good manual dexterity and will comply with proper care and use of the product. Skin breakdown, swelling, and strictures (scarring) can occur inside the urethra if a clamp is left in place too long.

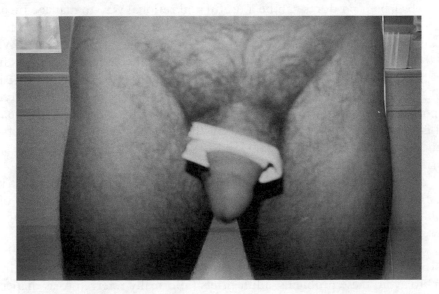

Figure 9.5. Incontinence clamp in place.

Men who use wheelchairs may place a clamp over their penis when they transfer from bed to chair and vice versa. Others will keep the clamp on their penis loosely and only compress the clamp when they move from position to position. Users must be told about potential complications associated with these devices and should be given written instructions on their correct use (see Appendix A: How to Safely Use an Incontinence Clamp).

ABSORBENT PRODUCTS

Absorbent products include innovative perineal pads or panty liners for slight leakage, undergarments and protective underwear for moderate to heavy leakage, guards and drip collection pouches for men, and traditional diaper-style products (called adult briefs) for moderate or heavy loss. These products absorb or contain urine and are either disposable or reusable. Reusables are made of cloth material with a rayon or polyester fiber core. The number, size, and arrangement of these fibers are factors in the absorption capacity. The urine-holding capacity of all absorbent products varies and is not standardized. The quality and materials used in these products vary widely. There are also underpads of differing sizes for bed and furniture protection that are washable or disposable. Advantages of the use of absorbent products to manage UI include the ability to

- Soak up or contain urine

- Provide protection for clothes, furniture, bedding, and floors

- Preserve the person's dignity and comfort

Absorbent products can be a useful and rational way to manage incontinence; however, few absorbent products have been subjected to user and clinician evaluation that has been published in the medical literature. When faced with choosing or recommending a product, the clinician often has little information about product performance on which to base a choice (Fader et al., 2001). Also, in LTC settings, product selection is an administrative or corporate decision that is primarily influenced by cost as opposed to quality and effectiveness. This is influenced by the fact that absorbent products account for significant costs to acute and LTC facilities. In nursing facilities, incontinence costs are the third highest resident care costs.

Absorbent products have made UI much more manageable for most people; however, early dependency on absorbent pads, especially in frail, older adults with chronic illness, may be a deterrent to continence, giving the wearer a false sense of security and acceptance of the condition. Their use may remove the motivation to seek evaluation and treatment for UI. In addition, improper use of absorbent products contributes to skin breakdown and infection. To avoid these problems, adult briefs (informally referred to as diapers in many LTC settings) and pads should be changed frequently to limit a person's exposure to the wet garment and eliminate build-up of odor.

Types of Absorbent Products

Similar to feminine hygiene products that are designed to absorb menstrual blood, absorbent incontinence products are designed specifically to absorb and contain urine. These products are designed so that the surface area that is against the perineum collects the urine and transmits it to an absorbent inner core. This absorbent inner core allows the urine to spread throughout the entire pad, facilitating absorption capacity while preventing urine leakage. Most of these products have a plastic layer for added protection. The technology in disposable absorbent products utilizes both wood pulp and a polymer that absorbs and bonds with the urine, changing it into a gel. The gel improves the pad's absorption capacity and minimizes urine leakage and odor. These products keep the urine away from the perineal skin (Brink, 1997). One study showed that there is less skin breakdown in people using disposable briefs with absorbing properties (Brown, 1994); however, despite the technology, the clinician and client must remember that every absorbent product has a saturation point, depending on the frequency, the quantity of urine loss, and the changing schedule.

Studies have shown that pad usage preference varies for women with stress UI and other types of UI. McClish, Wyman, Sale, Camp, and Earle (1999) reported that 77% of women who enrolled in a clinical trial for UI used a protective perineal pad at least once per week. This study also showed that women used lower cost products such as menstrual pads rather than specific incontinence pads. Women still chose a small, discreet pad such as a panty liner despite the need to change the product more frequently. One clinical study looked at usage of perineal pads in women with stress UI (Thornburn, Fader, Dean, Brooks, & Cottenden, 1997). They found that the most popular time for putting pads on was in the morning. Mean wear time was 6.6 hours. It is estimated that as much as 30% of all feminine hygiene pads are used by young women who have slight UI.

The most commonly used absorbent products are body-worn (pads, panty liners, undergarments, briefs, and washable pant/disposable pad systems).

- Products for light to moderate incontinence include perineal pads, male guards, shields, and inserts. These are attached to the underwear or panties with an adhesive strip and side gathers for fit (see Figure 9.6). Some are designed with a wide front or back for larger volumes of leakage. These are most appropriate for clients with light to moderate urine leakage and are preferred for their discreetness (Baker & Norton, 1996). These pads are similar in design to feminine hygiene pads but provide more effective protection.

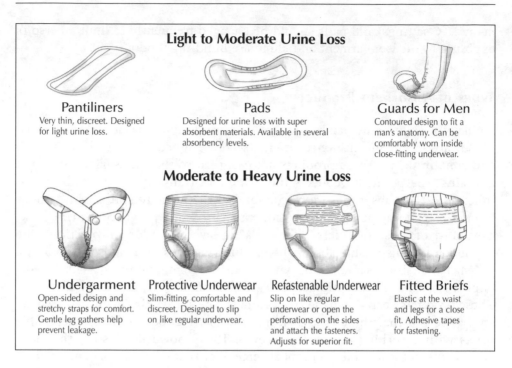

Figure 9.6.   Absorbent products. (Courtesy of Kimberly-Clark Corporation)

- For men, socklike drip-collecting pouches and guards are available that are comfortable and discreet. These pouches and drip collectors are held in place inside regular underwear, preferably briefs, and have guards with an adhesive strip (see Figure 9.6).

- Undergarments are very popular form-fitting large pads that extend to the waist and are held in place by elastic side straps using Velcro or buttons (see Figure 9.6). The button-type undergarment may be more difficult for older adults with arthritis. Most have a soft, breathable outer cover for a clean, comfortable feeling.

- Protective underwear is a disposable product similar to cloth underwear with added absorbent protection (see Figure 9.6). This is a very popular product used by both men and women.

- The adult brief (diaper) is used for moderate to severe UI and in people with both fecal incontinence and UI (see Figure 9.6). The brief can be easily placed on a person who is primarily bed bound.

- Pad-and-pant systems can be a combination of cloth (reusable) pants and disposable pads. They are useful for those people with moderate UI and allow for self-toileting in those who are more independent.

- Many people invent their own method of protection to minimize expense. These homemade products may include washcloths, paper towels, undershirts, and, most frequently, tissues. In some cases, people place these items in their own underwear or in a disposable product such as an undergarment. They will usually throw away the self-made product as it becomes saturated.

Product Selection

Little research has been done comparing absorbent products. At present, product selection is made by the consumer through trial and error and depends on budgetary constraints and availability in the practice setting. Clinicians and caregivers need to be aware of the characteristics of and indications for available products so they can counsel individuals on proper use.

- Select the most appropriate product designed for ease in self-toileting in those individuals who are "independent" continent, but need some protection for occasional urine leakage.

- Select a product that is designed to contain urinary leakage in those people who are not capable of maintaining continence independently or through regular toileting or other measures.

Personal preferences in products may vary. Considerations when choosing an absorbent product include the following:

1. The best product should be selected on the basis of comfort, ease of application/removal, and containment of urine and control of odor.

2. If the quantity of urine is small at any one time, then light thin pads or panty liners that attach to underwear will be adequate. This type of product will allow for easy removal when the person is attempting to toilet.

3. If urine leakage is severe, constant, or both, then a super-absorbent, larger product is needed. In these situations, many clinicians and caregivers choose wrap-around brief products. These products may be excellent at containing large amounts of urine leakage, but they can deter the person from self-toileting because they are difficult to remove and reapply. Protective underwear or a pant-and-pad system may be more appropriate because these products are similar to underwear.

4. If nighttime leaking is a problem, both bed pads and body-worn products may be necessary.

5. Soiled products should be disposed of in a sanitary manner. They should not be flushed down the toilet. Hands should be washed after handling the person and soiled absorbent product.

SKIN CARE

Skin problems associated with incontinence can range from irritations (contact dermatitis) to pressure ulcers (breakdown or opening of the skin; see Table 9.2). Causes of contact dermatitis include skin exposure to feces, urine,

Table 9.2. Definitions for common skin terms

Term	Definition
Maceration	Excess moisture in the epidermal cells such that there is separation of the skin tissues and denudation
Scaling, dry skin	Characterized by dryness and flaking; may appear fissured or cracked
Papules	Elevated, discolored flat area of skin, usually red and less than 0.5 cm in diameter
Erythema	Redness of the skin surface that varies in intensity from pale pink to bright red
Pressure (decubitus) ulcer	Any lesion resulting from prolonged pressure and involving loss of integrity of the skin, or damage to underlying tissue
Candidal (monilial) dermatitis	Red patches or plaques of *Candida albicans,* sometimes sparing skinfolds, found not only in the perineal area but also in the skinfolds of the upper thighs

chemicals, detergents, and allergens. Skin breakdown and erythema are directly related to exposure to urine and feces. Pressure ulcers are a costly problem in hospital, LTC, and home settings. Prevalence of pressure ulcers in nursing facility residents ranges from 2.4% to 23% (Schnelle et al., 1997). Residents at risk for developing skin problems include those with urinary and fecal incontinence, immobility, and dementia.

Development of Skin Problems

The skin is usually slightly acidic. This acidic pH is a major factor in helping to prevent the invasion of the skin by bacteria, particularly yeast and fungus. This is often referred to as the "protective acid mantle" of the skin. An alkaline pH adversely affects the skin, promoting the loss of normal skin integrity. Furthermore, the presence of excessive skin surface moisture can contribute to growth of bacteria that can lead to skin breakdown and infection. Potential sources of excessive moisture on the skin include

- UI
- Fecal incontinence
- Frequent washes
- Nonabsorbent or poorly ventilated padding on the skin
- Skin occlusion

When skin is subjected to moisture from urine in combination with fecal matter, further skin trauma results. Bacteria in the stool causes the urea (from the urine) to break down into ammonia. In the person whose skin is already compromised by exposure to urine and feces, the resulting change in skin pH (into the alkaline range) can be particularly devastating.

Prolonged exposure to urine and feces, moisture, and friction combine to macerate, abrade, and blister the skin over the buttocks and sacrum. Waste from UI can overhydrate the skin and promote the growth of microorganisms such as *Candida albicans*, resulting in candidiasis or yeast dermatitis. All of these factors work in concert to cause skin irritation, breakdown, and further skin problems. In addition, friction can cause skin abrasion to occur. Wet skin is more easily abraded by movement of skin against an object such as cloth, plastic in leg gathers, or tape fasteners on adult briefs. Tape cuts are commonly seen in obese adults who are wearing a tight-fitting brief.

Skin Care Products

Proper use of soaps, skin products, topical antimicrobials (agents that inhibit the growth of germs), gentle pH-balanced cleansers, and appropriate barrier products, as well as effective use of incontinence pads, are all important in skin care management. The use of disposable wipes or washcloths rather than toilet tissue may be more beneficial to the perineal skin. One must also consider the impact skin care products may have on efficacy of absorbent products. Petrolatum-based skin protectants are often used both prophylactically and as a treatment for incontinence dermatitis (Jeter & Lutz, 1996); however, there may be an incompatibility between petrolatum-based skin protectants and absorbent products such as adult briefs causing increased skin irritation.

Despite the availability of skin care products designed specifically to prevent skin breakdown, soap and water continues to be the most widely used skin regimen in LTC facilities. This is true despite the fact that there is research to show that a soap-and-water regimen alone is the least effective in preventing skin breakdown when compared with moisture barriers and no-rinse incontinence cleansers (Byers, Ryan, Regan, Shields, & Carta, 1995). Washing with regular soap and water has been found to be associated with problems such as dry skin, contact dermatitis, and *eczema* (Newman, Wallace, & Wallace, 2001). Because frequent washing with soap and water can dehydrate the skin, the use of a perineal rinse may be indicated.

Perineal cleansers are liquid solutions that remove bacteria or effluent. No-rinse perineal cleansers are more convenient and time saving, and are preferred over the popular bar soaps because the cleansing agents and antiseptics used in these formulations are gentler to the skin than those used in bar soaps. These cleansers also effectively remove urine and feces without personal discomfort because they can help emulsify and loosen stool and urine. In addition, no-rinse perineal cleansers are pH balanced for the skin, whereas bar soaps are almost always in the alkaline range. Some perineal cleansers are also formulated with topical antimicrobials that may decrease the bacteria on the skin. Fragrances, alcohol, and alkaline agents should be avoided when choosing a cleanser.

Moisturizers preserve the moisture in the skin by either sealing in existing moisture or adding moisture to the skin. Moisturizers can be creams, lotions, or pastes. Pastes are created by adding powder to an ointment, and do not need to be removed each time an area is washed.

Barrier products protect the skin from contact with moisture and decrease friction from absorbent products (Scardillo & Aronovitch, 1999); however, if the skin barrier product is easily removed with water during cleansing of an area, then it is not likely to provide a durable barrier to urine and feces. Clear, solvent-based, film-forming skin protectants are an even better alternative than creams, ointments, and pastes. Film-forming skin protectants are acrylate-based copolymers that quickly evaporate when applied to the skin, leaving the copolymer behind to form a protective film. This clear film allows for air flow but is impervious to external moisture and skin irritants.

Topical antifungal agents are available in ointments, powders, and creams. Some topical antifungals with anti-*Candida* activity are available as over-the-counter products (e.g., clotrimazole, miconazole). Topical antifungal cream should be applied after each incontinence episode and continued until any erythema is completely resolved. Other barrier products should not be used when using antifungals.

Skin Care Management

Careful and close attention to skin care reduces the occurrence of skin breakdown in people with incontinence. The key to preventing skin problems is to keep the perineal skin clean and dry. It is important for the caregiver to carefully select the appropriate absorbent product, preferably one that minimizes the possibility of dermatitis. It has been shown that products designed to absorb moisture and present a quick-drying surface to the skin keep the skin drier and are associated with a significantly lower incidence of skin rashes than cloth products (Kemp, 1994). The length of time an individual wears an adult brief should be limited because these products have a tight, permeable covering that can lead to perineal dermatitis.

All clients who have UI and wear absorbent products or use external or internal catheters to manage their UI need a perineal skin care program. The following is an example of a program for nursing care of perineal skin:

1. Put on gloves and remove soiled perineal pad or absorbent product, if indicated.

2. Inspect the skin of the buttocks, coccyx, rectal area, scrotum/perineum, genitalia, and upper thighs carefully every day. Assessment of the skin includes separation of skinfolds and wrinkles, looking for presence of rash, irritation, or skin breakdown. Assess perineal skin for signs of dermatitis, erythema, swelling, oozing, vesiculation, crusting, and scaling (see Figure 9.7).

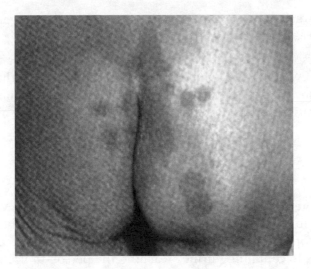

Figure 9.7.   Skin rash dermatitis.

3. Always wash the skin after any urine or bowel incontinence episode. Cleanse skin thoroughly with a mild soap (e.g., Dove), a no-rinse cleanser, or premoistened, alcohol-free towelettes in the following manner:

    a. Women—Position the woman on the bed, supine with legs apart and knees flexed. Clean the genitalia with a washcloth or wipes using a downward motion from the pubis (front) to the anus (back), using a different section of the washcloth or discarding wipes after each stroke to avoid contamination.

    b. Men—Cleanse the penis with special attention to the folds of the foreskin and glans (tip) of penis (particularly in the uncircumcised man). If the individual is not circumcised, pull back the foreskin and clean around the glans of the penis. Then, replace the foreskin back over the glans. Skin integrity is at risk in a man with scrotal edema.

4. After washing, let the skin air dry rather than rubbing with a towel to avoid irritation and skin tears.

5. Clean the groin, perineum, and buttocks thoroughly after removing a soiled absorbent product. Provide gentle cleansing with a mild cleansing agent immediately after soiling, and avoid force and friction during cleansing. Minimal use of any soap product reduces irritation, especially in the elderly woman who has atrophic perineal changes.

6. Skin care for people with urinary or bowel incontinence is as follows:

    a. With or without mild redness or chafing, use a barrier cream twice a day.

    b. With redness or minimal open, weepy skin lesions, use a barrier paste after each incontinence episode or with absorbent product changes and reapply as necessary.

c.   With rash but no open areas, use an antifungal cream and cover with a barrier cream at least three times a day.

7.   If the person is bed bound or uses a wheelchair, protect the skin from moisture. Avoid having the person sit or lie on any areas that are open or have a rash. Turn the individual frequently and support him or her in different positions by using pillows or wedges.

TOILETING DEVICES

Several hand-held, reusable urine collection containers and devices are available that can be successfully used by an individual or his or her caregiver as long as the proper device is identified. These devices have received little attention as aids to containing urine. Teaching the person to use a toileting device is an important part of rehabilitation and a valuable use of nursing staff time. The person can promote or maintain self-toileting through the independent use of these devices.

Types of Toileting Devices

Urinals   Urinals are bottle-shaped containers that can have two different types of necks. They are useful for people who have severe mobility restrictions, particularly when visiting places with inaccessible restrooms, when traveling, when bed bound, or when using a wheelchair (see Figure 9.8). Urinals have handles so they can be placed next to the person or hung on a bed rail, wheelchair, or walker. *Rehab urinals* have a flat bottom so that they can be laid flat on the bed. The openings in rehab urinals have a flange that

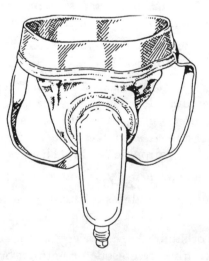

Figure 9.8.   Reusable male urinal.

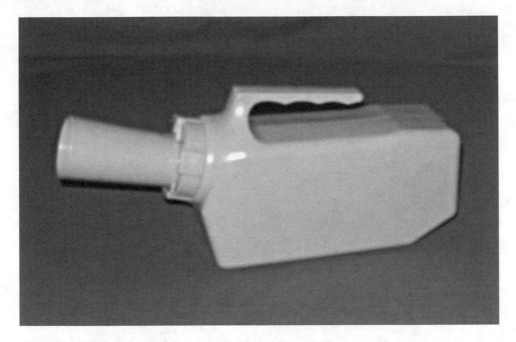

Figure 9.9.   Rehab male urinal.

extends into the urinal and does not allow backflow even when held almost upside down. For men, spill-proof urinals with large funnel openings are available to deal with a retracted penis (see Figure 9.9). Urinals for women have an opening designed to cup the perineal area and funnel the urine inside (see Figure 9.10). These are a better alternative for women who use wheelchairs or those who are bed bound. The following considerations are important when choosing a urinal:

- Material of the urinal—Lightweight plastic urinals are useful for people who have difficulty lifting. Steel urinals are very heavy and cumbersome.

- Handles to hold the urinal—If grip is a problem, rubber around the handle will increase grip. An extended handle may help if wrist movement is restricted.

- Ease of use and cleaning

- Spill-proof design

Bedpans   Often the use of a *fracture pan* enables women to urinate without pain, especially in the period after a fracture or hip repair. Sprinkling talcum powder or cornstarch on the bedpan will make sliding the pan under the person easier.

Toilets   A toilet seat that is a different color from the floor may be helpful for people with visual impairments. Raised toilet seats can be placed over a regular toilet to allow the person to get up and down on his or her own, thus

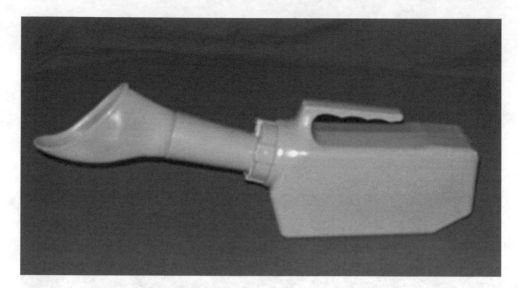

Figure 9.10.   Female urinal.

allowing for self-toileting. Seats with grab bars on either side are most often recommended to prevent falling and to aid with rising (see Figure 9.11).

Commode Chairs   If the person can get out of bed to urinate, a commode is a better alternative than a bedpan. Many different commodes exist that can ease toileting. A bedside commode can be placed close to the bed for easy use at night, or located on a floor of the house that does not have a bathroom. Some commodes have drop arms and adjustable heights to allow for individual needs. To minimize the odor and to make cleaning the bucket easier, keep water with a disinfectant in the bucket at all times. The commode can be camouflaged with an attractive cloth, or placed behind a screen. There are also wooden rather than metal commodes that can be disguised as an easy chair. General considerations when selecting a commode include the following:

- Height and weight of the person using the commode

- Mobility and dexterity, especially if the person will need to empty and clean the commode

- Cost, because most insurers will pay for a commode only when a physician writes a letter of medical necessity

Making Toilets Accessible   In a LTC facility, the location of toilets should be clearly indicated. Poorly designed signs to designate bathrooms or the use of terminology to identify the bathroom that residents do not understand can be a deterrent to self-toileting. Changes in bathroom architecture can also aid in toileting. For ease in toileting, bathroom size should be at least 5 feet by 5 feet. Grab bars in the right spot and a toilet seat adapter make the toilet safer. At least one grab bar should run parallel to the floor at a height of 33 inches. Bathrooms with gravity-assisted door closer mechanisms are help-

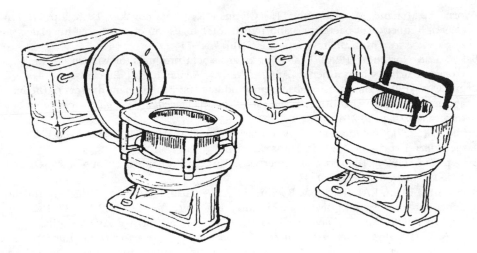

Figure 9.11.   Toilet risers.

ful; however, many people cannot open bathroom doors because they cannot grasp and turn the doorknob. To remedy this, doorknobs can be replaced with lever-type devices or the door can be disabled so that it opens and closes with a push. Removing the bathroom door and using a curtain or swinging doors makes access by a wheelchair possible.

CONCLUSION

Older people, family members, and clinicians are often confused about or unaware of various types of urine collection products, such as catheters, and their effectiveness in treating UI. Many urinary collection devices are available at local pharmacies, retail stores, and medical equipment dealers or directly from manufacturers. Medicare and other major insurers will usually pay for only a limited monthly supply of most of these products. Most health maintenance organizations (HMOs) and managed care insurers routinely do not pay for them, but some HMOs follow Medicare guidelines for payment. Absorbent products (pads, adult briefs) sold in retail stores and through mail-order catalogs are considered personal hygiene products, and their cost is not covered by insurers.

REFERENCES

Abrams, P., Cardozo, L., Fall, M., Griffiths, D., Rosier, P., Ulmsten, U., van Kerrebroeck, P., Victor, A., & Wein, A. (2002). The standardisation of terminology in lower urinary tract function: Report from the Standardisation Sub-Committee of the International Continence Society. *Neurourology and Urodynamics, 2*

Avorn, J., Monane, M., Gurwitz, J.H., Glynn, R.J., Choodnovskiy, I., & Lipsitz, L.A. (1994). Reduction of bacteriuria and pyuria after ingestion of cranberry juice. *Journal of the American Medical Association, 271*(10), 751–754.

Baker, J., & Norton, P. (1996). Evaluation of absorbent products for women with mild to moderate urinary incontinence. *Applied Nursing Research, 9*(1), 29–36.

Brink, C.A. (1996). The value of absorbent products and containment devices in the management of urinary incontinence [Guest editorial]. *Journal of Wound, Ostomy, and Continence Nursing, 22,* 2–4.

Brink, C. (1997). Containment of involuntary urine loss. In P.D. O'Donnell (Ed.), *Urinary incontinence* (pp. 436–438). St. Louis: Mosby.

Brown, D.S. (1994). Diapers and underpads. Part 1: Skin integrity outcomes. *Ostomy/Wound Management, 40,* 20–32.

Byers, P.H., Ryan, P.A., Regan, M.B., Shields, A., & Carta, S.G. (1995). Effects of incontinence care cleansing regimens on skin integrity. *Continence Care, 22*(4), 187–192.

ConvaTec. (1996). *National home care survey.* Princeton, NJ: Bristol Myers Squibb.

Day, A.N. (1996). *Characteristics of elderly home health care user: Data from the 1994 National Home and Hospice Care Survey.* Atlanta: Centers for Disease Control and Prevention.

Dignam, R.R., Ahmed, M., Kelly, K.G., Denman, S.J., Zaon, M., & Kleban, M. (1998). The effect of cranberry juice on urinary tract infection rates in a long-term care facility. *Annals of Long-Term Care, 6*(5), 163–167.

Diokno, A.C., Mitchell, B.A., Nash, A.J., & Kimbrough, J.A. (1995). Patient satisfaction and the Lofric catheter for clean intermittent catheterization. *Journal of Urology, 153,* 349–351.

Duffy, L.M., Cleary, J., Ahern, S., Kuskowski, M.A., West, M., Wheeler, L., & Mortimer, J.A. (1995). Clean intermittent catheterization: Safe, cost-effective bladder management for male residents of VA nursing homes. *Journal of the American Geriatrics Society, 43*(8), 865–870.

Easton, S. (2000). InstantCath from Hollister: Pre-lubricated self-catheterization. *British Journal of Nursing, 9*(6), 357–360.

Fader, M., Cottenden, A., & Brooks, R. (2001). The CPE network: Creating an evidence base for continence product selection. *Journal of Wound, Ostomy, and Continence Nursing, 28*(2), 106–112.

Fantl, J.A., Newman, D.K., Colling, J., et al., for the Urinary Incontinence in Adults Guideline Update Panel. (1996). *Urinary incontinence in adults: Acute and chronic management. Clinical practice guideline* (No. 2. Update; AHCPR Publication No. 96-0682). Rockville, MD: Agency for Health Care Policy and Research.

Fiers, S. (1994). Indwelling catheters and devices: Avoiding the problems. *Urologic Nursing, 14*(3), 141–144.

Jeter, K., & Lutz, J. (1996). Skin care in the frail, older, dependent, incontinence patient. *Advances in Wound Care, 9,* 29–34.

Kemp, M.G. (1994). Protecting the skin from moisture and associated irritants. *Journal of Gerontological Nursing, 20*(9), 8–14.

Kuzminski, L.N. (1996). Cranberry juice and urinary tract infections: Is there a beneficial relationship? *Nutrition Reviews, 54*(11), S87–S90.

McClish, D.K., Wyman, J.F., Sale, P.G., Camp, J., & Earle, B. (1999). Use and costs of incontinence pads in female study volunteers. *Journal of Wound, Ostomy, and Continence Nursing, 26*(4), 207–213.

McMahon-Parkes, K. (1998). Management of suprapubic catheters. *Nursing Times, 94*(25), 49–51.

Morris, N.S., Stickler, D.J., & Mclean, R.J.C. (1999). The development of bacterial biofilms on indwelling urethral catheters. *World Journal of Urology, 17,* 345–350.

Morris, N.S., Stickler, D.J., & Winters, C. (1997). Which indwelling urethral catheters resist encrustations by Proteus mirabilis biofilms. *British Journal of Urology, 80,* 58–63.

Moseley, C.B. (1994). Inappropriate clinical care in nursing homes. *American Journal of Medical Quality, 9,* 10–17.

Newman, D.K. (1998). Managing indwelling urethral catheters. *Ostomy/Wound Management, 44*(12), 26–28, 30, 32, 34–35.

Newman, D., & Blackwood, N. (1991, November 20). Applications and perspectives on the use of indwelling catheters. Paper presented at the National Multi-Specialty Nursing Conference, Kissimmee, FL.

Newman, D.K., Parente, C.A., & Yuan, J.R. (1997). Implementing the Agency for Health Care Policy and Research urinary incontinence guidelines in a home health agency. In M.D. Harris (Ed.), *Handbook of home health care administration* (2nd ed., pp. 394–403). Gaithersburg, MD: Aspen Publishers.

Newman, D.K., Wallace, D.W., & Wallace, J. (2001). Moisture control and incontinence management. In D. Krasner & D. Kane (Eds.), *Chronic wound care* (2nd ed., pp. 196–201). Wayne, PA: Health Management Publications.

Nicolle, L.E. (2001, May). The chronic indwelling catheter and urinary infection in long-term care facility residents. *Infection control and hospital epidemiology, 22*(5), 316–321.

Omnibus Budget Reconciliation Act of 1990, PL 101-508, 42 U.S.C. § 1396d *et seq.*

Ouslander, J.G., Kane, R.L., & Abrass, I.B. (1982). Urinary incontinence in elderly nursing home clients. *Journal of the American Medical Association, 248,* 1194.

Perrouin-Verbe, B., Labat, J.J., Richard, I., Mauduyt de la Greve, I., Buzelin, J.M., & Mathe, J.F. (1995). Clean intermittent catheterization from the acute period in spinal cord injury clients: Long term evaluation of urethral and genital tolerance. *Paraplegia, 33,* 619–624.

Rainville, N.C. (1994). The current nursing procedure for intermittent urinary catheterization in rehabilitation facilities. *Rehabilitation Nursing, 19*(6), 330–333.

Resnick, B. (1993). Retraining the bladder after catheterization. *American Journal of Nursing, 93*(11), 46–49.

Roe, B.H. (1990). Study of the effects of education on patients' knowledge and acceptance of their indwelling urethral catheters. *Journal of Advanced Nursing, 18,* 223–231.

Saint, S., Lipsky, B.A., Baker, P.D., McDonald, L.L., & Ossenkop, K. (1999). Urinary catheters: What type do men and their nurses prefer? *Journal of the American Geriatrics Society, 47*(12), 1453–1457.

Scardillo, J., & Aronovitch, S.A. (1999). Successfully managing incontinence-related irritant dermatitis across the lifespan. *Ostomy/Wound Management, 45*(4), 36–44.

Schnelle, J.F., Adamson, G.M., Cruise, P.A., Al-Sammarrai, N., Sarbaugh, F.C., Uman, G., & Ouslander, J.G. (1997). Skin disorders and moisture in incontinent nursing home residents: Intervention implications. *Journal of the American Geriatrics Society, 45,* 1182–1188.

Sedor, J., & Mulholland, S.G. (1999). Infections in urology: Hospital-acquired urinary tract infections with the indwelling catheter. *Urologic Clinics of North America, 26*(4), 821–828.

Sheriff, M.K.M., Foley, S., McFarlane, J., Nauth-Miser, R., Craggs, M., & Shah, P.J.R. (1998). Long-term suprapubic catheterisation: Clinical outcome and satisfaction survey. *Spinal Cord, 36,* 171–176.

Silverblatt, F.J., Tibert, C., Mikolich, D., Blazek-D'Arezzo, J., Alves, J., Tack, M., & Agatiello, P. (2000). Preventing the spread of vancomycin-resistant enterococci in a long term care facility. *Journal of the American Geriatrics Society, 48,* 1211–1215.

Terpenning, M.S., Bradley, S.F., Wan, J.Y., Chenoweth, C.E., Jorgensen, K.A., & Kauffman, C.A. (1994). Colonization and infection with antibiotic-resistant bacteria in a long-term care facility. *Journal of the American Geriatrics Society, 42*(10), 1062–1069.

Thornburn, P., Fader, M., Dean, G., Brooks, R., & Cottenden, A. (1997). Improving the performance of small incontinence pads: A study of "wet comfort." *Journal of Wound, Ostomy, and Continence Nursing, 24*(4), 219–225.

Verleyen, P., De Ridder, D., Van Poppel, H., & Beart, L. (1999). Clinical application of the Bardex IC foley catheter. *European Urology, 36,* 240–246.

Warren, J.W. (1997). Urinary tract infections: Catheter-associated urinary tract infections. *Infectious Disease Clinics of North America, 11*(3), 609–622.

Warren, J.W., Steinberg, L., Hebel, J.R., & Tenney, J.H. (1989). The prevalence of urethral catheterization in Maryland nursing homes. *Archives of Internal Medicine, 149,* 1535–1537.

Weld, K.J., & Dmochowski, R.R. (2000). Effect of bladder management on urological complications in spinal cord injured patients. *Journal of Urology, 163,* 768–772.

Zinn, J.S., Aaronson, W.E., & Rosko, M.D. (1993). The use of standardized indicators as quality improvement tools: An application in Pennsylvania nursing homes. *American Journal of Medical Quality, 8,* 72–78.

10

Drug Therapy for Incontinence and Overactive Bladder

Urinary incontinence (UI) may be treated with pharmacological agents, depending on the individual's symptoms and diagnostic evaluation. People whose overactive bladder (OAB) is secondary to excessive contractions of the bladder detrusor muscle (detrusor overactivity) may be treated with drugs that reduce excessive bladder (detrusor) contractions. Other individuals who have an underactive detrusor muscle will require treatment with drugs that stimulate contractions in the detrusor muscle. If the primary symptoms in the person result from excessive urethral sphincter contraction, drugs that relax the urethral sphincter may be indicated. The goal of drug therapy is for the person to reduce or even eliminate the number of UI and OAB symptoms through "independent continence" by following prescribed drug protocols. This type of treatment may also be classified as "dependent" continence if staff in a long-term care (LTC) facility or a caregiver in the home administers the medication. It is important to note that the majority of these medications have numerous and varied side effects, and their success diminishes with long-term use.

TREATMENT RECOMMENDATIONS

The recommendations for drug therapy in people with UI vary according to the type of incontinence.

Stress Incontinence

Stress incontinence is typically treated with surgery. Table 10.1 explains the types of surgery used for stress incontinence. Surgical correction of female stress incontinence (urethral hypermobility or intrinsic sphincter deficiency) is directed toward 1) repositioning the urethra and/or creating a backboard

Table 10.1 Surgical treatments for stress urinary incontinence

Procedure	Description	Complications
Colposuspension, Retropubic suspension	Retropubic procedures were long considered the gold standard surgical treatment for stress urinary incontinence (SUI). These operations elevate or stabilize the urethra and bladder neck into a well-supported retropubic position and may also provide a stable backboard on which the urethra and bladder neck are compressed during increases in intra-abdominal pressure. • The Marshall-Marchetti-Krantz (MMK) procedure involves an incision in the lower abdomen above the pubic bone. The urethra and the bladder neck are elevated and sutured to the pubic bone to prevent excessive displacement of the urethra during periods of increased physical stress. • The Burch procedure is another surgery performed through the lower abdomen. • Both procedures elevate and stabilize the urethra by suspending the anterior vaginal wall and periurethral tissues to fixed anatomic structures. The MMK fixes the tissues to the bone immediately anterior to the urethra (symphysis pubis) whereas the Burch fixes the tissues to iliopectineal (Cooper's) ligaments. Cooper's ligament is a strong, thick fibrous band that is located at the posterior and superior border of the superior ramus of the pubic bone. It is ideal for passing and holding the sutures. • There is a caution with this surgery because of continual gravitational pull on the urethra; the stitches can pull away from the tissue, causing the bladder neck and urethra to fall back into an abnormal position, especially if activity is resumed too early in the postoperative period. This is particularly true for physically active women who return to sports and exercising after surgery.	Urinary retention; urethral obstruction; new-onset pelvic prolapse (particularly enterocele formation); vesical, ureteral or bowel injury; urgency; frequency

Suburethral sling	The suburethral sling procedure stabilizes the urethra by placing it within a sling, suspending it to the rectus fascia or pubic bone. • The Pubo-vaginal sling uses a strip of fascia (the connective tissue covering muscles), usually taken from the abdominal wall or thigh, to add additional support to the bladder neck and to compress the urethra. Each end of the sling is secured to a fixed structure (the abdominal wall or pubic bone) with the middle portion of the sling supporting the urethra like a hammock. • TVT (Tension Free Support) is a mesh-like tape placed with minimal tension at the midurethra segment. It is inserted via a small vaginal incision. The aim is to have the tape lying free at rest (hence "tension-free") while exerting sufficient pressure on the urethra during a cough or laugh to prevent leakage of urine. TVT can be performed as an outpatient procedure.	Bladder overactivity, urinary retention, erosion of the sling material. TVT and slings can cause perforation of the bladder and bowel and retropubic bleeding. Overcorrection (e.g., too much tension applied to the sling or tape) may cause temporary or permanent lower urinary tract obstruction.
Periurethral injections of bulking agents	A substance is injected periurethrally to add bulk to the urethra and sphincter at the bladder neck to prevent urethral urine leakage by increasing outlet resistance. • Contigen is a collagen implant. A skin test is performed prior to injection to rule out allergy to the substance. • Durasphere is an injection of pyrolytic carbon beads that are not reabsorbable.	UTI, urinary retention, urgency, dysuria, hematuria, migration of the Durasphere beads into surrounding tissues.
Artificial urinary sphincter	A fluid-filled device is implanted inside the body but outside the bladder. The device consists of a cuff (bulb), a balloon, and a pump, all of which are connected by tubing. The cuff is placed around the outside of the urethra; the pump is placed in the labia majora in females and in the scrotal sac in males. The balloon is placed in the lower abdomen next to the bladder. There is fluid in the prosthesis, which is connected to the bulb or cuff through a small tube. The bulb or cuff gently squeezes the urethra shut to keep urine in the bladder. The man squeezes the pump in his scrotum to move the fluid from inside the cuff up to the balloon. The balloon will hold the fluid so urine may pass from the bladder. In 3–4 minutes, the fluid will return from the balloon down to the cuff to close off the urethra again and stop urinary leakage. After voiding, the pressure in the prosthesis returns to its normal level.	Urethral erosion, device malfunction, infection

of support or otherwise stabilizing the urethra and bladder neck in a well-supported retropubic (intra-abdominal) position that is receptive to changes in intra-abdominal pressure or 2) creating coaptation and/or compression or otherwise augmenting the urethral resistance provided by the intrinsic sphincter unit, with (i.e., sling) or without (i.e., periurethral injectables) affecting urethral and bladder neck support.

More than 100 different operations have been designed to treat female urethral incontinence. Surgeries directed toward repositioning or stabilizing the bladder neck and proximal urethra are often classified according to the operative approach: retropubic (transabdominal) or transvaginal. Sometimes, Tension Free Support is considered a separate entity. Unfortunately, the success rate for surgery may not be as high for older adults as it is for younger women if the woman has detrusor overactivity, urgency, and frequency in addition to stress UI. Long-term data indicate success (improvement/cure) rates of 80%–90% for sling procedures and slightly less for Burch and Marshall-Marchetti-Krantz procedures. Surgery for recurrent incontinence may have a poorer outcome.

For postmenopausal women with stress incontinence, α-adrenergic agonists (e.g., pseudoephedrine) may be recommended as adjunctive treatment. Adverse drug reactions (ADRs) with α-adrenergic agonists are infrequent but include anxiety, insomnia, agitation, dyspnea, headache, sweating, hypertension, and cardiac arrhythmia. These agents should be used cautiously in patients with hypertension, hyperthyroidism, cardiac arrhythmias, or angina. Patients with known or suspected breast, cervix, or uterine cancer or thromboembolic disorders should not receive estrogen.

Urge Incontinence

Anticholinergic agents such as tolterodine (Detrol/Detrol LA) and oxybutynin (Ditropan/Ditropan XL) are first-line pharmacotherapy for urge incontinence. Both drugs are associated with anticholinergic ADRs (e.g., dry mouth, blurred vision, constipation, mental status changes); however, Detrol has a greater affinity for bladder receptors and therefore may have a reduced incidence of anticholinergic ADRs. Surgical intervention for urge incontinence is used if conservative measures have failed, the person has interstitial cystitis, and the person has idiopathic chronic urinary retention. The procedure used is sacral nerve neuromodulation, or surgical implantation of a permanent device that modulates the neural pathways controlling bladder function. The device serves as a urinary bladder "pacemaker." The mechanism by which it exerts its effects are unknown, but it is theorized that the electrical signals from the device modulate the neural impulses that subserve micturition. The electrode is inserted into a sacral foramen and connected by a lead extension to the pulse generator, which is implanted in the subcutaneous area of the buttocks.

Mixed Incontinence

Therapeutic interventions are targeted at identifying and treating the most bothersome symptoms.

TYPES OF DRUGS

To Treat Urge Incontinence

Overactive bladder with urge incontinence and detrusor hyperreflexia are the two most common causes of urge UI that have been treated successfully by drug therapy. Drugs used to treat these conditions affect the central and peripheral neural control pathways or the detrusor muscle itself (Wien, 2001). Detrusor muscle overactivity may be treated with anticholinergics because of their ability to relax smooth muscle of the bladder. This treatment increases the bladder volume necessary to stimulate a detrusor contraction, while decreasing the strength of that contraction and increasing the total bladder capacity.

Various agents are used; the most commonly prescribed for OAB being antimuscarinic (anticholinergic) drugs. Historically, the tolerability and safety concerns that have accompanied antimuscarinic therapy have limited their use in the treatment of OAB, especially as this condition normally requires long-term treatment. The problem with antimuscarinic therapy is that it lacks receptor selectivity resulting in common anticholinergic side effects. The use of newer medications with improved selectivity causing fewer side effects and safety concerns has greatly improved the management of this condition.

Anticholinergics   Currently there are many anticholinergic preparations available for the pharmacological treatment of individuals with OAB and UI (see Table 10.2). In people with involuntary bladder contractions, anticholinergic agents will increase the volume of urine required to stimulate the first involuntary bladder contraction, decrease the amplitude of that contraction, and increase bladder capacity; however, the drug will not change the urgency. Thus, drug therapy must always be combined with behavior therapy to achieve optimal results in OAB (Wein, 1998). All anticholinergic agents are contraindicated in people with documented narrow-angle glaucoma (Lackner, 2000).

One of the most commonly used antimuscarinic preparation is oxybutynin (Ditropan), which was originally developed to treat gastrointestinal disorders. Oxybutynin is an anticholinergic and direct smooth muscle relaxant. It blocks the contraction of the bladder by relaxing the bladder muscles. Although oxybutynin is efficacious, the major drawback is its adverse effects, which are often severe enough to cause people to discontinue treatment. Of particular concern is bothersome dry mouth, which occurs in 61%–78%

Table 10.2. Drug therapy for urinary incontinence (UI)

Urge UI

Drug	Action	Dosage	Side effects	Comments
Tolterodine tartrate (Detrol, Detrol LA)	Anticholinergic agent that inhibits cholinergic muscarinic receptors in the bladder	2 mg twice daily (IR) 4 mg daily (ER) *In special populations:[a]* 1 mg twice daily (IR) 2 mg daily (ER, Detrol LA)	Dry mouth, somnolence, dyspepsia, headache, constipation, and xeropthalmia	Indicated for patients with an over-active bladder with symptoms of urinary frequency, urgency, or urge UI. May cause urinary retention. This agent may be better tolerated than others.
Oxybutynin (Ditropan, Ditropan XL)	Anticholinergic agent that blocks bladder contraction by relaxing the bladder muscles	5 mg two to three times a day 5 mg daily (Ditropan XL) *In special populations:[a]* 2.5–5 mg twice daily *Titrate:* Increase by 2.5-mg increments every 1–2 days as needed	Dry mouth, blurred vision, constipation, increased intraocular pressure, somnolence or confusion, and cardiac disturbances	Many patients discontinue therapy because of intolerable side effects. Sometimes useful at bedtime in patients with nocturia and nocturnal enuresis.
Imipramine (Tofranil) (can be effective in both stress and urge UI)	Tricyclic antidepressant and anticholinergic that decreases bladder contractions and increases urethral resistance to outflow	10–25 mg three times a day (but usually given at bedtime)	Postural hypotension, cardiac arrythmia, weakness, and fatigue	Food and Drug Administration has approved for enuresis in children but not in adults.

Propantheline (Pro-Banthine)	Tertiary amine that is a smooth muscle relaxant	15–30 mg every 4–6 hours	Dry mouth, confusion, agitation and orthostatic hypotension, constipation, and blurred vision	High incidence of side effects, especially in older adults. Use with caution in clients with glaucoma, coronary artery disease, or prostatism
Stress UI				
Phenylpropanolamine, phenylpropanolamine/chlorpheniramine (Ornade), pseudoephedrine (Sudafed)[b]	α_1-Adrenergic agents; increase bladder outlet resistance through actions on the bladder neck, bladder base, and proximal urethra. Produce urethral contraction and increase urethral pressure. Ornade is a combination antihistamine and decongestant; added anticholinergic effect may improve UI.	*Phenylpropanolamine:* Immediate release: 25–50 mg two or three times a day; extended release: 75 mg twice daily. *Ornade:* 1 capsule every 12 hours (75 mg phenypropanolamine and 12 mg chlorpheniramine per capsule) *Pseudoephedrine:* Immediate release: 15–30 mg three times a day; extended release: 120 mg every 12–24 hours	Tachycardia, elevated blood pressure, stomach cramping nervousness, respiratory difficulty, dizziness Signs of overdose or serious adverse effects include headache, confusion, seizures, and hallucinations.	Do not modify sustained-release forms to achieve dose. Components are found in over the counter (OTC) decongestants. Use with caution in clients with hypertension, angina, hyperthyroidism, or diabetes. Combination with β-blockers or digoxin may cause dangerous drug interactions. Sudafed and Ornade are OTC drugs. Use for UI constitutes an off-label use.

(continued)

Table 10.2. *(continued)*

Stress UI (*continued*)

Drug	Action	Dosage	Side effects	Comments
Conjugated estrogens (Premarin), oral estradiol, estradiol vaginal cream (Estrace and Premarin), estradiol vaginal tablets (Vagifem), estradiol vaginal ring (Estung)	Hormone replacement therapy restores the integrity of the urethral mucosa and increases resistance to outflow It is felt that estrogens may restore urethral mucosal coaptation and increase vascularity and tone	*Topical conjugated estrogens:* 0.3–1.25 mg/day topically every hour. Apply for 3 weeks on and 1 week off. *Oral estradiol:* 500 µg to 2 mg continuously or cyclically *Estradiol vaginal cream:* Insert 2- to 4-g (marked on applicator) dose for 1–2 weeks, then 1 g twice a week *Estradiol vaginal tablets:* Insert 25-µg tab every day for 2 weeks, then 1 tab twice weekly *Estradiol vaginal ring:* 7.5mg/24 hours. Silicone ring inserted every 90 days.	Uterine cancer (intact uterus), fluid retention, depression, nausea, vomiting, elevated blood pressure, gallstones, cardiovascular effects, and vaginal bleeding. Most effects are with oral dosage.	May benefit patients with stress UI and mixed UI. Women with a uterus need oppositional therapy with progesterone when oral estrogens are prescribed. Contraindicated in patients with known or suspected breast or uterine cancer. Women already taking oral hormones may benefit from topical application.

From Newman, D.K. (1998). Controversies in incontinence. *The Clinical Letter for Nurse Practitioners, 2*(6), 1–8; adapted by permission.

Key: IR—immediate release; ER—extended release

[a]Dosage adjustments are recommended for people with hepatic and renal failure.

[b]FDA recommended withdrawal of phenylpropanolomine from over the counter drugs, so check ingredients for inclusion.

of people receiving oxybutynin. Attempts to minimize the side effects of oxybutynin have included intravesically administered doses in patients with preexistent or intermittent catheters, use of transdermal patches (Oxytrol), and the development of a controlled-release delivery system incorporating the OROS osmotic drug delivery system (Ditropan XL). Research has shown that extended-release oxybutynin taken once daily has comparable efficacy to the immediate-release formulation (three times daily) at the same total daily dosage. The extended-release formulation has been associated with a significant reduction in dry mouth compared with the immediate-release formulation. Oxybutynin is also associated with gastrointestinal and central nervous system side effects. Oxybutynin should be used with caution in elderly people because of possible cognitive side effects.

A new drug, tolterodine (Detrol), has been introduced for the management of OAB. Tolterodine appears to lack many of the limitations of other antimuscarinic medications available for the treatment of OAB. Studies show that fewer patients taking tolterodine suffer from dry mouth and other gastrointestinal side effects when compared with oxybutynin at a therapeutically equivalent dosage (i.e., 5 mg three times per day). Tolterodine, at the normal dosage of 2 mg twice daily, is well tolerated and effective in the management of all symptoms of OAB, resulting in meaningful improvements for people with OAB. A new extended-release (ER) formulation of tolterodine, at a dosage of 4 mg daily, provided significant improvements in the symptoms of OAB in women and was 18% more effective than the immediate-release (IR) formulation in a comparative study (Chancellor et al., 2000). Moreover, compared with the existing IR tablet formulation, tolterodine ER is significantly more effective in reducing incontinence episodes and is better tolerated, with a lower frequency of dry mouth.

Hyoscyamine (Cystospaz) and hyoscyamine sulfate (Levsin, Cystospaz-M) are reported to have about the same anticholinergic actions and side effects as other drugs of this classification. Flavoxate (Urispas) has a direct spasmolytic as well as anticholinergic effect on smooth muscle. Research has not demonstrated the efficacy of these drugs. However, it is important to note that the newer ER formulations of both OAB drug (Detrol LA and Ditropan XL) control plasma drug fluctuations, thus reducing peak drug concentrations and lowering the risk of cholinergic side effects.

Bethanechol (Duvoid, Myotonachol, Urecholine) is a cholinergic drug that is used to treat bladder (detrusor) underactivity in those individuals with incomplete bladder emptying. This drug is contraindicated in people with asthma, bradycardia, and Parkinson's disease. Its side effects include sweating and excessive salivation, which are often considered intolerable.

Antidepressants   Imipramine, a tricyclic antidepressant, has a dual action when used to treat UI: It decreases bladder contractions through its anticholinergic effects and increases urethral resistance to outflow through its α-agonist properties. It should be noted that imipramine is officially approved by the Food and Drug Administration (FDA) for enuresis in children but not for adults. Side effects may include postural hypotension and cardiac conduction disturbances in older individuals. Older people with cardiac conduction problems should avoid treatment with this category of drugs unless the benefits outweigh the risks.

Tertiary Amines   Another commonly used agent is propantheline (Pro-Banthine), which has antimuscarinic and ganglionic blocking effects. Even in young people, the drug has a high incidence of side effects, and it must be used with caution in people with glaucoma, coronary artery disease, or prostatism. Elderly people are especially prone to confusion, agitation, and orthostatic hypotension when taking propantheline. When using this medication, postvoid urine residuals should be monitored to avoid urinary retention.

To Treat Stress Incontinence

α-Adrenergic Agents   In people with stress incontinence, pharmacological therapy should be focused on using agents that increase bladder outlet resistance through their actions on the bladder neck and base, and on the proximal urethra. Sympathomimetic drugs with α-adrenergic agonist actions are the agents of choice. The two most commonly used sympathomimetic agents are phenylpropanolamine (PPA), which can be found in agents such as Ornade, and pseudoephedrine, which can be found in Sudafed (see Table 10.2). Both of these over-the-counter drugs are commonly used as decongestants. Recently, the FDA recommended withdrawal of PPA from these OTC drugs. PPA is believed to stimulate α-adrenergic receptors and increase bladder outlet resistance. Side effects of this class of drug include tachycardia, elevated blood pressure, stomach cramping, nervousness, respiratory difficulty, and dizziness. These drugs should be used with caution in people with hypertension, angina, hyperthyroidism, and diabetes. Because of the possibility of additive side effects, sympathomimetic drugs of one class should not be combined with sympathomimetic drugs of another class.

Hormones   Another group of medications for women that are receiving more positive attention are hormones (estrogens). Estrogen therapy has the potential to treat urge and mixed UI and OAB symptomatology in postmenopausal women. Although there are multiple mechanisms by which estrogen might favorably affect lower urinary tract function, opinion is divided as to whether low-dose local (topical) therapy or systemic therapy can, per se, ameliorate irritative lower urinary tract symptoms in the postmenopausal woman (Cardozo, 1997). The increase in vaginal pH with aging is thought to change the entire urogenital environment, leading to urinary tract infections (UTIs), pelvic organ prolapse, UI, and OAB. Estrogen supports colonization of the vaginal vault by lactobacilli. Lactobacilli produce lactic acid, which keeps vaginal pH low, thus preventing the growth of bacteria (e.g., *Escherichia coli*). Studies have shown that estrogen therapy provides significant protection from UTIs (Cardozo, Bachmann, McClish, Fonda, & Bigerson, 1998; Maloney, 1997). It is believed that, when there is a vaginal response to estrogen, there will be a similar response in the urethra and bladder mucosa (Carson, Chaiken, Haney, & Staskin, 2000). Estrogens can restore the integrity of the urethral mucosa and thereby increase resistance to outflow.

Estrogens are either used systemically (orally) or topically (locally). The advantages to topical versus systemic hormone replacement therapy are that topical therapy has beneficial effects on vaginal and urinary symptoms and mucosal appearance without provoking withdrawal bleeding from the endometrium (Mouritisen & Frialoney, 1997). The following side effects of estrogens have been reported: endometrial cancer, fluid retention, depression, nausea, vomiting, elevated blood pressure, gallstones, and cardiovascular effects such as stroke and myocardial infarction. A cyclic topical application is preferred because of its decreased side effects. Local administration is believed to be more effective for reducing frequency of recurrent UTIs and other urogenital symptoms than oral therapy. In elderly women with diagnosed atrophic vaginitis, residing in nursing facilities or in their homes, a low dose of conjugated vaginal estrogen cream applied to urogenital tissues either intravaginally or externally for 6 weeks was found to be effective in reducing vaginal pH (Maloney & Oliver, 2001). Local application of estrogen may also prevent recurrent UTIs, especially in women with recurrent infections (Maloney, 1998). It is also believed that lower systemic absorption of estrogen results from intravaginal administration compared with oral administration.

The traditional form of local estrogen therapy is an estrogen vaginal cream (see Table 10.2). A fingertip's worth of estradiol cream weighs about 1 g, which equals 0.1 mg of estradiol; however, there are disadvantages to this form of topical application: Vaginal cream must be measured by the user and may be difficult to insert. The cream can also leave a residue on the vulva and undergarments and necessitate deferring coitus.

There are two relatively new low-dose estrogen drug delivery systems: an estrodial vaginal ring (Estring) and vaginal tablets (Vagifem). The ring is soft, slightly opaque, and flexible. It is inserted into the upper part of the vagina as a contraceptive diaphragm would be. The ring releases a steady, low dose of estrogen that is absorbed into the vaginal tissues over a period of 3 months. The estradiol release rate is determined by the silicone ring and remains constant at 7.5 μg/24 hours for a period of 90 days (Caspar et al., 1999). It normally takes 2–3 weeks after insertion to feel the full effects of the ring. Estradiol vaginal tablets are small, white, film-coated, hydrophilic tablets containing 25 μg of estradiol. The tablet is contained in a disposable single-use applicator used for insertion of the tablet into the vagina. A gel layer forms when the tablet comes in contact with the vagina. The estradiol is released from this gel layer.

REFERENCES

Cardozo, L. (1997). Discussion: The effect of estrogens. *Urology, 50*(Suppl. 6A), 85.

Cardozo, L., Bachmann, G., McClish, D., Fonda, D., & Bigerson, L. (1998). Meta-analysis of estrogen therapy in the management of urogenital atrophy in post-menopausal women: Second report of the Hormones and Urogenital Therapy Committee. *Obstetrics and Gynecology, 92*(4, Pt. 2), 722–727.

Carson, C.C., Chaikin, D., Haney, A.F., & Staskin, D.R. (2000). Urogenital consequences of estrogen deficiency. *Contemporary Urology*(Suppl.), 3–12.

Casper, F., Petri, E., and the Vaginal Ring Study Group. (1999). Local treatment of urogenital atrophy with an estradiol-releasing vaginal ring: A comparative and a placebo-controlled multicenter study. *International Urogynecology Journal, 10,* 171–176.

Chancellor, M., Freedman, S., Mitcheson, D., Antoci, A., Primus, G., & Wein, A. (2000). Tolterodine: An effective and well tolerated treatment for urge incontinence and bladder symptoms. *Clinical Drug Investigation, 19,* 83–91

Lackner, T.E. (2000). Pharmacologic management of urinary incontinence. *Annals of Long-Term Care, 8*(2), 29–37.

Maloney, C. (1997). Estrogen in urinary incontinence treatment: An anatomic and physiologic approach. *Urologic Nursing, 17*(3), 88–91.

Maloney, C. (1998). Hormone replacement therapy in female nursing home residents with recurrent urinary tract infection. *Annals of Long-Term Care, 6*(3), 77–82.

Maloney, C., & Oliver, M.L. (2001). Effect of local conjugated estrogens on vaginal pH in elderly women. *Journal of the American Medical Directors Association, 2,* 51–55.

Mouritisen, L., & Frialoney C. (1997). Estrogen in urinary incontinence treatment: An anatomic and physiologic approach. *Urologic Nursing, 17*(3), 88–91.

Newman, D.K. (1998). Controversies in incontinence. *The Clinical Letter for Nurse Practitioners, 2*(6), 1–8.

Wein, A.J. (Ed.). (1998). Urinary incontinence: The scope of the problem—the solutions on the horizon. *Urology, 51*(Suppl. 2A).

Wein, A.J. (2001). Pharmacological agents for the treatment urinary inconinence due to overactive bladder. *Expert Opinion on Investigational Drugs, 10*(1), 65–83.

11

Development of
Continence Services

Evaluation and treatment of urinary incontinence (UI), overactive bladder (OAB), and related pelvic disorders is a changing and expanding area of practice for doctors, allied health professionals, and nurses—especially advanced practice nurses (APNs). Almost every day, health care professionals encounter incontinent people despite the fact that UI is not always the reason for the initial professional contact. Surprisingly, physicians inquire about UI in only a minority of their at-risk patients (McFall, Yerkes, Bernard, & Le Rud, 1997), even though family doctors can be effective in treating incontinence by conservative measures when educated and motivated (Borrie, Bawden, Kartha, & Kerr, 1992; Lagro-Janssen, Debruyne, Smits, & VanWeel, 1992). A comprehensive service will only work well if those responsible for primary healthcare are educated about incontinence, learn to ask patients about the problem, and know how to refer appropriately.

Most doctors, nurses, and allied health professionals receive little if any basic training in fecal and urinary incontinence. Organizations such as the Agency for Health Care Policy and Research (AHCPR; now known as the Agency for Healthcare Research and Quality, AHRQ) have set guidelines for medical practitioners concerning urinary incontinence in adults, but these measures are largely ignored by the medical community.

GROWTH OF INCONTINENCE CARE SPECIALISTS

Despite this lack of formal training, there are a growing group of nurses—APNs—who have taken up the AHCPR's recommendations, incorporating them in evidence-based clinical practice and care pathways (Button et al., 1998; Sampselle et al., 2000). Advanced practice nurses are clinical nurse specialists, nurse practitioners, nurse midwives, and nurse anesthetists who have completed a master of science degree in nursing. These health care professionals are knowledgeable about a wide range of medical health conditions and work closely with a physician collaborator to maximize patient outcomes in acute, primary, home care, outpatient, and long-term care (LTC) settings. These APNs usually serve as clinical support for nurses who have incontinent patients. They also are catalysts for improved care and coordination of services. They provide comprehensive assessment and noninvasive treatment and act as educators and researchers. These APNs either practice independently or as part of a multidisciplinary team (McDowell, Burgio, Dombrowski, Loches, & Rodrequez, 1992). This situation has been aided by the broadening of authority for APNs, including 1) the ability to receive direct reimbursement from insurers such as Medicare, Medicaid, health maintenance organizations (HMOs), and other private insurers; 2) the implementation of prescriptive authority; and 3) the removal of barriers to independent practice (Newman, 1996). These changes have given APNs the opportunity to expand services for the management of UI (Mooney, Newman, Smith, & Grey, 1993; Newman & Palumbo, 1994).

Although small in number, some APNs are working in home care and LTC settings and providing expert consultation in UI and related disorders (Newman, Parente, & Yuan, 1997; see Profile 11.1). This author has provided UI consultation in both of these settings and developed the setting-specific materials found in Tables 11.1–11.3, which outline protocols and list types of referrals and steps used for implementing a bladder and bowel retraining program in the LTC setting. Some APNs have also been active in developing health promotion programs (e.g., *Dry Anticipations* by the Oklahoma State Health Department, *Dry Expectations* and *Bladder Health* by this author with Rutgers University School of Nursing and Philadelphia Corporation For Aging in Philadelphia) for community centers (McFall, Yerkes, Belzer, & Cowan, 1994; Newman, Palmer, O'Connor, Flynn, & Brown, 2001; Newman, Wallace, & Blackwood, 1996).

PROFILE 11.1: WELLSPRING PROGRAM

Leslie Saltzstein Wooldridge, MSN, RNCS, GNP
Owner, Adult Bladder Control Center
President, Diversified Nurse Consulting, Ltd., Ada, Michigan

In an effort to control the incidence and severity of UI in LTC, an organization called Wellspring Innovative Solutions developed a model for promoting quality of care in LTC settings. The model included a shared program of staff training, clinical consultation, and education from a geriatric nurse practitioner. The program, which was directed through the incontinence program, utilized an interdisciplinary approach to the care and treatment of incontinence.

This process began by having a 2½-day educational seminar where staff from nursing (registered nurses, licenses nurse practitioners, and certified nursing assistants), therapy, dietary, and even housekeeping came to-

Table 11.1. Bladder and bowel retraining protocol for long-term care (LTC)

The overall goal is for the consultant to assist the LTC staff in:

Assessing the resident's clinical and functional status, individual strengths, and personal and environmental factors that have an impact on the resident's risk of becoming or remaining incontinent or developing a related bladder problem (e.g., urinary tract infection [UTI])

Planning and implementing continuous individualized interventions to prevent urinary incontinence (UI) and UTIs

Maintaining normal bladder function or to achieve normal or improved bladder function and continence in all residents

Recognizing and addressing changes in the individual resident's status that may increase the resident's risk for incontinence or UTI or may signal attainment of the established goal regarding bladder function.

The consultant will provide:

Evaluation and assessment of residents with urinary incontinence and related problems to include comprehensive medical history, modified physical examination, determination of bladder function, and urinalysis

Environmental, functional, and mental status evaluation to determine deterrents to continence

Identification with staff assistance of daily habits, frequency, and circumstances of bladder or bowel dysfunction

Establishment of a diagnosis of the type of incontinence and contributing factors

Provision of assistance to nursing facility staff by participating in rounds or care plan conferences on identified residents

Assessment of bowel function with implementation of a bowel regimen

Development of a behavioral program to include toileting assistance or bladder retraining

Pelvic muscle rehabilitation training to appropriately motivated and cognitively intact persons with appropriate biofeedback training and/or pelvic floor electrical stimulation

Assessment of all residents with indwelling catheters and implementation of catheter removal or a voiding or intermittent catheterization program

Implementation of the use of appropriate collection devices or management strategies for individuals with chronic, long-term urinary incontinence who cannot be otherwise managed

Design an on-going care plan in partnership with the nursing facility staff to include revisions as needed

gether to learn about what incontinence was and how each member of the health care team contributed in the prevention and decrease in incidences. The different types of incontinence as well as how important the approach was to each type were discussed. Treatment options for the caregivers and what one might expect from the resident's provider, whether it be a physician or nurse practitioner, were identified. The staff took the lead in assessing the resident. Registered nurses did the physical assessment, including perineal observations. Licensed practical nurses

Table 11.2.   Types of referrals in long-term care

Assess residents with urinary incontinence and a variety of bladder related problems. The following are examples of appropriate referrals. Residents who:

Have complaints of urinary frequency, urgency, and "always running to the bathroom"

Have new onset of episodic urinary incontinence

Are using absorbent products and/or other toileting aids (e.g., bedpans)

May benefit from a structured toileting program

Have indwelling catheters and need assessment for alternative management and evaluation of catheter-related problems

Are cognitively impaired and need an appropriate care plan

Need complete history and physical examinations

Have pelvic prolapse and need a supportive device like a pessary

Have fecal incontinence, constipation, and other bowel problems

collected other information that was helpful in the final plan, and certified nurse assistants provided information related to results of urine dipsticks, postvoid residuals via bladder scanning, voiding patterns based on 3-day Bladder Records, fluid intakes, and mobility and dexterity observations. The team then assembled to review the problems, determine the type of incontinence, and develop a reasonable plan to get the resident on the road to recovery.

The monumental task of getting all the residents assessed and placing them on manageable plans took effort. Prior to leaving the seminar on the second day, teams developed a plan for getting all residents into the program over the next 6 months. This plan also included the process of teaching the rest of the staff what they had learned. The "Care Resource Team," as they were known, became the experts in the facility for this module of the program, called "urinary incontinence" or "elimination." The facility had access to an APN who specialized in geriatrics to provide guidance with difficult residents, their process of implementation, and staff management challenges. This APN made regular visits to the facility and met with the team to discuss progress. Problem solving utilizing the entire team was paramount to successful outcomes.

After about 4 months, the teams from each facility in an alliance (usually 10 facilities) met to discuss the implementation of their plans, their accomplishments, their challenges, and a case study of a resident success or a resident with whom they were looking for guidance. This session was facilitated by the APN who also discussed theory or gave a presentation on more advanced issues related to incontinence that he or she had noted to be a knowledge deficit in the progress of the program.

The final area of discussion was data collection. Knowing how each resident was progressing in an objective way was significant to the success of this program. It was this feedback to both staff and residents on how the plan was working that made for continued work toward making

Table 11.3. Steps to implementing a bladder and bowel retraining program in long-term care

Step 1

The key to success of the bladder and bowel retraining program includes a commitment by the administration of the facility. To meet that goal, a staff in-service on the bladder and bowel retraining program will be scheduled to include nursing staff on all three shifts. It is expected that all employees will participate in the education program. There will be ongoing continuing education to inform and educate new staff as to the techniques and principles of continence management.

Step 2

Meet with the medical director to discuss the bladder and bowel retraining program's assessment techniques, treatment, and management strategies. It is important that the medical director understands the concepts of this program and supports its implementation. If appropriate, a letter will be sent to the resident's family physician informing him of the implementation of the program. A chart order for a bladder and bowel evaluation of a resident should be obtained from the medical director or the resident's family physician by the nursing facility's nursing staff.

Step 3

It is the responsibility of the nursing facility's staff to notify residents and families about initiation of the program, citing goals and benefits of the program. Many residents and families are unaware of federal and state regulations that govern the development and implementation of programs for bladder and bowel retraining in nursing facilities. It is important that residents and families are notified of the program prior to implementation to allow for informed consent.

It is recommended that notification be given to the residents and/or families in the form of a letter or public announcement. A meeting with family members at a scheduled evening gathering to explain the program may be appropriate. This letter should be part of the facility's admission packet so all newly admitted residents and families are aware of the program.

It will definitely be considered an asset, both by the public and regulatory agencies, for a nursing facility to have in place an established and organized program for the treatment of this overwhelming problem.

each resident as dry as they could be. Each resident was reviewed with another 24-hour Bladder Record around the time of their quarterly staffing. This was reviewed with the previous record, and comparisons were done. Data were compiled and sent to a central data processing area each quarter where the numbers were calculated and the staff and administration received reports that indicated how each resident and unit had done on the program and how this impacted the prevalence and severity of incontinence in that facility. Plans were reviewed on a quarterly basis. Teams met with quality management teams in the facility to discuss the outcomes of the program and share cost savings in not only staff time but also supplies.

Elimination and urinary continence was one of seven clinical modules that each of these facilities went through. Completion of these modules as well as implementation took 2 years. During this time, there was an APN who was always available for consultation regarding clinical or systems issues in regards to the implementation of Wellspring.

Nurses have become the expert incontinence clinicians, educators, administrators, and researchers (Smith & Newman, 1990). However, no federal initiative has recommended formation of incontinence specialists. Therefore, a more formal structured movement in this nursing subspecialty is not likely in the near future. In 1994, Jacobs, Wyman, Rowell, and Smith (1998) surveyed nurses attending a national conference on UI about their educational preparation related to this condition. Respondents reported that less than half (40%) received academic education including course work in accredited post-baccalaureate or graduate programs related to UI. However, most nurses (76%) obtained instruction at professional conferences, continence clinics supervised by nurse practitioners or physicians, on-the-job training, self-study, and in-service programs. Another source of information was courses on the application of equipment and modality sponsored by companies who provide urodynamic and/or biofeedback equipment (e.g., The Prometheus Group, Hollister/Incare Medical Products, LifeTech, Laborie Medical Technologies, Circon Corporation).

Nurses have taken on certain activities to further their expertise in this area, including reading medical and nursing journals, attending professional meetings, observing clinical findings of other health care professionals (urologist, urogynecologist, or gynecologist), and joining professional organizations to discuss topics related to the care of incontinent patients. This author and her colleagues (Newman, Smith, et al., 1994) reported on a clinical and didactic training program held from 1987 to 1994 that trained 82 health care professionals on the identification, assessment, and evaluation of UI. The professionals attending this program completed hands-on training in the application of behavioral interventions including biofeedback and pelvic floor electrical stimulation. They were able to observe clinical practice in all settings, including hospital-based clinics, private practice, office, LTC, and home care. Participants included 76 nurses (6 nurses with Ph.D.s in nursing; 44 APNs, and 25 registered nurses), 2 physical therapists, 1 physician assistant, and 3 physicians. Time spent in training averaged 5 days but ranged from 3 to 21 days. Many of these professionals were able to expand an incontinence practice in their geographic area. One such practitioner is highlighted in Profile 11.2.

PROFILE 11.2: MULTI-SETTING PRACTICE FOR INCONTINENCE

Cindy Maloney, RNC, MS, FNP
Director, Seton Health Incontinence Treatment Center,
Troy, New York

Seton Health's Incontinence Treatment Center was established in 1993 as a specialty service of a large health system in Troy, New York. Seton Health includes an outpatient, hospital, skilled nursing, adult care, and other specialty services, as well as nine primary care practices, and it is a national member of Ascension Health. The center provides noninvasive evaluation and treatment of incontinence and related disorders in the outpatient, inpatient, skilled nursing, assisted living, and home care environments.

The Incontinence Treatment Center is staffed by nurse practitioners, one of whom is a certified wound, ostomy, and continence nurse. A urologist serves as the collaborating physician. The urologist and APN work collaboratively in the outpatient ambulatory center. The director and clinical supervisor lecture nationally on this subject and have published several articles related to noninvasive evaluation and treatment of urinary incontinence. The nurse practitioners' (NPs) mission is to provide individualized medical evaluation and care to patients with urinary incontinence. The NPs also play the role of educator and provide in-services to hospital, skilled nursing, and adult care staff as well as community audiences.

Referrals in the LTC facility (i.e., skilled nursing facility [SNF]) are initiated by the primary care provider. An important role of the NP is to educate SNF staff in becoming proficient in basic evaluation procedures including historical and physical assessments related to continence. Staff also request that a 3-day prompted voiding trial be done before referral to rule out functional incontinence. Outcomes are measured and usually reveal 65%–85% improvement or cure when behavioral and/or pharmaceutical intervention is implemented based on a differential diagnosis.

Urocare is a consultant service providing SNF evaluation in the New York City area that is similar to services provided by Seton Health. Utilizing the NP model, a focus on individualized assessment is done to produce recommendations specific to the resident.

INCONTINENCE PRACTICE MODELS

The organization of incontinence services depends on the organization and structure of health services generally. Urinary incontinence is so widespread and affects so many different types of people that those experiencing UI might ask literally any health care professional for help. It is impractical, therefore, to expect one portal of entry to a continence program. The challenge is to plan a service that ensures a systematic care pathway (i.e., a stepwise progression of investigation and treatment that each patient follows without overlaps or omissions) and the best use of limited resources (Newman et al., in press).

In some health systems, incontinence traditionally has been seen solely as a nursing problem, with little interest or input from other members of a multidisciplinary medical team. Except for a few isolated areas, the main intervention has been helping the individual and caregivers cope with symptoms rather than attempting to cure the incontinence. In fact, UI is often a complex and multi-faceted problem, particularly in frail or dependent individuals, and it may require input from a wide variety of disciplines (e.g., geriatrician, internal medicine, gastroenterologist) to tackle it effectively. While it may not be practical for all specialties to work in close proximity, careful consideration must be given to who does what, with protocols guiding appropriate referrals and ensuring good liaisons. Special attention must focus on avoiding gaps or overlaps in the service.

Members of the medical community understand the causes of and the urgency required to better address these conditions. Health care providers, specifically urologists, are treating UI more proactively, and companies, specifically the pharmaceutical and medical equipment industries, are investing significant resources in developing treatment alternatives. At the same time, aging baby boomers are demanding better solutions to many of the urological conditions awaiting them and are raising awareness and acceptance of urological problems. As the population worldwide expands, urological disorders will increase in prevalence. The population is aging, thus increasing the patient base of people who will require urologic services.

Urologists specialize in treating problems of the urinary tract in both men and women. In fact, a growing number of urologists collaborating with APNs are focusing solely on treating the genitourinary problems of women and men, particularly UI, OAB, interstitial cystitis, and related conditions (see Profile 11.3). Just as the patient population is seeking new treatment alternatives, the insurance industry, in general, and managed care organizations, in particular, are seeking providers who can provide all spectrum of services, especially for a condition as chronic and debilitating as incontinence.

PROFILE 11.3: COLLABORATIVE UROLOGIC PRACTICE FOR CONTINENCE AND PELVIC HEALTH

The Division of Urology, University of Pennsylvania Health System (UPHS), in Philadelphia created a Center of Excellence within the current urology department to address the problem of UI and pelvic disorders. The Penn Center for Continence and Pelvic Health has been a significant addition to the division, providing UPHS's physician and patient base with a comprehensive approach to this growing medical condition. The Division of Urology of the UPHS has an active clinical practice and research program and is, in fact, the busiest urologic practice in the region.

The center is a collaboration between two internationally known urologists, Dr. Alan Wein and Dr. Eric Rovner, and an internationally known incontinence APN, Diane Newman (the author). The center is a regional Center of Excellence for the diagnosis and treatment of all types of voiding dysfunction. The center offers complex diagnostic testing, all surgical treatments, and the latest advances in nonsurgical treatments such as behavioral modification, pelvic floor muscle rehabilitation using biofeed-

back, electrical stimulation, and magnetic therapy. The center also handles management for those individuals with chronic incontinence through use of products and devices.

This center does not replace current urologic services. Instead, by emphasizing labor intensive but effective alternative therapies and offering supportive care and excellent educational programs, it enhances current services by expanding to include patients who have not had success with previous treatments or have conditions that contraindicate the use of present services.

The center addresses the needs of those with all types of UI, OAB, interstitial cystitis (IC), pelvic floor dysfunction, prolapse, and neurogenic and nonneurogenic voiding dysfunction in both men and women. In addition to the comprehensive diagnostic evaluation and surgical treatments already provided, the Penn Center for Continence and Pelvic Health offers access to the latest advances in nonsurgical treatments such as behavioral modification, pelvic floor muscle rehabilitation using biofeedback, electrical stimulation, and magnetic therapy. In addition, for those people who, for medical or other reasons, are unable to benefit from these treatments, comprehensive and personalized management of the problem is provided.

This type of collaborative model is advantageous to the UPHS because it:

1. *Offers combined knowledge of three well-known and well-respected experts in the field of UI and pelvic floor voiding and dysfunction*

2. *Generates a secure revenue-producing service by*

   • *Providing increased referrals to urology and gynecology departments for more comprehensive urodynamic studies and surgical procedures*

   • *Generating increased patient volume through urology and gynecology departments as well as increased "down-stream" revenue generated by identifying concurrent medical problems requiring additional evaluation and treatment by others within UPHS*

   • *Providing a research site for treatments*

3. *Adds clinical training experience for residents and other providers*

4. *Offers alternative treatments for UI, OAB, IC and related disorders to UPHS's large network of primary care physicians who are looking for alternative treatments for these conditions*

5. *Is positioned at the forefront of a national trend to provide alternative treatments and management*

There are multidisciplinary models that target incontinence or pelvic floor disorders and combine the expertise of APNs and registered nurses working with urologists, geriatricians, gynecologists, and urogynecologists. These nurses may receive on-the-job training from a practicing physician whose background and interests lie in the care of women with urinary dysfunction, from preceptorships available from these physicians, and/or from attendance of instructional seminars or conferences on continence care. These collaborators will incorporate UI evaluation within an existing private practice, open a clinic within an outpatient hospital setting, or establish a free-standing practice separate from existing medical services. A trend for hospital systems is to establish Women's Centers, which typically include incontinence services. Usually, these centers are given names that identify the specifics of the services provided. Names such as Bladder Control Center, Pelvic Floor Dysfunction Center, Incontinence Treatment Center, Continence Center, Center for Continence and Pelvic Health, Bladder Wellness Center, Continence Management Program, Urofitness, Urology Wellness Center, and Urohealth are just a few examples. These centers will provide all-inclusive evaluation and treatment services, and will frequently serve as sites for research and professional training (see Table 11.4).

Changes in reimbursement for nonsurgical treatments such as biofeedback therapy and pelvic muscle electrical stimulation have allowed urologists, urogynecologists, and other professionals to consider the expansion of current treatments (pharmacologic and surgical) to alternative treatments such as pelvic muscle rehabilitation. In 2001, the Centers for Medicare & Medicaid Services (CMS), formerly the Health Care Financing Administration (HCFA), which administers Medicare (the insurer of the disabled and older adults), recommended biofeedback-assisted pelvic muscle exercises and pelvic floor electrical stimulation as a reimbursable service if certain criteria are met. It is important that professionals involved in continence care make funders aware of optimum clinical efficacy and of how funding arrangements can potentially distort clinical decisions. Identifying a management approach for UI that decreases patient dependency or caregiver burden can be a daunting task and requires a professional who has expertise in assessment of complex situations and environments. Management also includes the identification of the appropriate product or device, so professionals need to be knowledgeable about all products available. A range of professional organizations offer educational resources and catalogs that list appropriate products for the management of UI (see Appendix C: Resources).

Few studies exist that directly compare the effectiveness of specific health care delivery systems on continence care. Enthusiasts have conducted research, but the results may not generalize to the wider setting. Most models have combined the expertise of multidisciplinary providers to maximize service delivery (Abdelghany et al., 2001; Fiers & Silbert, 1993; Hesnan, 1985; Saltmarche, 1992). Although some might argue that a multidisciplinary approach is ideal, the reality is not always smooth. In some situations, rivalries and competition between disciplines and medical specialties surface. This may be caused by competition for patients and income or by disputes over the demarcation of the

Table 11.4. Outline of services in a continence center

A Continence Center is projected to have three main components:

1. Clinical services in an ambulatory office, home visits, and work with long-term care (LTC) settings
2. Research
3. Training of health care professionals

Clinical services

Evaluation and assessment of urinary incontinence

Ability to perform complex urodynamic (preferable videourodynamic) studies

Treatments including surgical, pharmacologic, and behavioral interventions

Behavioral treatment services:

Behavior modification and coping skills to maximize bladder control and related medical problems

Education on long-term transference of skills learned to the patient's daily life

Bladder retraining and urge inhibition techniques

Pelvic muscle rehabilitation to include biofeedback therapy

Pelvic floor electrical stimulation to increase strength, coordination, and control of bladder and pelvic muscles (in select patients)

Partnership with local long-term care facilities

Expert consultation to home care nurses and visits to clients who are homebound

Management of long term chronic incontinence that has not been amenable to standard treatments. This may involve working with families and caregivers

Expertise on the use of appropriate collection devices, catheters, or products that include management strategies

Behavioral treatments for fecal incontinence and other pelvic floor muscle disorders

Research

Large patient base and professional expertise for federally-funded or industry-supported research

Professional training

Resident and nursing clinical preceptorship enhanced through exposure to surgical and nonsurgical treatments as provided by a multidisciplinary team

---

scope of different disciplines (e.g., the boundary between urology and gynecology or between nursing and physical therapy). Ryden et al. (2000) demonstrated significantly improved outcomes for three clinical problems—UI, depression, and pressure ulcers—when advanced practice gerontological nurses worked with nursing facility staff to implement scientifically based protocols. This study also showed that consistent educational efforts with staff and residents produced interventions that improved or stabilized the level of UI in many people.

The trend being seen in health care practice today is for a more comprehensive medical approach to bladder and pelvic floor disorders. The most urgent educational need is being seen at the undergraduate medical and nursing level. Given these two changes, more professionals will be prepared to detect the problem of UI and make appropriate treatment or referral decisions.

REFERENCES

Abdelghany, S., Hughes, J., Lammers, J., Wellbrock, B., Buffington, P.J., & Shank, R.A. (2001). Biofeedback and electrical stimulation for treating urinary incontinence and voiding dysfunction: One center's experience. *Urologic Nursing, 21*(6), 401–405, 410.

Borrie, M.J., Bawden, M.E., Kartha A.S., & Kerr, P.S. (1992) A nurse/physician continence clinic triage approach for urinary incontinence: A 25 week randomized trial. *Neurourology and Urodynamics, 11,* 364–365.

Button, D., Roe, B., Webb, C., Frith, T., Colin-Thome, D., & Gardner, L. (1998). Consensus guidelines for the promotion and management of continence by primary health care teams: Development, implementation, and evaluation. *Journal of Advanced Nursing, 27,* 91–99.

Fiers, S., & Silbert, C. (1993). Urinary incontinence: A multidisciplinary approach. *Ostomy/Wound Management, 39*(7), 14–17.

Hesnan, K.D. (1985, March/April). Implementation of a hospital-based home care continence program. *Geriatric Nursing,* 100–102.

Jacobs, M., Wyman, J.F., Rowell, P., & Smith, D. (1998), Continence nurses: A survey of who they are and what they do. *Urologic Nursing, 18,* 13–20.

Lagro-Janssen, A.L.M., Debruyne, F.M.J., Smits, A.J.A., & Van Weel, C. (1992). The effects of treatment of urinary incontinence in general practice. *Family Practice, 9,* 284–289.

McDowell, B.J., Burgio, K.L., Dombrowski, M., Loches, J.L., & Rodrequez, E. (1992). An interdisciplinary approach to the assessment and behavioral treatment of urinary incontinence in geriatric outpatients. *Journal of Applied Gerontology, 40*(4), 370–374.

McFall, S., Yerkes, A.M., Bernard, M., & Le Rud, T. (1997). Evaluation and treatment of urinary incontinence: Report of a physician survey. *Archives of Family Medicine, 6*(2), 114–119.

McFall, S.L., Yerkes, A.M., Belzer, J.A., & Cowan, L.D. (1994). Urinary incontinence and quality of life in older women: a community demonstration in Oklahoma. *Family and Community Health, 17,* 64–75.

Mooney, R.A., Newman, D.K., Smith, D.A., & Grey, M. (1993). Establishing a Continence Service Using AHCPR Guidelines. *Ostomy/Wound Management, 39*(3), 28–30,32.

Newman, D., Smith, D., Blackwood, N., Wallace, J., Gerhard, C., & Manning, M. (1994, January). *Educating health care professionals about continence services* [Abstract] (p. 148–149). Phoenix, AZ: Multi-Specialty Nursing Conference on Urinary Incontinence.

Newman, D.K., & Palumbo, M.V. (1994). Planning an independent nursing practice for continence services. *Nurse Practitioner Forum, 5*(3), 190–193.

Newman, D.K., Parente, C.A., & Yuan, J.R. (1997). Implementing the agency for health care policy and research urinary incontinence guidelines in a home health agency. In M.D. Harris (Ed.), *Handbook of home health care administration* (2nd ed., pp. 394–403). Gaithersburg, MD: Aspen Publishers.

Newman, D.K. (1996). Program and practice management for the advanced practice nurse. In Hamric, A.B., Spross, J.A., & Hanson, C.M. (Eds.), *Advanced nursing practice* (pp. 545–568). Philadelphia: W.B. Saunders.

Newman, D.K., Denis, L., Gartley, C.B., Gruenwald, I., Lim, P.H.C., Millard, R., & Roberts, R. (in press). Promotion, education and organization for continence care. In P. Abrams,

S. Khoury, & A. Wein (Eds.), *Incontinence, proceedings from the second international consultation on incontinence.* Plymouth UK: Health Publication.

Newman, D.K., Wallace, J., & Blackwood, N. (1996). Promoting healthy bladder habits for seniors. *Ostomy/Wound Management, 42,* 18–28.

Newman, D.K., Palmer, M.H., O'Connor, M.P., Flynn, L., & Brown, D. (2001). *Health promotion needs of older adults concerning bladder control issues* [Abstract]. New Orleans: Sixth Multi-Specialty Conference on Urinary Continence.

Ryden, M.B., Snyder, M., Gross, C.R., Savik, K., Pearson, V., Krichbaum, K., & Mueller, C. (2000). Value-added outcomes: The use of advanced practice nurses in long-term facilities. *The Gerontologist, 40*(6), 654–662.

Saltmarche, A. (1992). Establishing a nurse continence service in Canada. *Urologic Nursing, 12*(2), 81.

Sampselle, C.M., Wyman, J.F., Thomas, K.K., Newman, D.K., Gray, M., Douglas, & Burns P.A. (2000). Continence for Women: A test of AWHONN's evidence-based protocol in clinical practice. *Journal of Obstetric, Gynecologic, and Neonatal Nursing, 29*(1), 18–26.

Smith D.A., & Newman, D.K. (1990). The role of continence nurse specialists in nursing for continence. In K. Jeter (Ed.), *Nursing for incontinence* (pp. 267–271). Philadelphia: W.B. Saunders.

A

Education Tools

These photocopiable handouts are designed for health professionals to use during staff training. They also may be used to educate consumers. The following topics are discussed:

- How to Prevent Bladder Infections
- Tips for Bowel Regularity
- Taking Care of Your Pessary
- Diet Habits that Can Affect Your Bladder
- Avoiding Foods and Liquids with Caffeine
- Bladder Retraining
- How to Do Pelvic Muscle Exercises
- Pelvic Muscle Exercises During Activities of Daily Living
- Care and Use of a Urinary (Foley) Catheter
- How to Care for Your Catheter Drainage Bag
- Clean Intermittent Self-Catheterization (CIC) for Women
- Clean Intermittent Self-Catheterization (CIC) for Men
- How to Use an External "Condom" Catheter
- How to Safely Use an Incontinence Clamp
- Using Topical Estrogen
- Pad Test

Tips for Bowel Regularity

Sometimes urinary incontinence may be aggravated by rectal pressure related to constipation or stool impaction (hard stool stopped in the bowel). Eating foods that have a lot of fiber helps overcome this problem. Fiber-rich foods include whole-grain breads, cereals, nuts, and raw fruits and vegetables. Another way to increase your fiber is by using a special bran recipe.

How to Make "Special Bran Recipe"

Mix together:

1 cup applesauce

1 cup coarse unprocessed wheat bran

¾ cup prune juice

You can buy unprocessed wheat bran in the grocery or health food stores. This type of bran is different from bran cereal.

Take 2 tablespoons of the mixture every day. Take the mixture in the evening for a morning bowel movement. Increase the bran mixture by 1 tablespoon per day until your bowel movements become regular. If the amount exceeds 4 tablespoons, take the mixture in split doses in the morning and evening. Always drink one large glass of water with the mixture.

What If I Don't Like the "Special Bran Recipe"?

Add unprocessed wheat bran to your diet. Start by taking 1–2 tablespoons every day. If necessary for regulation, increase bran slowly over several weeks to approximately 6 tablespoons every day. Mix bran in foods like applesauce, cereals, and sauces, or add it to gravies or puddings. Sprinkle bran on ice cream, vegetable and fruit salads, or cottage cheese. Add to muffins, breads, and cookies when baking.

Other "Natural Remedies" that May Help

Two natural laxative recipes have been shown to improve bowel function:

Fruit Spread

1 pound raisins

1 pound currants

1 pound prunes

1 pound figs

1 pound dates

1 28-ounce container undiluted prune concentrate.

Put fruit through a grinder. Mix with prune concentrate in large mixer (mixture will be very thick.) Store in large-mouthed plastic container. Refrigerate this mixture.

Power Pudding

½ cup prune juice

½ cup applesauce

½ cup unprocessed wheat bran flakes

½ cup whipped topping

½ cup stewed prunes (canned)

Blend ingredients. Take ¼-cup portions of recipe with breakfast. Regulate dose as needed. This mixture should be covered and refrigerated. You can keep mixture for 1 week.

When Will I Notice a Change?

You may notice effects on bowel function 3–5 days after starting bran or other natural remedies. You should continue to use these remedies for at least 1 month.

Will Bran and Other Natural Remedies Harm Me?

No! The normal reaction to bran, however, is stomach bloating and increased gas. To minimize this effect, you should gradually increase your amount of bran. These symptoms usually last for only the first week. If symptoms last longer, contact your nurse or doctor.

Remember, if you are taking bran, the bran absorbs water. Therefore, drink at least eight 8-ounce glasses of water every day.

What Type of Bowel Movement Schedule Should I Follow?

1. Try to have a bowel movement in a private place. The best time to move your bowels is after a meal, such as breakfast. Both eating and the smell of appetizing foods can cause your bowels to move. Drink something warm with your breakfast, such as warm water or warm prune juice. Warm food or a warm drink will stimulate the bowels to move.

2. Sit on the toilet or bedside commode 20 minutes after eating breakfast. Put your feet up on a footstool and push your body forward a little. Massage or rub your lower stomach to push the bowel movement into your rectum.

It may take about 20–30 minutes for you to have a bowel movement. A glycerin or Dulcolax suppository or digital stimulation technique (putting your finger in your rectal opening) may be used to make it easier to move your bowels. Put the suppository in your rectum around 20 minutes before you want to have the bowel movement. It will take time for the suppository to melt and work.

What Do I Do If I Have Severe Constipation?

Some people have severe constipation that may result in "impaction" (the stool hardens in your rectum and you can't get it out.) The following laxative can be used as a drink or an enema:

Laxative Drink

½ cup milk

½ cup molasses (Grandma's brand)

Heat until warm and drink in the morning.

Enema

1 cup milk

1 cup molasses

Heat until warm and pour in a standard enema bag with rectal-tube tip. Let the enema flow into your rectum and try to hold it for 15 minutes. Sit on the toilet or a bedpan and expel contents of the enema. The enema works best if you keep it in for 15 minutes.

Taking Care of Your Pessary

What Is a Pessary?

A pessary is put in the vagina to lift or support the pelvic organs: uterus, bladder, urethra, and/or rectum. Pessaries are made of silicone and are flexible. Most look like a contraceptive diaphragm, doughnut, or ring. Others look like a cube or mushroom or other shape.

Why Is it Used?

As women age, their pelvic organs may drop down or sag. This is called "prolapse." If this happens, women may find that they have to empty their bladders more often or have unwanted urine leakage. It has been found that, by placing a pessary into the vagina, these symptoms can sometimes be relieved.

What Does a Pessary Look Like?

Pessaries come in many shapes, but are usually round (see Figure A.1). They can also be cube or U shaped. A commonly used pessary looks like the contraceptive diaphragm with holes. There are several different types and sizes of pessary. It is not uncommon to have to change the type or size more than once after you are originally fitted, in order to provide optimal comfort.

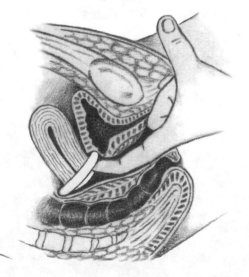

Figure A.1. Ring pessary in place. (Courtesy of Milex)

Can a Pessary Hurt Me?

Usually not; in fact, you should not be able to feel the pessary when it is placed inside you. Make sure you see your doctor and nurse as instructed. You must have regular follow-up visits to have the pessary removed and to have a pelvic exam. You should have it removed and cleaned at least every 4–6 weeks. The cube and inflato-ball pessary should be removed every night. Call and schedule an appointment if any of the following occurs:

- Vaginal discharge, bleeding, itching, foul odor, or pain
- Difficulty with voiding, emptying your bladder, or moving your bowels
- Back pain, vaginal pain or burning, and rectal pain

Will I Need to Douche When I Use a Pessary?

No, but if you have a discharge, a vinegar and water douche might be used so that the pessary will be more comfortable and less irritating. Trimo-san, a cleansing vaginal jelly, may be recommended. If Trimo-san jelly is recommended, insert ½ applicator-full three times during the first week, then ½ applicator-full two times a week for as long as the pessary is worn. You may also need to use estrogen cream. Estrogen cream will keep your vagina healthy.

How Do I Put in, Remove, and Care for My Pessary?

Your doctor or nurse will show you how to put in your pessary. If you ever used a diaphragm for birth control, then you know how. If not, follow these steps:

1. Empty your bladder before putting in or removing your pessary.
2. Find the position that is easiest for inserting and removing it. Usually women lie down with legs separated and knees bent, squat on a toilet, or lift and support one leg on a chair, a stool, or the toilet.
3. When putting in your pessary, fold the pessary and put water-soluble, lubricating jelly on the tip of the pessary that will enter the vagina first. Hold the pessary with one hand, and open your vagina with your other hand. Then, firmly push the pessary up and into your vagina. The pessary must be pushed far enough into the vagina so that it is under the cervix neck and behind the pubic bone. When it is properly placed, it should NOT be painful or uncomfortable.
4. When removing your pessary, put two fingers in your vagina, and grab the rim of the pessary. Slowly turn it as you pull it down and out. Try to fold the pessary into the shape it was in when you inserted it and carefully withdraw it.
5. Wash the pessary with soap and water. Then, dry it.

Diet Habits that Can Affect Your Bladder

Not Drinking Enough Fluids

Many people who have bladder control problems reduce the amount of liquids they drink in the hope that they will need to urinate less often. Although drinking less liquid does result in less urine in your bladder, the smaller amount of urine may be more highly concentrated and irritate the lining of your bladder. Highly concentrated (dark yellow, strong smelling) urine may cause you to go to the bathroom more frequently. It can also encourage bacteria to grow in your bladder. This can lead to infection. A bladder infection can cause incontinence. Do not limit your fluids to control your incontinence unless you are placed on specific fluid restriction by your doctor.

Certain Foods or Medications Can Affect Your Urine

Some foods, such as asparagus, can cause your urine to smell bad or peculiar. Some medications like those you may take for bladder inflammation may cause your urine to have a peculiar color or odor. Another cause of foul-smelling odor is a urinary tract (bladder) infection. So, if you notice that your urine has a strong odor and you have not eaten any foods that would cause this, you should see your doctor. Avoid alcohol! Alcohol causes rapid bladder filling and can cause urgency and frequency and also can dull your awareness of the need to void.

Common Bladder Irritants

Some foods and beverages are thought to contribute to bladder leakage. Their effect on the bladder is not always understood, but you may want to eliminate one or all of the following items and see if your bladder control improves:

Alcoholic beverages (e.g., beer, wine)

Citrus juices and fruits

Highly spiced foods

Carbonated beverages

Sugar, honey

Milk/milk products

Corn syrup

Soft drinks with caffeine, tea, coffee (even decaffeinated)

Artificial sweetener—Aspartame (e.g., Nutrasweet, Equal)

What to Drink

Grape, cranberry, apple, and cherry juices are thirst quenchers that usually are not irritating to a normal bladder. Cranberry juice may help control urine odor and makes the urine more acidic, thus preventing the spread of bacteria. Water is best!! Avoid drinking large volumes at one time by sipping 2–3 ounces every 20–30 minutes between meals.

Other Things that May Affect Your Bladder

- Women are more prone to developing bladder infections, so they should avoid nylon underpants and pantyhose. Cotton underpants are preferable. Avoid perfumed toilet tissue and sanitary napkins because the dyes and perfumes may be irritating. Also, do not take bubble baths or douche.

- Being overweight may be the cause of your incontinence and is also a dangerous health problem. Women especially may notice improved bladder control if they lose weight.

- Cigarette smoking is irritating to the bladder lining and is associated with bladder cancer. Coughing associated with smoking may lead to stress incontinence during repeated coughing spasms.

Avoiding Foods and Liquids with Caffeine

Many of the things you eat or drink contain caffeine. Caffeine is a bladder irritant and will make you go to the bathroom more frequently. The effect of caffeine may be seen within 30 minutes. Caffeine is found in chocolate, soft drinks, and over-the-counter medications and is used as a flavoring agent in many baked goods and processed foods. Americans average more than 200 mg (approximately 2 cups) of caffeine intake every day. The Food and Drug Administration (FDA) has identified more than 1,000 drugs that you can buy off the shelf in pharmacies and drug stores that contain caffeine. The fact that a drug, food, or drink contains caffeine is usually listed on the label. Table A.1 shows the most common caffeine sources.

Table A.1.   Common sources of caffeine

Source of caffeine	Serving size	Milligrams of caffeine
Coffee		
Brewed, drip	7.5 oz.	115–175
Brewed, percolated	7.5 oz.	80–135
Instant	7.5 oz.	65–100
Decaffeinated	5 oz.	2–4
Tea (black or green)		
1-minute brew	5 oz.	20–34
3-minute brew	5 oz.	35–46
5-minute brew	5 oz.	39–50
Instant tea	5 oz	30
Iced tea	12 oz.	67–76
Hot chocolate	5 oz.	2–15
Soft drinks		
Jolt Cola	12 oz.	71
Mountain Dew	12 oz.	54
Coca-Cola	12 oz.	60
Diet Coke	12 oz.	46
Pepsi-Cola	12 oz.	43
Diet Pepsi	12 oz.	36
Dr. Pepper	12 oz.	60
Chocolate desserts		
Brownie (with nuts)	1.25 oz.	8
Cake	⅟₁₆ of 9″	14
Ice cream	⅔ cup	5
Pudding	2 cups	6

Table A.1. Common sources of caffeine

Source of caffeine	Serving size	Milligrams of caffeine
Chocolate candy		
Milk chocolate	1 oz.	1–15
Sweet, dark chocolate	1 oz.	20
Baking chocolate	1 oz.	25–35
Painkillers		
Anacin	2 tablets	64
Excedrin	2 tablets	130
Vanquish	2 tablets	66
Midol	2 tablets	64
Darvon Compound	2 tablets	65
Fiorinal	2 tablets	80
Norgesic	2 tablets	30
Cold/allergy medications		
Coryban-D	1 tablet	30
Dristan	2 tablets	32
Sinarest	1 tablet	30
Stimulants		
No-Doz	2 tablets	200
Vivarin	1 tablet	200

Data from Bunker, M.L., & McWilliams, M. (1979). Caffeine content of common beverages. *Journal of The American Dietetic Association, 74,* 28–32; and Lamarine, R.J. (1994). Selected health and behavioral effects related to the use of caffeine. *Journal of Community Health, 19,* 449–466.

Bladder Retraining

Controlling Urgency and Frequency

Urgency is the sudden need to go to the toilet immediately that may result in urine leakage on the way to the bathroom.

Frequency is going often to the bathroom to void (more than 8 times a day) and passing only small amounts of urine.

Urgency and frequency happen when the bladder muscle starts to contract before going to the toilet. This can happen if you get into the habit of going to the toilet "just in case," which means that the bladder only has to hold a small amount of urine, instead of waiting until the bladder is full.

Urgency follows a wave pattern: it starts, grows, peaks and then subsides until it stops (See Figure A.2).

The key to controlling urinary urge is not to respond by rushing to the bathroom. Rushing causes movement, which jiggles your bladder, which in turn increases the feeling of urge.

Controlling the Urge

The goal is for you to be voiding no more than every ____ hours. If you get the urge to void and it is not yet your scheduled voiding time, stop all activity and sit down, if possible. Then try to do the following:

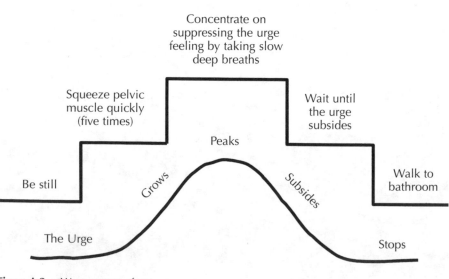

Figure A.2. Wave pattern of urgency.

Managing and Treating Urinary Incontinence. Copyright © 2002 by Diane Kaschak Newman.
Health Professions Press, Inc., Baltimore.

- Take some slow, deep breaths through your mouth, concentrating on your breathing.

- Concentrate on an activity, such as taking a vacation, visiting a friend, counting backward from 100, or reciting the words of a favorite song or nursery rhyme.

- Use self-statements such as " I can wait" or "It's not time yet to go." Make up something that fits your situation.

- Perform five quick, strong pelvic muscle contractions several times in a row. This will quiet the bladder long enough for the urge to lessen.

When to Toilet

After this urge goes away, try to wait until your scheduled voiding time or at least several minutes longer. Then go to the bathroom whether you feel you have to go or not. Never rush or run to the bathroom—walk slowly!

When to Try Bladder Retraining

Begin by practicing this only at home, where you are relaxed and the bathroom is nearby. Empty your bladder immediately before going to sleep to reduce the chances of awakening to urinate. Remember to cut down on caffeine and drinks containing alcohol.

When You Will Notice a Change

Do not despair or get discouraged. In time, you will see improvement, and you will be urinating every 3–4 hours during the day and will be up less often at night to urinate.

How to Do Pelvic Muscle Exercises

Finding the Pelvic Muscles

Without tensing the muscles of your leg, buttocks, or abdomen, imagine that you are trying to control the passing of gas or pinching off a stool. Or imagine you are in an elevator full of people and you feel the urge to pass gas. What do you do? You tighten or pull in the ring of muscles around your rectum—your pelvic muscles. You should feel a lifting sensation in the area around the vagina or a tightening of your rectum.

Exercise Regimen

One exercise consists of both "tightening and relaxing." It is equally important to control when your muscles tighten and relax. Therefore, you should relax for the same amount of time you tighten. Be sure to relax completely between each muscle tightening. Tighten your pelvic muscles and hold for a count of 3 seconds, then relax the muscles completely for a count of 3 seconds. Over time you will increase tightening the muscles to 5–10 seconds and even longer.

Where to Practice

You can practice these exercises anywhere and anytime. You should do the exercises in these positions:

- *Sitting:* Sit upright in a firm seat and straight-backed chair, knees slightly apart, feet flat on the floor or legs stretched out in front and crossed at the ankles.

- *Lying down:* Lie on your back, flat or with your head on a pillow, knees bent and feet slightly apart. It is helpful to support your knees with a pillow.

- *Standing:* Stand by a chair, knees slightly bent with feet shoulder-width apart and toes slightly pointed outward. You can also lean on the kitchen counter with your hips flexed.

It is recommended that you do at least 20 exercises in each position. Do 10 sets of each in the morning, then again at night.

When to Increase the Exercises

If you experience urine loss in one specific position only, such as when you stand, then follow these steps:

- Increase the number of exercises for that position only, *or*
- Add an additional set of exercises each day with the focus on doing all the exercises in that position only.

Common Mistakes

- DO NOT tighten leg muscles (thighs), buttocks, or abdomen. If you feel your stomach move, then you are also using these muscles. Concentrate and tighten (lift) only the pelvic floor muscles.
- DO NOT hold your breath. Breathe normally and/or count out loud.

Can These Exercises Be Harmful?

No, these exercises cannot harm you in any way. You should find them easy and relaxing. If you get back pain or stomach pain after you exercise, you are probably trying too hard and using your stomach muscles. If you experience headaches, then you are also tensing your chest muscles and probably holding your breath.

When You Will See a Change

After 4–6 weeks of daily exercise, you will begin to notice less urine leakage. Make the exercises part of your daily lifestyle. Tighten the muscles when you walk, as you stand up, and on the way to the bathroom.

Pelvic Muscle Exercises During Activities of Daily Living

In addition to doing your sets of daily pelvic muscle exercises, you should start doing your exercises during activities of daily living (activities you do on a daily basis).

1. Any activity that increases pressure in your abdomen may cause you to lose urine. Examples of such activities are coughing, sneezing, laughing, bending/lifting, carrying objects, sitting down, standing up, and going up/down stairs. During these activities, pressure is placed on the bladder, forcing it to empty.

    *   To prevent urine loss, tighten your pelvic muscles just before these activities.

    *   For short activities like a cough, tighten your muscles until you finish, then relax.

    *   For prolonged activities, tighten during the most stressful moments, or tighten them on and off during the entire activity.

    *   Contract your pelvic muscles prior to standing up and keep muscles contracted until you are in an upright position.

2. Do your exercises when

    *   Standing at the sink and brushing your teeth

    *   Washing dishes

    *   Putting on your makeup

    *   Sitting in the car at a stoplight

    *   Sitting down at dinner

    *   Reading a book in bed

    *   Going for a walk

    *   Talking on the phone

3. Try to always tighten your muscles when you get a strong urge that you cannot control. Tighten your muscles on the way to the bathroom.

4. Do both types of exercises, short and long holds, during your activities of daily living. You do not have to keep a formal count of the number of times you do each exercise—just do it several times in a row. Do them often enough to make them a habit.

Remember, the more exercising you do:

- The stronger your pelvic muscles will get
- The faster they will get stronger
- The easier it will be to maintain muscle strength

YOU MUST PRACTICE THESE EXERCISES SO THAT EXERCISING BECOMES A HABIT!

Care and Use of a Urinary (Foley) Catheter

What Is an Indwelling Urinary (Foley) Catheter?

Some people need help to pass urine from their bladder because certain medical problems do not let the bladder empty completely. If this happens, a tube called a "catheter" is put into the bladder to drain the urine.

A catheter is a soft tube that drains the urine from your bladder. The catheter is made from latex or silicone material. The catheter is attached to a long tube and a "drainage" bag, which collects the urine. The catheter is held in place in the bladder by a balloon filled with water. The balloon sits at the base of your bladder. The catheter and bag, once placed, is a "closed system" and should never be opened unless you are told to do so by your nurse or physician. Minimizing the opportunity for infections is extremely important.

How Does the Catheter Feel?

You may sometimes feel "burning" or "spasms" when urine passes through the catheter. This is a normal reaction, and there is no cause for alarm. These "spasms" may cause some urine to leak out around the catheter. If they continue without stopping, call your doctor or nurse. A mild painkiller or medication to relieve the spasms may be prescribed. Spasms may also indicate that the catheter needs to be changed.

How Do I Care for My Catheter?

ALWAYS wash your hands before and after touching the catheter or drainage bag. Wash the skin around the catheter with soap and water every day and after you move your bowels. Empty the drainage bag at least every 4–8 hours or if it becomes filled before 4 hours. Do not touch the end of the drainage spout.

Do not disconnect any portion of the drainage system unless your doctor or nurse has allowed you to use a leg bag during the day and an overnight bag at night. If the tubing does become disconnected, clean the ends with an alcohol pad and reconnect immediately. Then, call the nurse because the catheter may need to be changed.

How Do I Position My Catheter?

Women anchor the catheter securely to the upper thigh by using the Velcro strap, but should not pull the catheter tightly. Men should anchor the catheter to the lower abdomen below the belly button. Leave some "slack" on the catheter to prevent pressure in the bladder.

Prevent kinks or loops in the catheter and tubing that might stop the flow of urine. Do not clamp the catheter or drainage tube.

What Can I Do to Prevent Infections?

Drink plenty of fluids (at least 6–8 glasses of nonalcoholic liquids) daily, unless your doctor tells you otherwise. Nonalcoholic liquids include water, tea, coffee, fruit juice, Kool-Aid, lemonade, and the like. Ice cream, sherbet, and Popsicles also provide fluid. Take vitamin C (true ascorbic acid), 500 to 1,000 mg daily, or drink three 8-ounce glasses of cranberry juice, or take the equivalent cranberry tablets, each day. For persistent or repeated infections, you should call the doctor.

Special Instructions

You may shower with the catheter in place but always keep the drainage bag connected to the catheter while in the shower. Do not irrigate the catheter. If it becomes clogged and stops draining, call your nurse or doctor.

Remember, a catheter may occasionally leak. This is normal and is caused by bladder spasms. There is no reason to be alarmed unless the catheter leaks continuously or if there is no urine in the drainage bag.

Always call your nurse or doctor if any of the following occurs:

- The urine has a strong odor or becomes cloudy or turns red.
- You experience chills, fever above 99.4°F, lower back pain, and/or leakage around the catheter.
- There is swelling at the catheter insertion site.
- The catheter is not draining any urine (make sure the catheter or tubing is not blocked or kinked).
- The catheter falls out.

How to Care for Your Catheter Drainage Bag

What Is a Drainage Bag?

There are two types of drainage bags:

1. An overnight drainage bag is a bag with a long tube connected to your catheter that is used during the night. The bag should be hung over the side of the bed below the level of your catheter so that the urine will flow easily.

2. A leg drainage bag is a smaller collection bag for use at home during the day or when you go out of your house (see Figure A.3). The smaller bag can be strapped to your leg (thigh or calf) or held in place with a net sleeve or stocking, and is easy to hide under your clothing. If you use straps, make sure they are not too tight around your leg. Take care of the leg bag as you would the larger drainage bag.

How to Position Your Drainage Bag

The position of your drainage bag is important. You must have good drainage and prevent backflow of urine. Urine must always drain "down-

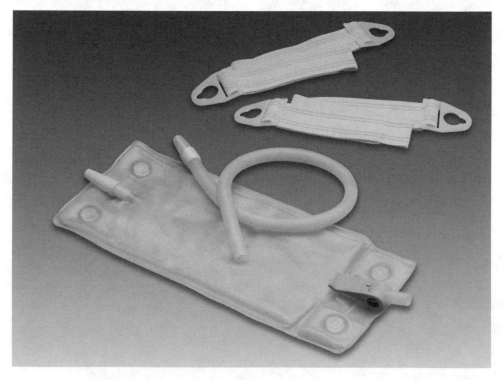

Figure A.3. Example of a leg bag. (Courtesy of Hollister)

Managing and Treating Urinary Incontinence. Copyright © 2002 by Diane Kaschak Newman.
Health Professions Press, Inc., Baltimore.

hill," so keep the urine drainage bag below the level of the bladder at all times. This allows the urine to drain by gravity and will prevent the urine from flowing back into the bladder. As the drainage bag fills with urine, it becomes heavy and could drag uncomfortably if not supported. You can support your overnight bag by hooking it on a hanger attached to the bed frame.

How to Disconnect or Change Your Drainage Bag

Pinch the catheter tubing above the drainage bag connection between your fingers to stop the flow of urine. Using a twisting motion, disconnect the tubing and bag from the catheter. Take an alcohol pad and clean the end of the new tubing and the connection site of the catheter. Insert the new tubing into the catheter. Using an alcohol pad, clean the end of the tubing that was removed and replace the protective cap. Save caps to drainage bags to cover ends of tubing when not in use.

How to Clean Your Drainage Bag

Drainage bags can be cleaned and deodorized by filling the bag with a solution of two parts vinegar and three parts water and letting it soak for 20 minutes. Dry the bag by hanging it with the emptying spout pointing downward. Do not hang the bag over the heat of an oven or radiator. When dry, recap the bag until ready for reuse. If your bag starts to wear out or deteriorate, get a new bag. To avoid infections, clean the bag every 5–7 days and use a new bag at least monthly.

What to Do If You Get an Infection

If you get repeated bladder infections, spasms, and pain, you may be told by your nurse or physician not to disconnect the catheter from the bag. You should only use the overnight drainage bag.

Clean Intermittent Self-Catheterization (CIC) for Women

Gather your equipment together before you start, so that you can easily reach it.

Procedure to Follow

1. Arrange your clothing so that it does not get in your way. Try to urinate before the catheterization. Wash your hands with soap and water. However, never skip a catheterization because you do not have access to soap and water. It is more important to empty your bladder.

2. Sit far back on the toilet or bedside commode with legs spread, or stand with one foot on the toilet seat.

3. With your nondominant hand, separate your labia with your first and third fingers and identify your clitoris, urethra, vaginal opening, and rectum (see Figure A.4). If necessary, use a mirror to help locate these structures. Place your index (second) finger on your clitoris and place your third and fourth finger at the opening to your vagina. Rest this hand there.

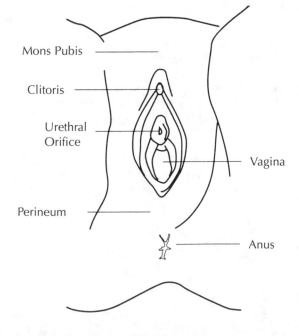

Mons Pubis

Clitoris

Urethral Orifice

Vagina

Perineum

Anus

Figure A.4. Female genitalia. (Courtesy of Hollister)

4. With your dominant hand, hold the catheter like a pencil, about 1–2 inches from the tip. Put it in the urethra (the opening that is found directly above the opening to your vagina and below the clitoris; see Figure A.5). When putting in the catheter, point it upward.

5. When the urine starts to flow, put the catheter in another inch or two. Let the urine drain until it stops. Push with your hand on your lower stomach to completely empty your bladder.

6. Wait until urine stops draining before slowly removing the catheter.

Catheterization should be done four times a day, or approximately every 6 hours and at bedtime. Record the amount you void and the amount of urine that comes from the catheterization. Do not let your bladder hold more than 13 ounces (400 ml) of urine. This must be avoided at all costs and is the reason you have been placed on CIC. It is believed that infections occur when the bladder has been allowed to become too full with urine.

Taking Care of Your Catheter

After using the catheter, wash it with hot, soapy water. Rinse with hot water. You can also clean the catheter by boiling it for 10–15 minutes. Place the catheter on a paper towel to air dry. Store the dry catheter in a plastic bag or clean container. Each catheter should be put in a separate bag.

Replacing Catheters

One catheter can be used for at least 1 week. Always replace the catheter if it becomes discolored, hard, or brittle or isn't draining. The catheter should also be replaced if it becomes too soft to insert.

Helpful Tips

- Make the catheter work for you; do not work for it!
- Control the amount of liquids you drink. Only drink between 48 and 64 ounces each day.
- Do not drink after 7:00 P.M. This may help you sleep through the night without needing catheterization.
- If any problems occur, call your nurse or physician, especially if you are having trouble doing the catheterization.

What Problems Might Occur?

- *Bleeding at the time of catheterization:* There may be a slight amount of bleeding when you insert the catheter because it may have irritated

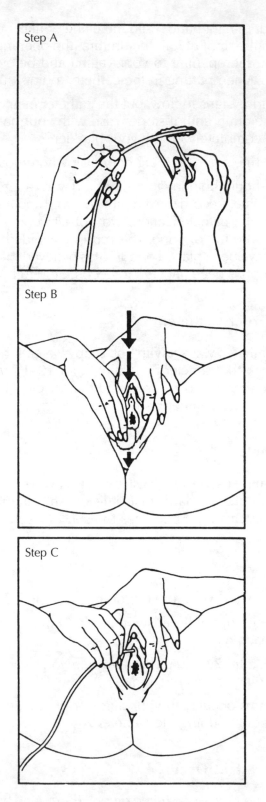

Figure A.5. Female clean intermittent self-catheterization.

Managing and Treating Urinary Incontinence. Copyright © 2002 by Diane Kaschak Newman.
Health Professions Press, Inc., Baltimore.

your urethra. Do not be alarmed; it should stop. If it does not stop, call your doctor or nurse.

- *Infection:* As long as you wash your hands and perineum (area between the anus [or your rectum] and the vagina) before catheterization, you will not likely get an infection. Catheters can be boiled between use or washed with soap and water. Do not place catheters in the microwave to clean them. One or two bladder infections per year, especially when beginning catheterization, is normal.

What Catheter to Use

Size _____

Length _____

Manufacturer _____

- ☐ Clear plastic—straight
- ☐ Coudé—curved tip
- ☐ Red rubber—coudé
- ☐ Coudé—olive curved tip
- ☐ Red rubber—straight
- ☐ Other

Clean Intermittent Self-Catheterization (CIC) for Men

Gather your equipment together before you start, so that you can easily reach it.

Procedure to Follow

1. Try to urinate before the catheterization. Wash your hands with soap and water. However, never skip a catheterization because you do not have access to soap and water. It is more important to empty your bladder.

2. Sit on the toilet or bedside commode, or in front of the commode. If this is the first catheterization of the day, hold up your penis with one hand and wash the penis from the top to the bottom with soap and water (see Figure A.6).

3. Put a lot of water-soluble lubrication (K-Y Jelly) along the entire length of the catheter. Do not use Vaseline jelly.

4. With your nondominant hand, hold your penis firmly directly under the head, lifting the penis up straight. Holding the penis makes insertion of the catheter easier.

5. If you are right-handed, hold the catheter in your right hand 2–3 inches from the tip. Put the catheter in slowly. Some resistance may be felt halfway (at the site of the prostate). If this happens, stop and take a few deep breaths, then continue to pass the catheter, gently but firmly. Do not force the catheter by pushing down on the penis. Put the catheter in 1–2 inches more after urine starts to flow out.

6. Let the urine drain until it stops. Pushing down on the bladder may help the bladder empty completely.

7. Remove the catheter slowly, allowing any remaining urine to drain out. Hold the catheter tip up as you pull it from your penis so that urine does not spill.

Catheterization should be done four times a day, or approximately every 6 hours and at bedtime. Record the amount you void and the amount of urine that comes from the catheterization. Do not let your bladder hold more than 13 ounces (400 ml) of urine. This must be avoided at all costs and is the reason you have been placed on CIC. It is believed that infections occur when the bladder has been allowed to become too full of urine.

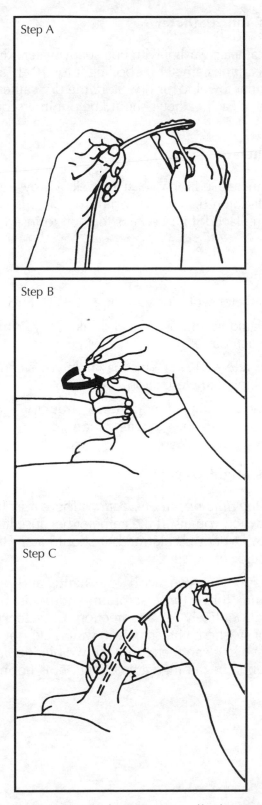

Figure A.6.   Male clean intermittent self-catheterization.

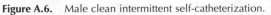

Taking Care of Your Catheter

After using the catheter, wash it with hot, soapy water. Rinse with hot water. You can also clean the catheter by boiling it for 10–15 minutes. Place the catheter on a paper towel to air dry. Store the dry catheter in a plastic bag or clean container. Each catheter should be put in a separate bag.

Replacing Catheters

One catheter can be used for at least 1 week. Always replace the catheter if it becomes discolored, hard, or brittle or isn't draining. The catheter should also be replaced if it becomes too soft to insert.

Helpful Tips

- Make the catheter work for you; do not work for it!
- Control the amount of liquids you drink. Only drink between 48 and 64 ounces each day.
- Do not drink after 7:00 P.M. This may help you sleep through the night without needing catheterization.
- If any problems occur, call your nurse or doctor, especially if you are having trouble doing the catheterization.

What Problems Might Occur?

- *Bleeding at the time of catheterization:* There may be a slight amount of bleeding when you insert the catheter because it may have irritated your urethra. Do not be alarmed; it should stop. If it does not stop, call your doctor or nurse.
- *Infection:* As long as you wash your hands and perineum (area between the anus [or rectum], scrotum, and penis) before catheterization, you will not likely get an infection. Catheters can be boiled between use or washed with soap and water. Do not place catheters in the microwave to clean them. One or two bladder infections per year, especially when beginning catheterization, is normal.

What Catheter to Use

Size _____

Length _____

Manufacturer _____

- ☐ Clear plastic—straight
- ☐ Coudé—curved tip
- ☐ Red rubber—coudé
- ☐ Coudé—olive curved tip
- ☐ Red rubber—straight
- ☐ Other

How to Use an External "Condom" Catheter

What Is an External Condom Catheter?

An external condom catheter is used by men to collect urine leakage (see Figure A.7). This catheter fits over the penis and connects to a drainage bag that is strapped to your leg. The catheter has adhesive inside so that it sticks to the penis.

Another type of external catheter is called a retracted penis pouch. This pouch has adhesive and a pouch that is attached to the drainage bag. This pouch can be used by men whose penis may have "retracted" or those who cannot or will not be fitted with a condom catheter.

Getting Started

Wash your hands. Then, gather your equipment: correct-sized condom catheter, leg drainage bag with extension tubing, manicure scissors, soap, washcloth, towel, and protective ointment.

Trim the hairs on the shaft and base of your penis so they won't stick to the adhesive tape on the inside of the catheter. Do not shave the hairs with a razor. Before each catheter change, wash, rinse, and dry your penis. To protect your skin from urine, coat your penis with a skin barrier product and let the product dry (it will feel sticky). The purpose of this product is to protect your skin from perspiration and urine moisture so your skin will not tear open when you remove the catheter.

Putting on the Catheter

First, tightly roll the condom sheath (balloonlike part) to the edge of the connector tip (see Figure A.8). Hold your penis and place the catheter

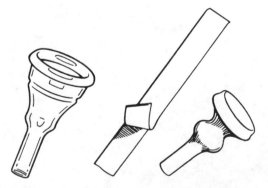

Figure A.7. Condom catheter with adhesive and condom catheter with separate adhesive strip. (Courtesy of ConvaTec)

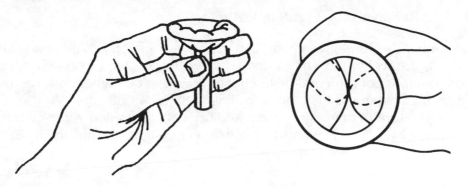

Figure A.8. Condom catheter application. (Courtesy of Hollister)

sheath on the end of your penis, leaving about half an inch of space between the tip of your penis and the connector tip so your penis does not rub against the end of the catheter. If you are not circumcised, leave your foreskin in place. Swelling of your foreskin may result if the foreskin is not kept over the head of the penis.

Gently stretch your penis as you unroll the condom. When the condom is unrolled, gently press it against your penis, so that it sticks. Put pressure on your penis for several minutes to be sure any wrinkles are sealed together and to get rid of air bubbles. If there are a lot of wrinkles, the condom catheter may be too large.

How to Connect the Drainage Bag

Connect one end of the tubing to the connector tip and the other end to the extension tube attached to the drainage bag. If the extension tube is too long, cut it to the length you want. Strap the drainage bag to your thigh. Do not use too large a leg bag because this will put too much weight on the condom catheter, causing the device to fall off your leg.

How to Empty the Drainage Bag

To remove the drainage bag, squeeze the tube closed. Release the leg straps and disconnect the extension tubing at the top of the bag.

How to Care for the Drainage Bag

Empty the bag every 3–4 hours and do not let it fill completely to the top. You'll need to clean the bag about twice a day. Use a solution of one part vinegar and seven parts water. Do not use the same drainage bag longer than 1 month.

How to Remove Your Condom Catheter

Remember the condom catheter is disposable, and you should change it every 1–2 days. In hot and humid weather, it will need to be changed more often. A convenient time to change is when you bathe. Remove the condom catheter and the tape by rolling them forward.

Make sure to thoroughly wash and dry your penis and your scrotum between changes. It is worth trying different systems to find the system that best fits your needs.

Special Instructions

- If the catheter doesn't stick to your skin, make sure that your penis is completely dry and that the protective ointment is completely dry, too.

- If the catheter pulls away from your skin, you may need to apply some adhesive ointment (e.g., Stoma adhesive). Also, make sure the catheter is snug (but not tight).

- If urine leaks when you're wearing the catheter, squeeze the sheath to get a better seal.

- If the catheter sheath wrinkles in contact with the tape, the sheath may be too large. If so, select a smaller size sheath.

- Use only skin products and adhesives prescribed by your doctor or nurse. Don't wash with Betadine because this can irritate your skin.

- Check your penis every 2 hours for swelling or unusual color. If it feels uncomfortable or doesn't look normal, take off the condom catheter and call your doctor.

- Call the nurse or doctor if you feel pain or burning when you urinate, have the urge to urinate very frequently, smell an unpleasant odor from your urine, or see blood or pus (cloudiness) in your urine.

What Catheter to Use

Size _____

Type _____

Manufacturer _____

How to Safely Use an Incontinence Clamp

What Is a Clamp?

An incontinence clamp is a compression device that is placed around the penis to prevent urine leakage.

What Do the Clamps Look Like?

There are several kinds of clamps. The Cunningham clamp is the one most often used and is pictured in Figure A.9. The inside of the clamp has a flexible, soft part made of foam that conforms to fit your penis. The outside is made of metal with several notches on the side to adjust the tightness.

How Is it Used?

You open the clamp and place it around the penis about halfway down the shaft. The hump side of the clamp is placed on the underside of your penis. The clamp flexes to fit comfortably over your penis. You then squeeze the clamp shut, making sure it is not too tight.

To release the catch, press inward on both the spring wire loops. Make sure the clamp is not so tight that it stops blood circulation.

YOU MUST RELEASE THE CLAMP EVERY 1–2 HOURS TO URINATE, WHETHER YOU FEEL YOU HAVE TO OR NOT.

Can the Clamp Hurt You?

Yes, the clamp can hurt you if it is not used properly! You should look at your penis—top to bottom and underneath, especially the skin—from time to time, and stop using the clamp if the skin is torn open. Check your penis to see if the skin is pale, blue, reddened, or broken. You can apply a skin cream to the penis for protection before you put on the clamp. If you do not release the clamp at least every 1–2 hours, you may develop bladder problems such as an infection. *Try not to use the clamp continuously throughout the day* (e.g., only use for several hours in the morning and then again in the evening if you go out). Contact your nurse or doctor if you

- Have any discharge (drainage) from your penis, itching, foul urine odor, or pain.

- Find you cannot void or empty your bladder when you release the clamp.

Managing and Treating Urinary Incontinence. Copyright © 2002 by Diane Kaschak Newman. Health Professions Press, Inc., Baltimore.

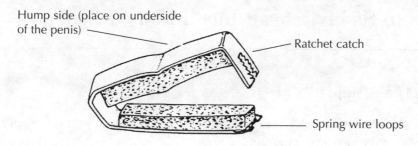

Hump side (place on underside of the penis)

Ratchet catch

Spring wire loops

Figure A.9. Cunningham clamp.

How to Care for the Clamp

Wash the clamp with soap and warm water. Rinse well in cool, clean water. Squeeze the soft foam to remove the water. Let the clamp air dry in a cool place, away from heat or direct sunlight. Make sure it is dry before you reuse the clamp.

Using Topical Estrogen

What Is Menopause?

Menopause is the transition time in a woman's life from the reproductive stage to the nonreproductive stage. During this transition period, your ovaries stop functioning and your menses or "period" stops. The word *menopause* refers to the complete or permanent stopping of menstruation and is indicated by your final menstrual period. The average age of menopause is 51 years. Menopause happens because of a drop in levels of the hormone estrogen and an increase in other hormones from your pituitary gland. These changes in your hormone levels are normal, and the decreases can be replaced through hormone medication.

Can Estrogen Help Incontinence, Urgency, and Frequency?

Estrogen receptors are found in the tissue in your vagina, urethra, and bladder. When your estrogen hormone levels drop, the tissue starts to weaken, causing symptoms such as urgency, frequency, painful intercourse, burning when urinating, vaginal dryness, itching, and vaginal discharge. The loss of estrogen may make you more susceptible to bladder infections. It may also cause your pelvic organs, bladder, uterus, and rectum to sag or fall. This is called "prolapse." Applying topical estrogen can strengthen the tissue in the pelvic support area, thereby providing more support to the organs.

What Is Topical Estrogen?

Topical estrogen is an estrogen cream that is applied over the opening of and into the vagina, or a tablet or ring that is placed into the vagina.

How to Use Topical Estrogen Products

Wash your hands with soap and water, and dry them.

1. TO USE THE CREAM (Estrace brand or Premarin brand):
    *   You can use the applicator that comes with the cream. Or, you can squeeze some cream to cover your fingertip and then rub it on the opening to your vagina, toward your urethra.
    *   Squeeze 1 gram of cream (about enough to cover ⅓ of your index finger) from the tube.

- Locate the opening to your vagina. Carefully spread the cream onto the external vaginal/urethral area. As the cream is spread, some may be gently inserted into the vagina.

- Usually your doctor or nurse will instruct you to use the cream nightly for 10 days, then twice a week.

2. TO USE THE TABLETS (Vagifem brand)

- You can insert the tablet either lying down or standing with your foot raised onto a short stool.

- Hold the applicator so that the finger of one hand can press the applicator plunger.

- The other hand should be used to guide the applicator gently and comfortably through the vaginal opening.

- One half of the applicator should be put inside your vagina. Do not force the applicator into your vagina.

- Gently press the plunger until it is fully depressed and the tablet will be ejected.

3. TO USE THE RING (Estring brand)

- The ring is usually inserted the first time by your doctor or nurse.

- Once inserted, the ring should only be removed for intercourse.

- It may take 2–3 weeks after insertion to feel the full effect of the estrogen ring.

- The ring loses the estrogen effects after 90 days, and it will need to be replaced.

Pad Test

What Is a Pad Test?

You have been asked by your doctor to perform a Pad Test. A Pad Test is a very simple test to accurately determine the amount of urine leakage (incontinence) that you experience during a regular, routine day. The amount of urine is determined by weighing the pad. This test is very important to the doctor in determining the appropriate treatment for your condition.

How Do I Perform a Pad Test?

Follow these steps:

1. One day prior to your next office visit with the doctor, please save ALL of the pads (pantiliners, pads, tissues, towels, undergarments, disposable protective underwear, adult briefs, or diapers) that you use for an entire 24-hour period (day and night). Figure A.10 shows some of the pads you may be using.

2. Put the pads for each day in SEALED plastic bags. Only include the pads in the bags.

3. Label each plastic bag with the date and time the pad was used.

4. Bring the sealed plastic bags with you to your next office visit with the doctor.

5. You will also need to bring one unused (dry) pad to the office visit.

What Will Be Done with the Pads?

The doctor or nurse will weigh the pads on a scale. First, the dry pad will be weighed to determine the baseline "dry" weight of the pad. Then, each wet pad will be weighed separately. The weight of the dry pad is subtracted from the total weight of the wet pads. The difference is an objective measurement of your urine leakage.

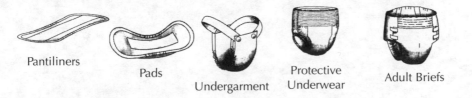

Pantiliners
Pads
Undergarment
Protective Underwear
Adult Briefs

Figure A.10.   Absorbent products. (Courtesy of Kimberly-Clark)

B

Forms

These photocopiable forms are designed for health professionals to use for evaluation and consultation. Forms include

- Initial Consultation
- Pelvic Muscle Assessment
- Past Medical History
- Incontinence Patient Profile
- Bladder and Bowel Record (used in long-term care facilities)
- Bladder and Bowel Retraining Preassessment (used in long term care facilities)
- Findings and Recommendations
- Daily Voiding Record (or Frequency Volume Chart)

Initial Consultation

Name: _____ Date of birth: _____ Date: _____

Caregiver: _____ Allergies: _____ Condition of home: □Good □Fair □Poor

Chief complaint: _____

□ Urine loss   □ Cough   □ Sneeze   □ Exercise   □ Lift objects   □ Change position   □ Urinary urgency

□ Fecal loss   □ On way to the bathroom   □ Walking   □ While asleep/night   □ Without warning

□ Other: _____   □ Foley catheter _____ #FR _____ Balloon

Fecal incontinence: □No □Yes _____ Day/Wk. # of pads used/24 hrs. _____ Type of pad _____

Frequency of voids: ___ daytime ___ nighttime   UI episodes: ____ /day ____ /night   Amount: □Sm □Med □Lg

---

MEDICAL HISTORY	Relevant Surgery: _____

□ Alzheimer's disease/dementia

□ Anemia

□ Arthritis

□ Back injuries/back compression fractures

□ Bladder suspension surgery

□ Bleeding problems

□ Cancer

□ Cataracts   □ Glaucoma

□ Chest pain

□ Congestive heart failure

□ Constipation/impaction

□ COPD   □ Asthma

□ Diabetes

□ Falls

□ Fractures/joint replacements

□ Head injuries

□ Heart attack   □ Murmurs

□ Heart disease (CAD, arrhythmia, atrial fibrillation)

□ Hemorrhoids   □ Polyps

□ High blood pressure

□ Hysterectomy

□ Irritable bowel

□ Kidney stones/bladder stones

□ Mental health/depression

□ Mitral valve prolapse

□ Multiple Sclerosis

□ Osteoporosis

□ Pacemaker

□ Parkinson's disease

□ Prostate cancer

□ Prostatitis/BPH

□ Renal disease

□ Seizures

□ Skin sensitivities or conditions

□ Stroke

□ UTI

□ Vascular disease/PVD

□ Other–specify: _____

_____

Typical fluid intake: _____ Caffeine intake: _____

Special nutritional needs: _____

Current medications: (*Name/Dosage/Frequency*)

_____   _____   _____

_____   _____   _____

Smoker? □yes □no **ETOH?** □yes □no **Safety problems:** □yes _____ □no ADLs–general ability _____

Equipment and prostheses: □cane □walker □wheelchair □commode □urinal □bedpan

Frequency of bowel movement: □one per day □more than one per day □2-3 times/week □other _____
(specify)

Comments: _____

Vital signs: T_____ P_____ R_____ **BP** _____ sitting _____ standing

General appearance: Peripheral edema □yes □no Site: _____ Wt _____ □WNL □Obese

Comments: _____

Abdomen   Bowel sounds: □present □decreased   Tenderness/pain: □present □absent

Suprapubic/bladder distention: □yes □no   Masses: □no □yes

Hernia present: □yes □no   Scars: □no □yes

Comments: _____

Genito-urinary — Women

External genitalia: □dry □moist □vaginal discharge   Labia/vaginal mucosa: □dry □moist □atrophic changes

Perineal Sensation: □yes □no   Lesions: □yes □no

Urethra: □fixed □hypermobile □normal   Urethral caruncle: □yes □no

Urethral prolapse: □yes □no   Cystocele: □no □yes Degrees: □1st □2nd □3rd □4th

Uterine prolapse: □none □removed □yes Degrees: □1st □2nd □3rd □4th

Vaginal Stenosis: □yes □no   Muscle wasting/disuse atrophy: □yes □no

Rectocele: □no □mild □moderate □large   Muscle tone: □strong □moderate □weak ___ grade (0-5)

Comments: _____

Genito-urinary—men

Penis
Circumcised: ☐ Yes ☐ No   Retracted Penis: ☐ Yes ☐ No   Comments: _____
Freely moveable foreskin: ☐ Yes ☐ No   Penile Discharge: ☐ Yes ☐ No   Comments: _____
Scrotum
General appearance: ☐ Normal   ☐ Abnormal
Tender: ☐ Yes   ☐ No   Comments: _____
Prostate gland
Size: ☐ WNL ☐ Enlarged   Symmetry: ☐ Yes ☐ No   Nodules present: ☐ Yes ☐No   Tenderness: ☐Yes ☐ No

Rectum

Hemorrhoids: ☐ Yes   ☐ No   Anal tone: ☐ Strong   ☐ Moderate ☐ Weak
Anal wink: ☐ Yes   ☐ No   Stool: ☐ None ☐ Soft   ☐ Hard   ☐ Impaction
Guaic: Test done ☐ Yes ☐ No   Results: ☐ Positive ☐ Negative
Comments: _____

Perineal skin integrity

Rashes: ☐ Yes   ☐ No   Lesions: ☐ Yes ☐ No   Ulcers: ☐ Yes   ☐ No
Comments: _____

Neurological

DTRs: ☐ Patellar   ☐ Ankle
Sensory: ☐ Position sense   ☐ Sharp   ☐ Dull
Gait: ☐ WNL   ☐ Abnormal:

Musculoskeletal

Dexterity: ☐ Normal   ☐ Abnormal: _____
Transfer independent: ☐ Yes   ☐ No

Urinalysis performed

Last urinalysis performed: _____ Results: _____
Leukocytes: _____ Nitrites: _____ Protein: _____ Glucose: _____ RBC: _____ PH: _____
Micro: _____ Culture sent: ☐ Yes   ☐ No
Post Void Residual Volume Analyzed _____ cc   Report attached: ☐ Yes ☐No ☐ Catheterized ☐ Scan

Bladder and bowel assessment				
Assessment	3	2	1	0
Voids correctly without UI	Always	Yes, at least one per day	Yes, but less than once per day	No
Fecal incontinence	No	Yes, 1–3 times per week	Yes, 1–4 times per week	Daily
Walks to the bathroom or transfers to toilet/commode. Can manage clothing, wipe, and so forth	Alone, with reasonable speed	Alone, but slowly	Needs assistance for one side	Completely immobile or needs assistance from more than one side
Mental status	Alert and oriented	Forgetful but can follow commands	Confused, needs physical prompting Mini -Mental Score: _____	Very confused, comatose, or combative. Depressed/ psychotic
Aware of urge sensation and need to toilet	Always	Usually	Sometimes	Never
Perineal/genitalia/gluteal skin condition	No redness	Some redness, predecub	Stage I–II decub	Stage III–IV decub
Predisposing diseases	Absent	Minor	Serious	Debilitating, terminal
Predisposing medical conditions: _____				

Potential bladder and bowel training

15–21   Good candidate for individualized training (pelvic muscle rehabilitation)

8–14   Fair candidate for toileting scheduling (timed voiding; prompted voiding); may be candidate for pelvic muscle rehabilitation

0–7   Poor candidate for schedule or retraining (management)   **Score:** _____

Comments: _____
_____
_____

Diagnosis: _____

☐ 728.2   Muscle wasting/disuse atrophy   ☐ 596.51 Overactive bladder   ☐ 787.6   Fecal incontinence
☐ 788.32 Stress UI male   ☐ 625.6   Stress UI female   ☐ 788.43 Nocturia
☐ 596.59 Detrusor instability   ☐ 788.41 Frequency   ☐ 625.9   Pelvic pain
☐ 564.0   Constipation   ☐ 599.0   Urinary tract infection   ☐ 788.36 Nocturnal enuresis
☐ 788.21 Incomplete bladder emptying   ☐ 728.31 Urge UI
☐ 728.85 Spasm of muscle   ☐ 788.33 Mixed UI

Recommendations: _____
_____

Follow-up visit: ☐ Yes   ☐ No   Visit time: _____

Signature: _____

Pelvic Muscle Assessment

Check one: ☐ Vaginal exam   ☐ Rectal exam

Circle one:

Score	Description
0/5	No contractions
1/5	Trace contractions: less than 1 second
2/5	Weak contraction: with or without posterior elevation of fingers, held for greater than 1 second but less than or equal to 3 seconds
3/5	Moderate contraction: with or without posterior elevation of fingers, held at least 4–6 seconds, repeated three times
4/5	Strong contraction: with posterior elevation of fingers, held for at least 7–9 seconds, repeated 4–5 times
5/5	Unmistakably strong contraction: with posterior elevation of fingers, held at least 10 seconds, repeated 4–5 times

Use of accessory muscle groups

Abdominal	☐ Yes	☐ No
Gluteal	☐ Yes	☐ No
Thigh/abductor	☐ Yes	☐ No

Evaluation—Muscle hypertonus/spasm

Circle one:

0	No pressure or pain associated with exam
1	Comfortable pressure associated with exam
2	Uncomfortable pressure associated with exam
3	Moderate pain associated with exam, intensifies with contraction
4	Severe pain associated with exam; patient unable to perform muscle contraction because of pain

EMG evaluation   ☐ Yes   ☐ No

Results: _____

Diagnosis: Muscle wasting/disuse atrophy   ☐ 728.2

Muscle spasm   ☐ 728.85

Muscle weakness/dysfunction   ☐ 728.9

Comments: _____
_____
_____

Signature: _____   Date: _____

Past Medical History

Name:_____ Date:_____

Instructions: Please answer each question making a checkmark (✓) in appropriate boxes, unless otherwise directed.

1. Education:
   - ☐ Less than high school
   - ☐ Completed high school
   - ☐ More than high school

2. Occupation (now or last job):
   _____

3. Date of last complete medical exam:
   - ☐ Within last month
   - ☐ Within last 6 months
   - ☐ More than 6 months

4. Allergies (medications, foods, or other):

   Substance
   allergic to   Reaction
   _____   _____
   _____   _____
   _____   _____
   _____   _____

5. Do you drink alcohol?
   - ☐ Yes   ☐ No

   If yes, indicate number of glasses per week:
   _____ Beer (glasses)
   _____ Wine (glasses)
   _____ Spirits (ounces)

6. Indicate what amount you drink of the following in a typical day:
   _____ Water (8 oz. glasses)
   _____ Juice (8 oz. glasses)
   _____ Coffee (cups)
   _____ Tea (cups)
   _____ Soda (8 oz. glasses)

7. Have you ever been diagnosed or treated for cancer, a tumor, or noticed any lumps or swelling?
   - ☐ Yes   ☐ No

   Please describe. _____
   _____
   _____

8. Have you ever been treated for any of the following:

	Yes	No
Anxiety	☐	☐
Depression	☐	☐
Nervous problems	☐	☐
Alcoholism	☐	☐
Drug addiction	☐	☐

9. Do you have trouble with:

	Yes	No
Feeling of tingling or numbness in any parts of your body	☐	☐
Weakness in your arms and legs	☐	☐
Weakness of one side of your body	☐	☐

10. Please check the appropriate box(es) if you use any of the following:
    - ☐ Cane   ☐ Wheelchair   ☐ Walker

11. Do you smoke?
    - ☐ Yes   ☐ No

    If yes, how many every day?
    _____ Cigarettes
    _____ Cigars
    _____ Pipe
    _____ Chew tobacco
    _____ Recreational drugs

Comments: _____
_____
_____

Managing and Treating Urinary Incontinence. Copyright © 2002 by Diane Kaschak Newman.
Health Professions Press, Inc., Baltimore.

Name: _____ Date: _____

12. List all medications you are currently taking (prescription and over-the-counter):

Name	Dosage	Reason for taking

13. Which, if any, of the following have you been treated for?

☐ Alzheimer's disease/dementia   ☐ Falls   ☐ Osteoporosis

☐ Anemia   ☐ Fractures/joint replacements   ☐ Pacemaker

☐ Arthritis   ☐ Glaucoma   ☐ Parkinson's disease

☐ Asthma   ☐ Head injuries   ☐ Polyps

☐ Back injuries/back compression fractures   ☐ Heart disease (CAD, arrhythmia, atrial fibrillation)   ☐ Renal disease

☐ Bleeding problems   ☐ Heart attack   ☐ Seizures

☐ Cancer   ☐ Heart murmurs   ☐ Skin sensitivies or conditions

☐ Cataracts   ☐ Hemorrhoids   ☐ Stroke

☐ Chest pain   ☐ High blood pressure   ☐ Vascular disease/PVD

☐ Congestive heart failure   ☐ Irritable bowel   ☐ Other–specify

☐ Constipation/impaction   ☐ Kidney stones/bladder stones   _____

☐ COPD   ☐ Mitral valve prolapse   _____

☐ Diabetes   ☐ Multiple Sclerosis   _____

Urological Review - Both Men and Women

14. Prior Genitourinary history:

☐ Hysterectomy ____ yr.   ☐ Bladder tumor
     ☐ Vaginal   ☐ Bladder surgery
     ☐ Abdominal
     ☐ Ovaries removed   ☐ Pelvic radiation
☐ Urethral stricture/ dilatation   ☐ Prostatitis/BPH
     ☐ Prostate Cancer
☐ Discharge - genital area
☐ Urinary tract infection   ☐ Collagen infections
   Date and type   ☐ Other–specify
   _____   _____
☐ Itching/odor–genital area/vagina

Gynecological Review - Women Only

15. Gynecological review

Prolapse:
☐ Bladder   ☐ Uterus
☐ Rectum

Menstrual cycle Information
_____ Date of last period
_____ Date of last pap smear

Pregnancy and childbirth information
Use of: ☐ Pessary   ☐ IUD   ☐ Diaphragm
     ☐ Birth Control   Specify _____
_____ # of Pregnancies
_____ # of Vaginal deliveries
_____ # of Cesarean sections
_____ # of Episiotomies

Previous surgery: _____

Reviewed by: _____ Date: _____

Incontinence Patient Profile

Name:_____ Date:_____

Instructions: Please answer each question below by making a checkmark (✓) in the appropriate box. Bring this form with you to your first appointment.

1. How long have you had a problem with urinary leakage (incontinence)?

□ 1 week to 3 months

□ 3 to 12 months

□ 1 to 5 years

□ 5 to 10 years

□ More than 10 years

2. Did the urine leakage

□ Begin suddenly □ Develop gradually over time

3. How often do you lose urine/water during a typical week?

□ Less than once a week

□ Once a week

□ More than once a week

□ Once a day

□ More than once a day

4. When does the leakage occur?

□ Mainly during the day

□ Mainly at night

□ Both day and night

5. When you leak/lose, how much do you leak?

□ Damp/a few drops

□ Wet enough to wet underpants

□ Quite wet, a cupful (soak pads/other protection)

6. When your bladder feels full, how long can you hold your urine?

□ Less than a minute or two

□ Just a few minutes

□ More than a few minutes

□ Cannot tell if bladder is full

7. Do you experience urinary leakage during any of the following?

□ Coughing   □ Nervousness

□ Sneezing   □ Rushing

□ Laughing   □ Running water

□ Lifting heavy objects □ Cold weather

□ Active exercise   □ Continual leakage

□ "Key in door" when □ Dribbling
trying to open door   after urination

□ Sleeping   □ Walking

□ On the way   □ Without being
to the bathroom   aware

□ Changing position □ Other _____

8. Do you have strong urinary urges you cannot always control?

□ Yes   □ No, never

9. Do you have trouble getting to the toilet on time?

□ Yes   □ No, never

10. How often do you urinate during the day?

□ More often than every hour

□ About every 1 to 2 hours

□ About every 3 to 5 hours

□ Frequency varies

□ Unknown

11. Do you wake up at night to urinate?

□ Never or rarely

□ About one to two times

□ Three or more times

12. When urinating, do you experience

□ Problem starting stream

□ Weak, slow stream/dribbling

□ Pain   □ Discomfort   □ Burning

□ Blood in the urine

□ Bladder not emptying fully

□ Loss of urine in sudden large amounts

□ Stopping and starting urine stream

□ None of the above

Managing and Treating Urinary Incontinence. Copyright © 2002 by Diane Kaschak Newman.
Health Professions Press, Inc., Baltimore.

13. Do you use any of the following for protection during urinary leakage?

- ☐ Panty liner
- ☐ Sanitary napkins—feminine hygiene pads
- ☐ Minipads
- ☐ Guards for men
- ☐ Undergarments (with straps and buttons)
- ☐ Protective underwear—disposable
- ☐ Adult briefs/diapers
- ☐ Bed or furniture pads
- ☐ Cloth garments
- ☐ Larger pads in underwear
- ☐ Homemade pads, tissues
- ☐ Bedside commode/urinal
- ☐ Other, please note below:

_____

14. How many times per day do you need to change pads or other products?

- ☐ 1 or fewer   ☐ 3   ☐ 5
- ☐ 2   ☐ 4   ☐ 6 or more

15. Have you ever seen a urologist or other doctor for your problem?

- ☐ Yes   ☐ No
- ☐ Name (if, yes): _____
  What did he/she do?

  _____

  _____

16. Are you avoiding certain activities because of a urine loss problem?

- ☐ Yes   ☐ No

17. Are you sexually active now?

- ☐ No   ☐ Yes (answer a, b, c)

a. Do you have difficulty with urination after intercourse?

- ☐ Yes   ☐ No

b. Do you have pain/discomfort with intercourse?

- ☐ Yes   ☐ No

c. Do you ever leak/lose urine during intercourse?

- ☐ Yes   ☐ No

18. For men: Are you having problems with impotence and maintaining an erection for intercourse?

- ☐ Yes   ☐ No

19. How often do you have a bowel movement?

- ☐ Once a day
- ☐ More than one per day
- ☐ 2-3 times a week
- ☐ Less than 1 time once a week

20. Do you have any of the following?

- ☐ Constipation
- ☐ Diarrhea
- ☐ Bloody stools
- ☐ Bowel incontinence
- ☐ None of the above

21. Do you use laxatives?

- ☐ No   ☐ Yes (which ones?)
  Describe _____

22. Do you ever lose control of your bowels?

- ☐ Yes   ☐ No
  Describe _____

23. Has there been a change in the pattern of your bowel movements in the past year?

- ☐ Yes   ☐ No

24. Have you previously tried pelvic muscle exercises or Kegel exercises?

- ☐ Yes   ☐ No

  If you have tried pelvic muscle or Kegel exercises, describe how you have done them.

  _____

  _____

Comments: _____

_____

Reviewed by: _____   Date: _____

Bladder and Bowel Record

Name: _____ Date: _____

Time of day	Voided in toilet (✓)	Aware of urge to void?	Did resident leak urine?*	Activity when leakage happened (coughing, on way to the bathroom)	Bowel movement +	Fluid intake in cups
7:00 A.M.		Yes No	S M L		F H L	
8:00 A.M.		Yes No	S M L		F H L	
9:00 A.M.		Yes No	S M L		F H L	
10:00 A.M.		Yes No	S M L		F H L	
11:00 A.M.		Yes No	S M L		F H L	
12:00 NOON		Yes No	S M L		F H L	
1:00 P.M.		Yes No	S M L		F H L	
2:00 P.M.		Yes No	S M L		F H L	
3:00 P.M.		Yes No	S M L		F H L	
4:00 P.M.		Yes No	S M L		F H L	
5:00 P.M.		Yes No	S M L		F H L	
6:00 P.M.		Yes No	S M L		F H L	
7:00 P.M.		Yes No	S M L		F H L	
8:00 P.M.		Yes No	S M L		F H L	
9:00 P.M.		Yes No	S M L		F H L	
10:00 P.M.		Yes No	S M L		F H L	
11:00 P.M.		Yes No	S M L		F H L	
12 MIDNIGHT		Yes No	S M L		F H L	
1:00 A.M.		Yes No	S M L		F H L	
2:00 A.M.		Yes No	S M L		F H L	
3:00 A.M.		Yes No	S M L		F H L	
4:00 A.M.		Yes No	S M L		F H L	
5:00 A.M.		Yes No	S M L		F H L	
6:00 A.M.		Yes No	S M L		F H L	

Product worn: ☐ Pad   ☐ Pant/pad   ☐ Brief   ☐ Other (specify): _____

*	S = Slightly wet	M = Wets most of pad	L = Outside of clothing is wet
+	F = Formed	H = Hard	L = Loose/liquid

Reviewed by: _____

Bladder and Bowel Retraining Preassessment

Name:_____ Room:_____ Date:_____

Primary diagnosis: _____ Date of birth:_____

Diagnosis or history of: □ Urinary incontinence □ Fecal incontinence □ Constipation

□ Fecal impaction □ Chronic UTI □ Prostate problems

□ Psychiatric disorder □ Memory deficit: □ Minimal □ Severe

Other significant medical conditions: _____

Present medications: □ Diuretics □ Antihypertensives □ Psychotropics □ Narcotics □ Sedatives

Bladder and bowel records obtained for 3 days? □ Yes (please attach) □ No

Average daily activity: □ Sedentary □ Ambulatory □ Bedbound □ Other_____

Average 24-hour fluid intake for 3 days:_____ ounces

Average dietary fiber intake per day: □ Poor □ Adequate—describe _____

1. Urine loss on way to bathroom? □ Yes □ Sometimes □ No

2. Urine loss with coughing, changing position, exertion, laughing? □ Yes □ Sometimes □ No

3. Continually incontinent? □ Yes □ No

4. Aware of urge (need to urinate)? □ Yes □ Sometimes □ No

5. Bowel movement pattern: □ Daily □ Every other day □ 2-3 times/week □ 1 time/week

6. Laxative use? □ Yes □ No

   If yes, please list _____

7. Use of perineal pads/briefs for protection? □ Yes □ No

   If yes, please list type _____

Assessment of toileting

□ Toilets self or with minimal assist:

   □ Uses grab bar □ Toilet elevation

   □ Uses device: □ Bedside commode □ Urinal type_____

   □ Catheter (size and type)_____

   □ Absorbent pads/products_____

□ Needs assistance with transfer

   □ One person

   □ Two people

   □ Total care

Plan of care — Bladder and bowel movement program

□ A Can toilet self or with minimal assistance—may benefit from retraining

□ B Needs toileting assistance—poor candidate for retraining

□ C Needs management system:_____

Comments: _____

_____

Bladder and bowel evaluation requested: □ Yes □ No Date performed: _____

Signature: _____ Date:_____

Findings and Recommendations

Name: _____ Date: _____

Impressions/findings: _____

_____

The following includes instructions given verbally and in written form to the a patient and/or caregiver.

General information

Anatomy of   ☐ Genitourinary system   ☐ Gastrointestinal system

Physiology of   ☐ Bladder function   ☐ Bowel function

      ☐ Skin care   ☐ Odor control   ☐ Other hygiene measures

Medications: _____

Activities of daily living

      Use of daily   ☐ Voiding diary   ☐ Bowel diary

      ☐ Specific toileting program _____

      ☐ Prompted voiding program _____

Behavior modification, therapeutic activities, and self-care activities

      ☐ Facilitation of bladder emptying and voiding   ☐ Postvoid dribble technique

      ☐ Techniques to decrease nocturia and nocturnal enuresis

      ☐ Facilitation of activity level to promote toileting and bowel regularity

      ☐ Education in urge inhibition techniques, relaxation techniques, and bladder retraining

      ☐ Dietary restriction of caffeine   ☐ Other bladder irritants   ☐ Overall fluid management

      ☐ Dietary changes to: ☐ Improve bowel irregularity   ☐ Decrease fecal incontinence

      ☐ Use of pelvic muscle during symptoms of urgency, frequency, and stress/urge incontinence

      ☐ Pelvic muscle exercise for home therapy program   ☐ Demonstration   ☐ Audiocassette tape

Self-care management activities

      ☐ Use of protective/absorbent products   Type:_____ Size:_____

      ☐ Indwelling catheter care   Type: _____ Size: _____

      ☐ Intermittent self-catheterization   Type: _____ Size: _____

      ☐ External penile clamp   Type: _____ Size: _____

      ☐ Pessary   Type: _____ Size: _____

      ☐ Use of urinal or other toileting device   Type: _____

      ☐ Skin care product recommended   Type: _____

      ☐ Other (specify) _____

Instructions reviewed with: _____ (patient's name)

Patient's response: _____

Recommendations: _____

_____

Signature: _____ Visit time: _____

Daily Voiding Record (or Frequency Volume Chart)

Name: _____ Date: _____

It is important for you to record your voiding pattern every day. This will allow us to better understand your condition so recommendations can be made that will best assist you.

Instructions:

Fill in the day and date.

1. In the second column, next to the correct time interval, place a check each time you urinate in the toilet. Also, record the amount in ounces or millimeters.
2. In the third column, mark every time you leak, have an incontinent episode or urine leakage, and indicate whether it is a large (L) or small (S) amount.
3. In the fourth column, record the reason for the urine leakage such as sneezing, lifting, coughing, laughing, couldn't make it to the bathroom, and so on.
4. In the fifth column, place a check in the correct time interval each time a wet pad is changed. Mark how wet: "D" if the pad is slightly wet or damp, "W" if wet, and "S" if the pad is saturated or very wet.
5. In the sixth column, in the correct time interval, describe your liquid intake (e.g., coffee, water, orange juice), and estimate the amount (e.g., one cup, six ounces).

Time interval	Urinated in toilet/ amount	Incontinent episode amount L/S	Reason for urine leakage	Changed wet pad D/W/S	Type/amount of liquid intake
6:00 A.M.					
7:00 A.M.					
8:00 A.M.					
9:00 A.M.					
10:00 A.M.					
11:00 A.M.					
12:00 NOON					
1:00 P.M.					
2:00 P.M.					
3:00 P.M.					
4:00 P.M.					
5:00 P.M.					
6:00 P.M.					
7:00 P.M.					
8:00 P.M.					
9:00 P.M.					
10:00 P.M.–MIDNIGHT					
MIDNIGHT–2 A.M.					
2:00–4:00 A.M.					
4:00–6:00 A.M.					

Type of pad used: _____ Number of pads used: _____

C

Resources

MANUFACTURERS OF DRUGS AND PRODUCTS

This is a list of the major manufacturers of products, catheters, and devices for urinary incontinence (UI) management. Most of these products are mentioned throughout the book. These manufacturers have additional educational material on UI and their products.

3M Health Care
3M Center Building
St. Paul, MN 55144
(800) 228-3957
http://www.mmm.com/healthcare
Skin care and perineal cleanser products (e.g., Cavilon no-sting barrier film)

A+ Medical Products, Inc.
442 Mitchell Hollow Road
Post Office Box 10
Haines Falls, NY 12436
(888) 843-3334
http://www.aplusmedical.com
Female catheter guide, urinal

A-T Surgical Mfg. Co., Inc.
115 Clemente Street
Holyoke, MA 01040
(800) 225-2023
http://www.a-tsurgical.com
Reusable pads, catheter straps and holders

American Biffy Company
674 Wells Road
Boulder City, NV 89005
(877) 422-4339
http://www.biffy.com
Bidet attachment that can be mounted along toilet providing complete perineal care

American Medical Systems
10700 Bren Road West
Minnetonka, MN 55343
(800) 328-3881
http://www.visitams.com
Artificial urinary sphincters

Americare (Aldan) Products
115 Woodbine Drive
Danville, PA 17821
(800) 220-2273
http://www.aldanonline.com
http://www.priva-inc.com/
Incontinence/main.htm
Reusable pads and products

Astra Tech, Inc.
21535 Hawthorne Blvd., Suite 525
Torrance, CA 90503
(877) 456-3742
http://www.astratechusa.com
Hydrophilic straight catheters for
self-catheterization

Aventis Pharmaceuticals
300 Somerset Corporate Boulevard
Bridgewater, NJ 08807
(800) 981-2491
http://www.aventispharma-us.com
Nasal Spray/Tablets (DDAVP) for
nocturnal enuresis

Bard Medical Division
C.R. Bard, Inc.
8195 Industrial Blvd
Covington, GA 30014
(800) 526-4455
http://www.bardmedical.com
Large variety of indwelling,
intermittent, and external catheter
and drainage bag products. Also
carries skin care and perineal
cleanser products called "Special
Care" and periurethral bulking
agent (Contigen).

Calmoseptine, Inc.
16602 Burke Lane
Huntington Beach, CA 92647
(800) 800-3405
http://www.calmoseptine.com
Skin care ointment

**Carbon Medical Technologies,
Inc.**
1290 Hammond Road
St. Paul, MN 55110
(888) 207-0262
http://www.durasphere.com
Injectible periurethral bulking
agent (Durasphere)

Care-Tech Laboratories, Inc.
3224 South Kingshighway Blvd
St. Louis, MO 63139
(800) 772-4610
http://www.caretechlabs.com
Skin care and perineal cleanser
products (Barri-Care)

Carrington Laboratories, Inc.
2001 Walnut Hill Lane
Irving, TX 75038
(800) 527-5216
http://www.carringtonlabs.com
Skin care, perineal cleanser, and
deodorizer products (Carrington)

Chester Labs, Inc.
1900 Section Road, Suite A
Cincinnati, OH 45237
(800) 354-9709
http://www.chester-labs.com
Skin care products, perineal
cleansers, and odor eliminators
(April Fresh)

Circon Corporation/ACMI
300 Stillwater Ave
Stamford, CT 06902
(888) 524-7266
http://www.circoncorp.com
Urodynamic UI evaluation system
and biofeedback system

Coloplast Corporation
1955 West Oak Circle
Marietta, GA 30062
(800) 533-0464
http://www.us.coloplast.com
Large variety of external and
intermittent catheters and drainage
bags (Conveen). Skin care and
perineal cleanser products (Baza).

ConvaTec
Professional Services
Post Office Box 5254
Princeton, NJ 08543
(800) 422-8811
http://www.convatec.com
Skin care and perineal cleanser
products (Aloe Vesta and Sensi-Care,
catheter anchor adhesive fastener)

Cook Wound/Ostomy/Continence
1100 West Morgan Street
Post Office Box 266
Spencer, IN 47460
(800) 843-8451
http://www.cookwoc.com
Penile compression device (penile
clamp), pessaries, and catheters

Dale Medical Products, Inc.
Post Office Box 1556
7 Cross Street
Plainville, MA 02762
(800) 343-3980
http://www.dalemed.com
Catheter anchor strap

DesChutes Medical Products, Inc.
1011 SW Emkay Drive
Suite 104
Bend, OR 97702
(800) 383-2588
http://www.deschutesmed.com
Pelvic muscle strengthening home
trainer (Myself)

**Diagnostic Ultrasound
Corporation**
21222 30th Drive, SE
Bothell, WA 98021
(800) 331-2313
http://www.dxu.com
Portable ultrasound (BladderScan)

Dumex Medical
825 Franklin Court, Unit G
Marrietta, GA 30067
(877) 796-8637
http://www.woundcaredirect.com
Skin care and perineal cleanser and
deodorizer products (PrimaDerm).
Reusable absorbent pads and
products.

E.K. Johnson, Industries
4869 "G" Street
Springfield, Oregon 97478
(541) 746-6126
Spill-proof Rehab Urinal

Empi, Inc.
599 Cardigan Road
St. Paul, MN 55126
(888) 367-3674
http://www.empi.com
Portable pelvic floor exerciser and
electrical stimulator for home use
(Minnova, Innova, InnoSense)

First Quality Products, Inc.
80 Cuttermill Rd, Suite 500
Great Neck, NY 11021
(800) 227-3551
http://www.fqnet.com
Disposable absorbent products

Geri-Care Products
252 Wagner Street
Middlesex, NJ 08846
(732) 469-7722
http://www.geri-careproducts.com
Reusable absorbent products

GOJO Industries, Inc.
Post Office Box 991
Akron, OH 44309
(800) 321-9647
http://www.GOJO.com
Skin care and perineal cleanser
products (Provon)

Greenwald Surgical Co., Inc.
2688 DeKalb Street
Lake Station, IN 46405
(888) 926-1829
http://www.greenwaldsurgical.com
Cunningham and Baumrucker penile
clamps

Gynecare, Division of Ethicon, Inc.
Post Office Box 151
Somerville, NJ 08876
(888) 496-3227
http://www.gynecare.com
Surgical tape for stress UI

Healthpoint Ltd.
3909 Hulen Street
Fort Worth, TX 76107
(800) 441-8227
http://www.healthpoint.com
Skin care and perineal cleanser and
deodorizer products (Proshield)

Hollister, Inc.
InCare Medical Products
2000 Hollister Drive
Libertyville, IL 60048
(800) 323-4060
http://www.hollister.com
Wide variety of external male
catheters and pouches (e.g., for
retracted penis), external female
pouches, catheter drainage bags,
odor eliminator products, skin care
(Restore) and perineal cleansers
products. Sophisticated EMG/
biofeedback equipment.

Humanicare International, Inc.
9 Elkins Road
North Brunswick, NJ 08816
(800) 631-5270
http://www.humanicare.com

Disposable and reusable absorbent
products (Dignity)

Hygienics Industries
3968 194th Trail
Miami, FL 33160
(888) 463-7337
http://www.hygienics.com
Reusable absorbent products (Safe &
Dry)

J & J Engineering, Inc.
22797 Holgar Court, NE
Poulsbo, WA 98370
(888) 550-8300
http://www.jjengineering.com
Customized EMG/biofeedback
equipment

J.T. Posey Company
5635 Peck Road
Arcadia, CA 91006
(800) 447-6739
http://www.posey.com
Reusable catheter supplies/tube
straps/drainage bag holders

Kendall Company
Tyco Healthcare
15 Hampshire Street
Mansfield, MA 02048
(800) 962-9888
http://www.kendallhq.com
Indwelling (Curity) and external
catheters, collection bags, skin care
products (Vaseline)

Kimberly-Clark Corporation
Adult Care Division
2001 Marathon Ave
Neenah, WI 54956
(888) 233-7363
http://www.depend.com
http://www.poise.com

Retail supplier of absorbent products (Depend). Introduced protective underwear and pantiliners for incontinence (Poise).

Laborie Medical Technologies, Inc.
310 Hurricane Lane
Williston, VT 05495
(800) 522-6743
http://www.laborie.com
Catheter straps, home wetness monitor, complex urodynamic and biofeedback equipment

Life-Tech, Inc.
4235 Greenbriar Drive
Stafford, TX 77477
(800) 231-9841
http://www.life-tech.com
Abdominal leg bag for indwelling or suprapubic catheters, urodynamic equipment

Maddak, Inc.
6 Industrial Road
Pequannock, NJ 07440
(973) 628-7600
http://www.maddak.com
Bathroom toileting aids

Mallinckrodt, Inc.
675 McDonnell Blvd
Hazelwood, MO 63042
(888) 744-1414
http://www.mallinckrodt.com
Tofranil (imipramine HCL) drug treatment for overactive bladder (OAB), nocturia and stress UI

McKesson Medical-Surgical
8741 Landmark Road
Richmond, VA 23228
(800) 446-3008
http://www.mckgenmed.com

Skin cleansers, creams (StayDry), and absorbent products

Medline Industries, Inc.
One Medline Place
Mundelein, IL 60060
(800) 633-5463
http://www.medline.com
Indwelling and intermittent catheters, drainage bags, disposable absorbent products, skin creams, and cleansers

Medtronic
710 Medtronic Parkway
Minneapolis, MN 55421
(800) 328-2518
http://www.interstim.com
Implantable electrical stimulator for urgency and frequency

Mentor Healthcare-Urology
201 Mentor Drive
Santa Barbara, CA 93111
(800) 328-3863
http://www.mentorcorp.com
Indwelling, external (including McGuire reusable external catheter/urinal), and intermittent (large selection) catheters; collection bags; large selection of pessaries

Milex Products, Inc.
4311 North Normandy Ave
Chicago, IL 60634
(800) 621-1278
http://www.milexproducts.com
Large selection of pessaries and vaginal weights

Nature Plus, Inc.
555 Lordship Blvd
Stratford, CT 06615
(203) 380-0316
http://www.nature-plus.com
Odor eliminator

Neurodyne Medical Corp.
52 New Street
Cambridge, MA 02138
(800) 963-8633
http://www.neumed.com
EMG/biofeedback equipment

North American Distributors
4482 Barranca Parkway, No. 180-175
Irvine, CA 92604
(800) 995-0510
http://www.nadinc.com
EMG/biofeedback equipment,
neuromuscular stimulators

Ortho-McNeil Pharmaceutical
1000 Rt. 202, Box 300
Raritan, NJ 08869
(888) 395-1232
http://www:ditropanxl.com
Ditropan XL (oxybutynin chloride;
drug treatment for OAB)

Paper-Pak Products, Inc.
1941 White Ave
LaVerne, CA 91750
(800) 635-4560
http://www.paperpak.com
Disposable absorbent products
(Confidence)

Pharmacia Corporation
100 Route 206 North
Peapack, NJ 07977
(888) 768-5501
http://www.detrolla.com
Detrol (tolterodine tartrate) for OAB,
Vagifem vaginal tablets

Principle Business Enterprises
Post Office Box 129
Dunbridge, OH 43414-0129
(800) 467-3224
http://www.gopeach.com
Disposable absorbent products
(Tranquility)

The Prometheus Group
1 Washington Street, Suite 303
Dover, NH 03820
(800) 442-2325
http://www.theprogrp.com
EMG/biofeedback equipment,
neuromuscular stimulators

Rochester Medical Corporation
One Rochester Medical Drive
Stewartville, MN 55976
(800) 243-3315
http://www.rocm.com
Specially coated intermittent
catheters, indwelling and external
catheters, and FemSoft urethral
insert

Rusch, Inc.
2450 Meadowbrook Parkway
Duluth, GA 30096
(800) 553-5214
http://www.ruschinc.com
Indwelling and intermittent
catheters, collection bags, pessary,
Cunningham penile clamp

SCA Incontinence Care
500 Baldwin Tower
Eddystone, PA 19022
(800) 992-9939
http://www.tena-usa.com
Disposable absorbent products
(Tena) and skin cleansers

Salk, Inc.
Park Seneca Building
1515 Mockingbird Lane
Charlotte, NC 28209
(887) 553-9594
http://www.healthdri.com
Reusable absorbent products
(HealthDri)

Smith & Nephew, Inc.
11775 Starkey Rd
Post Office Box 1970
Largo, FL 33773
(800) 876-1261
www.snwmd.com
Skin care products (Triple Care)
and cleansers

Standard Textile Company
1 Knollcrest Drive
Post Office Box 371805
Cincinnati, OH 45222
(800) 999-0400
http://www.standardtextile.com
Reusable absorbent products

Summit Industries, Inc.
Lantiseptic Division
Post Office Box 7329
Marietta, GA 30065
(800) 241-6996
www.lantisepseptic.com
Body wash and skin cream
(Lantiseptic)

Sunrise Medical, Inc.
7477 East Dry Creek Parkway
Longmont, CO 80503
(800) 333-4000
http://www.sunrisemedical.com
Raised toilet seats

Swiss-American Products, Inc.
4641 Nall Road
Dallas, TX 75244
(800) 633-8872
http://www.elta.net
Skin care products (Elta)

Timm Medical Technologies
6585 City West Parkway
Eden Prairie, MN 55344
(800) 438-8592
http://www.timmmedical.com

Urodynamic evaluation equipment,
penile compression device (C3),
vaginal weights (StepFree)

Tyco Healthcare Retail Group
(formerly Kendall Confab Retail
Group)
601 Allendale Rd
King of Prussia, PA 19406
(800) 326-6322
http://www.confab.com
Disposable absorbent products

Urocare Products, Inc.
2735 Melbourne Ave
Pomona, CA 91767-1931
(800) 423-4441
http://www.urocare.com
External catheter (reusable latex bag)
and supplies (Uro-Cath)

Utah Medical Products, Inc.
7043 South 300 West
Midvale, UT 84047
(800) 533-4984
http://www.utahmed.com
Pelvic floor electrical stimulator

Warner Chilcott Company
Rockaway 80 Corporate Center
100 Enterprise Drive, Suite 280
Rockaway, NJ 07866
(800) 524-2624
http://www.estrace.com
Estrace (vaginal cream)

Wyeth-Ayerst Laboratories
Division of Home Products Corp
Post Office Box 8299
Philadelphia, PA 19101
(800) 999-9284
http://www.premarin.com
Premarin (vaginal cream)

MAIL-ORDER CATALOGS

These companies send catalogs upon request, so clients can purchase products directly.

Byram Healthcare Centers, Inc.—Home Health Supplies
11400 47th Street North, Suite A
Clearwater, FL 33762
(800) 354-4054 (CT, NY, NJ)
(800) 649-9882 (MA, VT, RI, ME)
(800) 234-1779 (All other states)

Edgepark Surgical, Inc.
1810 Summit Commerce Park
Twinsburg, OH 44087
(800) 321-0591
http://www.edgepark.com

Home Delivery Incontinent Supplies Co, Inc. (HDIS)
9385 Dielman Industrial Drive
Olivette, MO 63132
(800) 269-4663
http://www.hdis.com

PROFESSIONAL ORGANIZATIONS

These professional organizations and consumer groups provide education or information on incontinence, OAB, and related disorders.

Agency for Healthcare Research and Quality
(Formerly Agency for Health Care Policy and Research)
2101 E. Jefferson Street, Suite 501
Rockville, MD 20852
(301) 594-1364
http:www.ahrq.gov

American College of Obstetricians and Gynecology
409 12th Street, SW
Post Office Box 96920
Washington DC 20024
(800) 762-2264
http://www.acog.org

American Foundation of Urologic Disease
Bladder Health Council
1128 North Charles Street
Baltimore, MD 21201
(800) 242-2383
http://www.afud.org

American Physical Therapy Association
Section on Women's Health
111 North Fairfax Street
Alexandria, VA 22314
(800) 999-2782
http://www.APTA.org

American Urogynecologic Society
2025 M Street, NW
Suite 800
Washington DC 20036
(202) 367-1167
http://www.augs.org

American Urological Association,
Inc.
1120 North Charles Street
Baltimore, MD 21201
(410) 727-1100
http://www.auanet.org

Association of Women's Health,
Obstetric and Neonatal Nurses
2000 L Street, NW
Suite 740
Washington DC 20036
(800) 673-8499
http://www.awhonn.org

International Foundation for
Functional Gastrointestinal
Disorders
Post Office Box 170864
Milwaukce WI 53217
(888) 964-2001
http://www.iffgd.org

National Association For
Continence (NAFC)
Post Office Box 8310
Spartanburg, SC 29305-8310
(800) 252-3337
http://www.nafc.org

National Institute On Aging
National Institutes of Health
Building 31, Room 5C27
31 Center Drive, MSC 2292
Bethesda, MD 20892
(301) 496-1752
http://www.nih.gov/nia

National Institute of Diabetes and
Digestive and Kidney Diseases
Information Clearinghouse
3 Information Way
Bethesda, MD 20892
http://www.niddk.nih.gov

Simon Foundation for Continence
Box 835-F
Wilmette, IL 60091
(800) 237-4666
http://www.simonfoundation.org

Society of Urologic Nurses
and Associates
East Holy Avenue, Box 56
Pitman, NJ 09071
(888) 827-7862
http://www.suna.org

US TOO! International, Inc.
Prostate Cancer Survivor Support
Groups
5003 Fairview Avenue
Downers Grove, Il 60515
(800) 808-7866
http://www.ustoo.org

Wellness Partners, LLC
237 Old Tilton Rd
Canterbury, NH 03224
web site for consumers
http://www.seekwellness.com/
incontinence

Wound, Ostomy and Continence
Nurses Society
4700 West Lake Ave
Glenview, IL 60025
(800) 224-9626
http://www.wocn.org

PRODUCT RESOURCE GUIDES

These guides list products available through specific companies.

Bruce Medical Supply
411 Waverly Oaks Road
Waltham, MA 02454
(800) 225-8446
http://www.brucemedical.com

Express Medical Supply, Inc.
200 Seabold Spur
Fenton, MO 63026
(800) 633-9188
http://www.exmed.net

Kestrel Incontinence Product Sourcebook
73-4519 Kohanaiki Road, Ste. B15
Kailua-Kona, HI 96740
(808) 325-5200
www.kestrelhealthinfo.com
www.incontinencesource.com

Resource Guide: Products and Services for Incontinence
NAFC
Post Office Box 8310
Spartanburg, SC 29305
(800) 252-3337
http://www.nafc.org

Glossary

Absorbent products Pads and garments, either disposable or reusable, worn to contain urinary incontinence or uncontrolled urine leakage. Absorbent products include shields, guards, undergarment pads, combination pad–pant systems, diaper-like garments, and bed pads.

Acetylcholine Substance (neurotransmitter) that plays an important part in the transmission of nerve impulses in the parasympathetic nervous system. These transmitters control smooth muscles, including those of the bladder and urethra, and stimulate the bladder to contract.

Acontractile detrusor Detrusor muscle that cannot be demonstrated to contract during testing (urodynamic studies).

Activities of daily living Activities necessary to meet essential human needs, such as bathing, grooming, toileting, and social interactions.

Acute incontinence Incontinence that comes on suddenly, usually caused by a new illness or condition, and is often easily reversed with appropriate treatment of the condition that caused it.

Anal sphincters Two rings of muscles surrounding the rectum and anus, which help control passage of bowel movements.

Antibiotics Substances that inhibit the growth of or kill microorganisms (bacteria and viruses); used to treat infections

Anticholinergic Drug that interferes with the effects of acetylcholine, thus impeding the action of the parasympathetic nervous system. An anticholinergic drug will facilitate storage of urine by increasing bladder capacity and decreasing bladder overactivity.

Anus Final two inches of the rectum, surrounded by the internal anal sphincter and the external sphincter.

Artificial urinary sphincter Mechanical device surgically implanted into the patient that consists of a cuff placed around the bulbar urethra or bladder neck, a pressure-regulating balloon, and a pump. The device is used to control opening and closing of the urethra manually and is the most commonly used surgical procedure for the treatment of male urethral insufficiency.

Atonic bladder   Often caused by peripheral neuropathies, such as diabetes mellitus. The bladder is flaccid and overdistended with urine. Overflow incontinence may occur. Also referred to as a lower motor neuron bladder.

Autoimmune   Condition in which the body produces antibodies to its own tissue.

Bacteria   Microscopic organisms that can cause infection and are usually treated with antibiotics.

Bacteriuria   Bacteria present in the urine—100,000 colony forming units (cfu).

Bedside commode   Portable toilet used by individuals who have difficulty ambulating to standard facilities.

Behavioral techniques   Specific interventions designed to alter the relationship between the patient's symptoms and his or her behavior and/or environment for the treatment of maladaptive urinary voiding patterns. This may be achieved by modification of the behavior and/or environment of the patient.

Benign prostatic hyperplasia (BPH)   Common disorder of men older than 50 characterized by enlargement of the prostate which may press against the urethra and interfere with the flow of urine, causing overflow incontinence. BPH is the most common cause of such anatomic obstruction in elderly men.

Biofeedback therapy   Behavioral technique in which a person learns how to consciously control involuntary responses such as muscle contractions. The person receives a visual, auditory, or tactile signal (the feedback) that indicates how well the person's muscles are responding to the commands of the person's nervous system. The signal is derived from a measurable physiologic parameter, which is subsequently used in an educational process to accomplish a specific therapeutic result. The signal is displayed in a quantitative way, and the patient is taught how to alter it and thus control the physiologic process.

Bladder   Hollow, muscular organ that lies in the pelvis and is supported by the pelvic floor muscle. The bladder has only two functions: to stretch to allow the storage of urine and to contract to enable the expulsion of urine. The term detrusor is used to refer to the smooth muscle structure of the bladder.

Bladder cancer   Carcinoma of the transitional-cell epithelium that lines the bladder. Tumors in the bladder may be benign or cancerous. Bladder cancers account for 2%–6% of all cancers in the United States and are three times more prevalent in men than in women. Bladder cancer can spread throughout the body, so early detection is critical. After prostate cancer, bladder cancer is the most common urinary tract cancer.

Bladder catheterization   Procedure in which a catheter is passed through the urethra and into the bladder for the purpose of draining urine and performing diagnostic tests of bladder or urethral function.

Bladder diary or record   Daily record of bladder habits documenting urination and episodes of incontinence.

Bladder training   Behavioral technique that requires the patient to resist or inhibit the sensation of urgency (the strong desire to urinate), to postpone voiding, and to urinate according to a timetable rather than the urge to void.

Bowel movement   Act of passing feces through the anus.

Bowels   Another word for intestines.

Caruncle (urethral caruncle)   Small, red benign tumor that is visible at the posterior part of the urethral meatus. Occurs chiefly in postmenopausal women and usually causes no symptoms.

Cathartics   Medications that increase the clearing of intestinal contents. Also known as laxatives.

Catheter   Narrow, flexible rubber, latex, or silastic tube that is inserted or passed through the urethra or lower abdomen and into the bladder for the purpose of draining urine or performing diagnostic tests of bladder or urethral function.

Catheterization   Techniques for bladder emptying employing the use of a slender tube (catheter) inserted through the urethra or through the anterior abdominal wall into the bladder to drain the bladder.

Cervix   Lower portion of the uterus that connects with the vagina.

Cholinergic   Relating to fibers in the parasympathetic nervous system that release acetylcholine.

Clinical practice guidelines   Set of systematically developed statements or recommendations designed to assist practitioner and patient in making decisions about appropriate health care for specific clinical circumstances. Such guidelines are designed to assist health care practitioners in the prevention, diagnosis, treatment, and management of specific clinical conditions.

Compression device   Device used to put direct pressure on the urethra, causing it to remain closed until the device is removed and the bladder is allowed to drain. Also known as a penile clamp.

Condom catheters   Condom-like device placed over the penis to allow bladder drainage and collection of urine. See External (condom) catheters.

Continence   Ability to exercise voluntary control over the urge to urinate or defecate until an appropriate time and place can be found.

Continuous urinary incontinence   Report that a person has leaked urine without sensation or precipitating factors such as exertion or effort. Absence of sensation may be due to neurological disease.

Coudé catheter   Curved-tip catheter that allows for the passage of the catheter beyond certain urethral, prostatic, or bladder neck impediments that may pose problems for a straight catheter.

Credé maneuver   Method of applying direct pressure with one or two hands to the abdomen over the bladder while voiding in order to empty the bladder.

Cystitis   Irritation or inflammation (swelling) of the bladder usually caused by an infection.

Cystocele Intrusion or bulging of the bladder into the vagina, usually caused when the vaginal muscles that support the bladder and urethra are stretched or damaged.

Cystometry Test used to assess the function of the bladder by measuring the pressure or volume as the bladder is slowly being filled. Cystometry is used to assess detrusor activity, sensation, capacity, and compliance. There are different variations of the test depending on the problem being investigated, but regardless of the technique, cystometry involves insertion of a catheter into the bladder.

Cystoscopy Procedure used to diagnose urinary tract disorders and provide a direct view of the urethra and bladder by inserting a thin, flexible telescopelike instrument into the urethra and then into the bladder.

Daytime frequency Number of voids recorded during waking hours, including the last void after waking and rising in the morning.

Decreased bladder compliance Failure to store urine in the bladder caused by the loss of bladder wall elasticity and of bladder accommodation. This condition may result from radiation cystitis or from inflammatory bladder conditions such as chemical cystitis, interstitial cystitis, and certain neurologic bladder disorders.

Decubitus ulcer Area of local tissue necrosis (death or damage) that usually develops where soft tissues are compressed between bony prominences and any external surface for prolonged periods.

Defecation Act of emptying the bowels or having a bowel movement.

Dehydration State that occurs when not enough fluid is present to fulfill the body's fluid needs.

Dementia General loss of short- and long-term memory and mental deterioration. It may affect emotions, abstract thinking, judgment, impulse control, and learning and can cause functional incontinence.

Detrusor Smooth muscle bladder wall that stretches to accommodate and store urine and contracts uniformly to expel the urine.

Detrusor hyperactivity with impaired bladder contractility (DHIC) Condition characterized by involuntary detrusor contractions in which patients either are unable to empty their bladders completely or can empty their bladders completely only with straining, due to poor contractility of the detrusor.

Detrusor overactivity Urodynamic observation characterized by involuntary detrusor contractions during bladder filling, which may be spontaneous or provoked.

Detrusor overactivity incontinence Incontinence due to an involuntary detrusor contraction.

Detrusor sphincter dyssynergia (DSD) Inappropriate contraction of the urethral and/or periurethral striated sphincter concurrent with an involuntary contraction of the detrusor. Occasionally voiding may be prevented altogether.

Detrusor underactivity Contraction of reduced strength and/or duration, resulting in prolonged bladder emptying and/or failure to achieve complete bladder emptying within a normal time span.

Diabetic neuropathy   Condition in which portions of the spinal cord and its nerves have degenerated as a result of diabetes.

Disimpaction   Act of removing stool from the rectum, which could not be eliminated normally.

Diuresis   Production of excessive amounts of urine that may precipitate urinary incontinence or overactive bladder. Can be caused by medical problems such as diabetes mellitus and edema.

Diuretic   Agent (e.g., drug, alcohol, caffeine) that increases urination by causing the kidneys to secrete more fluid from the blood.

Diverticula   Pouches in the walls of organs that, if found in the bladder or urethra, can hold excess urine and become infected or inflamed.

Eczema   Pruritic dermatitis that occurs as a reaction to a drug or some other skin contact. Characterized in the acute state by an erythema; edema associated with serious exudates between the cells of the epidermis; and an inflammatory infiltrate in the dermis, causing oozing, vesiculation, crusting, and scaling of the epidermis.

Electrical stimulation   Application of electric current to stimulate or inhibit the pelvic floor muscles or their nerve supply in order to induce a direct therapeutic response.

Electromyography (EMG)   Diagnostic test used to measure the electrical activity of muscles.

Enterocele   Prolapse or falling down of the intestines into the vagina.

Enuresis   Involuntary loss of urine (urinary incontinence).

Epididymitis   Seminal vesicle infection that causes inflammation of the ejaculatory duct and vas deferens, resulting in pain, dysuria, urinary frequency, and occasional fever.

Episiotomy   Surgical incision into the perineum between the vagina and anus to ease childbirth through the vagina.

Established (chronic) incontinence   Pattern of incontinence that is chronic or long standing in nature.

Estrogen   Hormone produced primarily by the ovaries. Estrogen is believed to play a major role in maintaining the strength and tone of the pelvic floor.

Evacuation   Another word for bowel movement.

External (condom) catheters   Devices made from latex, rubber, polyvinyl, or silicone that are used for externally draining the bladder. They are secured on the shaft of the penis by some form of adhesive and connected to urine collecting bags by a tube. Also called penile sheaths.

External sphincter   Band of muscle downstream from the internal sphincter that is responsible for maintaining urinary and fecal continence.

Fecal impaction   Large amount of hardened stool in the rectum that an individual is unable to pass. A fecal impaction may present as small amounts of watery and incontinent stool.

Fecal incontinence   Accidental and involuntary loss of liquid or solid stool or gas from the anus.

Feces   Waste material from the intestines. Feces are composed of bacteria, undigested food, and material sloughed from the intestines.

Fistula   Abnormal passage or connection between a hollow body cavity or organ and the surface of the body.

Flatulence   Release of gas through the anus.

Fracture pan   Specially-designed bedpan for individuals who are unfit to lift their hips to position themselves on the bedpan. A handle allows the caregiver to remove the pan gently, without turning or lifting the user.

Frequency   Voiding more than eight times in a 24-hour period.

Frequency Volume Chart   Records the volumes voided as well as the time of each micturition, day and night, for at least 24 hours.

Gas   Material that results from swallowed air or that is created when bacteria in the colon break down waste material. Gas that is released from the rectum is called flatulence.

Habit training   Behavioral technique that calls for scheduled toileting at regular intervals on a planned basis to prevent incontinence.

Hematuria   Blood in the urine, which may only be detected using a microscope.

Hesitancy   Difficulty or delay in initiating voiding, resulting in delay in the onset of voiding after the person is ready to pass urine.

Hydronephrosis   Dilation of the renal pelvis and calices and sometimes the collecting ducts. Hydronephrosis is secondary to obstruction of urine flow by calculi, tumors, neurologic disorders, or any various congenital anomalies.

Hydrophilic-coated catheter   One-time use tube devices that are coated with a substance that absorbs water and binds it to the device's surface.

Idiopathic   Occurring without known cause.

Impaction   Blockage in the rectum composed of a large amount of dried stool that is difficult to evacuate.

Incontinence   Accidental or involuntary loss of urine or feces (stool). A person may have urinary or fecal incontinence or both (sometimes called double incontinence.)

Indwelling catheters   Tube device inserted into the bladder to drain the urine continuously. Sometimes called a Foley catheter.

Indwelling urethral catheterization   Process of inserting a tube device into the bladder through the urethra to drain urine continuously.

Intermittency   Term used when the individual describes urine flow that stops and starts on one or more occasions during voiding. Also called intermittent stream.

Intermittent (in/out) catheterization   The use of catheters inserted through the urethra into the bladder every 3–6 hours for bladder drainage in persons with urinary retention. Intermittent catheterization performed by the patient at home is called clean intermittent catheterization (CIC).

Intravesical pressure Pressure within the bladder.

Intrinsic sphincter deficiency (ISD) Cause of stress urinary incontinence in which the urethral sphincter is unable to contract and generate sufficient resistance in the bladder, especially during stress maneuvers. ISD may be due to congenital sphincter weakness, such as myelomeningocele or epispadias, or it may be acquired subsequent to prostatectomy, trauma, radiation therapy, or sacral cord lesions.

Introitus External vaginal opening.

Kegel exercises Exercise named after Dr. Arnold Kegel, who first prescribed a specific set of pelvic-floor exercises to women in the 1940s. See Pelvic muscle exercises.

Kidney One of two paired urine-making organs that lie in the back behind the 13th rib. The principal function is to filter the blood to separate out waste products, which are combined with excess water to form urine.

Lower urinary tract Consists of the bladder, prostate gland (in men), urethra, and urinary sphincters.

LUTS Abbreviation for lower urinary tract symptoms: a group of symptoms including 1) incontinence, 2) weak stream, 3) hesitancy, 4) urgency of urination, 5) nocturia, 6) postvoid dribbling, and 7) intermittency, an interrupted urinary stream.

Meatus Opening to the urethra.

Micturition Another term for urination or voiding.

Minimum Data Set (MDS) Federally mandated screening and assessment form for Medicare- and Medicaid-certified long-term care facilities in the United States. This form is completed within 14 days of admission to the facility, quarterly, and when there is a significant change in the resident's status. An annual update is also required. The information collected in the MDS is used in planning the care of the individual.

Mixed urinary incontinence Combination of involuntary leakage associated with urgency and also with exertion, effort, sneezing, and coughing. A person has both urge and stress urinary incontinence.

Nervous system Voluntary nervous system and the involuntary nervous system are composed of the brain, the spinal cord, and sensory nerves, which provide messages to the brain from the body, and motor nerves, which provide messages from the brain to the muscles and help muscles function.

Neurogenic bladder dysfunction Condition in which there is an abnormality of the nerve supply to the lower urinary tract.that results in incontinence or the inability to completely empty the bladder (urinary retention). It is usually caused by neurological conditions, such as diabetes, stroke, or spinal cord injury.

Nighttime frequency Needing to void one or more times per night between the time the person goes to bed with the intention of sleeping and the time the person wakes with the intention of rising.

Nocturia   Complaint that the individual has to wake at night one or more times because of the need or urge to urinate.

Nocturnal enuresis   Complaint of loss of urine during sleep. In children it is called bedwetting.

Nocturnal polyuria   Present when more than one third of the 24-hour output occurs at night (normally 8 hours while person is in bed). The nighttime urine output excludes the last void before sleep but includes the first void of the morning.

Overactive bladder   Condition characterized by involuntary detrusor contractions during the bladder filling phase, which may be spontaneous or provoked and which the patient cannot suppress.

Overflow incontinence   Involuntary loss of urine associated with overdistension of the bladder. Overflow incontinence results from urinary retention that causes the capacity of the bladder to be overwhelmed. Continuous or intermittent leakage of a small amount of urine results.

Painful bladder syndrome   Complaint of suprapubic pain related to bladder filling, accompanied by other symptoms such as increased daytime and nighttime frequency, in the absence of proven urinary tract infection or other obvious pathology. This term is used in place of interstitial cystitis.

Palpate/palpation   To feel with the palmar surface of the hands and fingers to delineate organs, masses, and tenderness during a physical examination.

Parasympathetic nerves   Maintenance component of the autonomic nervous system. Stimulation of the parasympathetic nervous system that innervates the bladder promotes voiding by stimulating the bladder muscle to contract, causing the urge sensation, and indirectly relaxing the internal urethral sphincter, which allows urine to enter the urethra. Stimulation of the parasympathetic nervous system that innervates the intestinal tract will increase motility and secretion.

Pelvic diaphragm   Levator ani group.

Pelvic muscle exercises (PMEs)   Repetitive active exercise of the levator ani muscle to improve urethral resistance and urinary control by strengthening the periurethral and pelvic muscles. Also called Kegel exercises, pelvic-floor exercises, or pelvic-floor muscle training.

Pelvic muscles   General term referring to the muscles of the pelvic diaphragm and urogenital diaphragm as one unit. These muscles form a "hammock" slung from the front of the pelvis to the back. They support the organs of the pelvis: the bladder, uterus, and rectum. Also referred to as pelvic floor.

Pelvis   Ring of bones at the lower end of the trunk in which the pelvic organs lie.

Perineum   Area between the anus and vagina in women and anus and base of penis in men.

Pessary   Devices for women that are placed intra-vaginally to treat pelvic relaxation or prolapse of pelvic organs by supporting or lifting these organs.

Pharmacological treatment   Use of medications to treat urinary incontinence.

Phimosis   When the orifice of the foreskin is constricted, preventing retraction of the foreskin over the glans of the penis.

Polyuria   Excretion of a large volume of urine (usually > 2.5 liters in 24 hours). Can be a result of uncontrolled diabetes mellitus or the administration of a diuretic.

Postmicturition dribble   Involuntary loss of urine immediately after a person has finished voiding.

Postvoid residual (PVR) volume   Amount of fluid remaining in the bladder immediately following the completion of urination. Estimation of PVR volume can be made by abdominal palpation and percussion or bimanual examination. Specific measurement of PVR volume can be accomplished by catheterization, pelvic ultrasound, radiography, or radioisotope studies.

Pressure sore   Lesion resulting from prolonged pressure and involving loss of integrity of skin or damage to underlying tissue.

Prevalence   Number of cases of a disease existing in a population at a given time.

Prolapse   To slide forward or downward, usually referring to the pelvic organs, such as the falling down of the bladder, uterus, or rectum through the vagina. Prolapses are staged, using objective criteria, by the severity of the maximum protrusion of the prolapse during examination.

Prompted voiding   Behavioral technique for use primarily with dependent or cognitively impaired persons. Prompted voiding attempts to teach the incontinent person awareness of his or her incontinence status and to request toileting assistance, either independently or after being prompted by a caregiver.

Prostate   Walnut-shaped gland found only in men that surrounds the urethra between the bladder and the pelvic floor.

Prostatitis   Irritation or inflammation of the prostate.

Proximal urethra   Portion of the urethra closest to the bladder.

Pubic symphysis   The center front portion of the pelvic bone.

Pubococcygeus muscle   Another name for the levator ani muscle, one of the pelvic muscles that holds the pelvic organs in place.

Pudendal nerve   Main nerve that innervates all of the muscles of the pelvic floor, including the external urinary sphincter. The pudendal nerve originates at S2–S4 (the sacral micturition center) and causes the external urinary sphincter to contract, retaining urine in the bladder.

Pyuria   Pus cells present in the urine, which is a hallmark of an inflammatory response.

Rectocele   Bulging of the rectum into the space normally occupied by the vagina, suggesting weakness of the pelvic floor.

Rectum   Last segment of colon, or large intestine, the lowest part of the bowel found right before the anus.

Rehab urinals   Portable receptacles for collecting urine, usually made of plastic or metal, that are specifically designed to aid individuals who have decreased dexterity or functional ability.

Resident Assessment Protocol (RAP)   Part of the Minimum Data Set that assists the nurse to assess the cause of various disruptions or conditions. The RAP provides a systematic method of assessment and is used in the development of the care plan for the individual residing in a nursing home.

Residual urine   Retention of urine in the bladder after voiding due to incomplete emptying.

Restraints   Medications or devices (e.g., belts, straps, jackets, chairs) used to immobilize a person.

Retention   Inability to empty urine from the bladder, which can be caused by atonic bladder or obstruction of the urethra.

Retracted penis   Penis with a penile shaft of decreased length. The penis retracts into the pelvic area and can resemble an uncircumcised penis.

Risk factor   Quality that makes a person more susceptible to a specific disease.

Scheduled toileting   Assistance to toilet or use of bedpan or urinal offered on a fixed schedule, for example, every 2–4 hours.

Scrotal abscess   Bacterial infection of the scrotum, causing swelling and pain.

Sepsis   Presence of organisms or bacteria in the blood. Sepsis in the genitourinary tract is referred to as urosepsis.

Sphincter   Muscular structure that opens and closes to allow the bladder to store or empty urine.

Straining to void   Muscular effort used to either initiate, maintain, or improve the urinary stream.

Stress maneuvers   Activities that increase pressure in the bladder, such as coughing and laughing. They are used as a diagnostic test to check for stress urinary incontinence.

Stress urinary incontinence   Involuntary loss of urine from the urethra due to effort or physical exertion; for example, during coughing and laughing.

Suppositories   Medication adapted for introduction into the rectum, vagina, or urethra. Suppository bases are solid at room temperature but melt or dissolve at body temperature.

Suprapubic   Above the pubic bone.

Suprapubic catheterization   A surgical procedure involving insertion of a tube or similar instrument through the anterior abdominal wall above the symphysis pubis into the bladder to permit urine drainage from the bladder.

Sympathetic nerves   Fight or flight component of the autonomic nervous system, which originates in the thoracic and lumbar region of the spinal cord. Stimulation of the sympathetic nervous system that innervates the bladder will promote bladder filling by relaxing the bladder (detrusor) muscle and contracting the internal proximal portion of the urethral sphincter to prevent urine from entering the urethra. Sympathetic fibers that innervate the intestine will cause reduced motility and reduced secretions.

Topical When a medication (e.g., cream, ointment) is applied to a specific site or location, usually on the skin or external mucosa.

Transient (acute) urinary incontinence Temporary episodes of urinary incontinence that are reversible once the cause or causes of the episode(s) are identified and treated.

Trigone Triangle-shaped muscle that extends up from the urethra to the posterior bladder wall and to the urethral openings. The trigone is the most sensitive area of the bladder muscle because of its high concentration of nerves.

Ureters Two very thin muscular tubes about 8 or 9 inches long that transport urine from the kidneys to the bladder.

Urethra Narrow tube through which urine flows from the bladder to the outside of the body; the opening of the urethra is at the end of the penis in men and just above the vaginal opening in women.

Urethral dilatation Procedure in which a metal rod, called a dilator, is passed through the urethra for the purpose of opening a urethral stricture.

Urethral obstruction Blockage of the urethra causing difficulty with urination, usually caused by a stricture or, in men, by an enlarged prostate.

Urethral pressure profilometry (UPP) Test used to measure pressures in the urethra.

Urethral sphincter mechanism Segment of the urethra that influences storage and emptying of urine in the bladder. It controls bladder voiding by relaxing, which opens the outlet from the bladder, allowing urine to flow from the bladder to the outside of the body. A deficiency of the urethral sphincter mechanism may allow leakage of urine in the absence of a detrusor contraction.

Urethral stricture Narrowing of the urethra.

Urethrocele Prolapse or falling down of the urethra into the vaginal wall.

Urge Sensation from the bladder producing the desire to void.

Urge incontinence Involuntary and accidental loss of urine when the person is aware of the need to get to the bathroom but is not able to hold the urine long enough to get there. Usually, it is accompanied by or immediately preceded by urgency.

Urgency Strong, intense, and often sudden desire to void. Urgency, with or without urge incontinence, usually with frequency and nocturia, can be described as overactive bladder syndrome, urge syndrome, or urgency-frequency syndrome.

Urinary incontinence (UI) Involuntary or accidental loss (leakage) of urine.

Urinary system Part of the body (kidneys, ureters, bladder, and urethra) that produces, stores, and eliminates urine.

Urinary tract   Passageway from the pelvis of the kidney to the urinary orifice through the ureters, bladder, and urethra.

Urinary tract infection (UTI)   Infection in the urinary tract caused by the invasion of disease-causing micro-organisms that proceed to establish themselves, multiply, and produce various symptoms in their host. UTI in women is known as cystitis. In men, infection is usually associated with obstruction to the flow of urine, such as prostate gland enlargement.

Urinate   To void or to pass urine.

Urination   Act of passing urine.

Urine   Waste products filtered from the blood and combined with excess water by the kidneys.

Urine culture   Test to determine whether bacteria is present in the urine. It is performed by placing a drop of urine on a culture plate containing agar, a jellylike substance full of nutrients that promote the growth and multiplication of bacteria. If there are bacteria in the urine, they will start to grow and form colonies on the agar and, within a few days, they'll be visible to the naked eye. The type of bacteria can be determined by the color and appearance of the colonies. The number of bacteria are determined by estimating the number of colonies per milliliter.

Urodynamic tests   Tests designed to duplicate as nearly as possible the symptoms of incontinence in the way that people actually experience them. These tests determine the anatomic and functional status of the urinary bladder and urethra. See Cystometry, Electromyography, Urethral pressure profilometry, and Uroflowmetry.

Uroflowmetry   Urodynamic test that measures urine flow either visually, electronically, or with the use of a disposable flowmeter unit.

Urosepsis   Infection of the urinary tract that causes bacteria to enter the bloodstream, causing tissue destruction.

Uterine prolapse   Uterus has dropped from its normal position, and the cervix is closer to or may protrude outside the vagina.

Vagina   Collapsible tube of smooth muscle with its opening located between the urethral orifice and the anal sphincter of women. Also known as the birth canal.

Valsalva maneuver   Action of closing the airways and straining down on the abdominal muscles (such as when straining to have a bowel movement).

Void   Synonym for urination.

Voiding or Bladder Diary (Record)   Record maintained by the patient or caregiver that is used to record the frequency, timing, amount of voiding, and/or other factors associated with the patient's urinary incontinence. Also called an incontinence chart.

Voiding reflex   Reflex in which the bladder indicates to the spinal cord that it is full of urine, and the spinal cord signals the bladder to contract and empty.

Index

Page numbers followed by *f* indicate figures; those followed by *t* indicate tables.